Exercise Science

by Steve Glass, PhD, FACSM; Brian Hatzel, PhD, AT, ATC; and Rick Albrecht, PhD

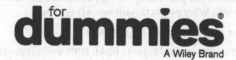

A Wiley Brand

Exercise Science For Dummies®

Published by: **John Wiley & Sons, Inc.**, 111 River Street, Hoboken, NJ 07030-5774, www.wiley.com

For general information on our other products and services, please contact our Customer Care Department within the U.S. at 877-762-2974, outside the U.S. at 317-572-3993, or fax 317-572-4002. For technical support, please visit https://hub.wiley.com/community/support/dummies.

Wiley publishes in a variety of print and electronic formats and by print-on-demand. Some material included with standard print versions of this book may not be included in e-books or in print-on-demand. If this book refers to media that is not included in the version you purchased, you may download this material at http://booksupport.wiley.com. For more information about Wiley products, visit www.wiley.com.

Library of Congress Control Number is available from the publisher.

ISBN 978-1-394-32389-0 (pbk); ISBN 978-1-394-32391-3 (ebk); ISBN 978-1-394-32390-6 (ebk)

SKY10100827_032425

Contents at a Glance

Table of Contents

Introduction

Life is movement. Starting from the smallest living cells to the most dynamic athletic skill, all aspects of the human body are in a constant state of movement. Exercise science is a field that studies the acute responses of the body to physical activity and exercise, as well as the chronic adaptations of the body to exercise as a student, within or beyond the classroom, you'll study how the body initiates and controls movement, starting with the brain and involving all the different body systems, including neuromuscular, cardiovascular, and metabolic.

About This Book

This book contains the primary principles of the field of exercise science, a vast field. Textbooks within even the subdisciplines contain so much information that you can get lost in the details. This book, on the other hand, covers the major concepts you need to know — the key aspects of exercise science across all the major systems of the body, the primary subdisciplines, and so on — in a much easier-to-read and easier-to-understand format than you'll find in other textbooks in the field.

Exercise Science For Dummies is an excellent introductory text to the entire field of exercise science. Here, we show you the forest rather than force you to focus too much on the trees. To make information easy to understand, we use the following conventions:

>> Throughout the book, we introduce you to the jargon you'll hear as an exercise science student to help ease you into the complexity of the information. Understanding these basic concepts will help you confidently pursue deeper study in the field of exercise science, if you want.

>> We've sprinkled sidebars and paragraphs accompanied by Technical Stuff icons throughout the book. You can skip these tidbits if you like, but if you're hungry for more information or deeper understanding, these discussions can help point the way.

Finally, within this book, you may note that some web addresses break across two lines of text. If you're reading this book in print and want to visit one of these web pages, simply key in the web address exactly as it's noted in the text, pretending as though the line break doesn't exist. If you're reading this as an e-book, you've got it easy — just click the web address to be taken directly to the web page.

Foolish Assumptions

You may be an aspiring student of the exercise sciences. Maybe you're interested in a health profession, such as physical therapy, occupational therapy, physician assistant studies, athletic training, or public health. Maybe you want to work in the exercise science field as a cardiac rehab specialist, exercise physiologist, or strength and conditioning specialist. Maybe you want to work in corporate wellness or some environment that allows you to work one-on-one with clients trying to change their health and fitness using exercise as a tool. This book is for you!

Although we assume you don't have a substantial background in the exercise science field, we do assume that you have some knowledge of anatomy and basic physiology — things like the anatomy of muscle, the skeletal system, the heart and circulatory system, as well as the basic physiology of how these systems function within the body.

Here are a few other assumptions we've made about you:

>> **If you're an avid exerciser,** you may be reading this book for your personal use, because you want to know more about how the body works. We assume you want the main points, the big picture, and useful information that will help you in your training.

>> **If you're a budding exercise science student,** this book is an excellent way to get a broad view and some key information about exercise science and its many subdisciplines. Reading this text as part of an introductory course in the exercise sciences is a very good first step in your training.

>> **If you're a coach or personal trainer,** you have a background in one or more aspects of exercise science, but you're trying to broaden the scope of your knowledge. Consider this book a refresher in material you may have learned already and an introduction to topics you may not have previously been exposed to.

Icons Used in This Book

You'll notice some images in the margins throughout this book. These icons clue you in to particular types of information:

TIP

This icon points you in the direction of understanding. Sometimes just a simple statement can make you think, "Aha! Now I get it!"

REMEMBER

This icon summarizes and reiterates important information that you need to know. Keep these tidbits filed away for later.

WARNING

An important aspect of studying movement is being able to recognize when an activity or situation increases the likelihood of an injury. We highlight these situations with this icon. When you see it, pay close attention so that you can avoid potentially dangerous situations.

TECHNICAL STUFF

This icon highlights information that we just had to share! We consider these points important enough to include but a bit technical or slightly beyond the scope of the text. You can read these for added information or skip them.

Beyond the Book

In addition to what you're reading right now, this product also comes with a free access-anywhere Cheat Sheet that explains how aerobic training strengthens the cardiovascular system, keys to building muscle, tips on avoiding injuries, and information on how to use exercise as medicine. To get this Cheat Sheet, simply go to www.dummies.com and enter **Exercise Science For Dummies Cheat Sheet** in the Search box.

Where to Go from Here

This book is designed so you can jump in anywhere. You don't need to begin at the beginning. Do you see a chapter that interests you? Start there! If you're not sure where to start, head to the table of contents or the index to find specific topics that may interest you.

The key thing to remember is that this book is designed so that you can jump in anywhere, get the info you need, and jump back out. Jumping, as you'll soon discover, is a great way to approach both this book and the study of movement.

1

Getting Started with Exercise Science

Chapter 1

Introducing Exercise Science

The human body was made to move. Your health depends on it, your survival is supported through it, and your ability to engage and interact with the world requires it. *Exercise science* is the science behind exercise, how the body adapts to exercise, and using exercise as therapy to improve the body's condition.

Because the human body is complex, the study of exercise and exercise itself is complex as well. In this chapter, we offer a quick overview of the science, the field, and the options available to you as a student — official or not — of exercise science.

Getting Familiar with Key Areas of Study

Exercise science grew out of the areas of physiology, medicine, and physical education. It has only been around as a field since the 1970s, and it's connected to many disciplines that examine the human body at rest, during motion, and as it adapts and changes because of exercise and physical activity.

Forming the foundation of exercise science

Before you can understand how the body moves and adapts to exercise, you must understand the human body at rest. These basics — knowing important biological processes, explaining the function of the body's structural components and its systems, knowing the chemical reactions that occur in the body, being familiar with principles governing matter in motion, and so on — give you a working knowledge of the human body and how it works.

Here's a quick rundown of the subjects you need to know *before* you get into exercise science, arranged in a way to give you a glimpse of how the body works:

>> **Biology:** Learning about living organisms and what makes them tick sets you on the right path. Biology helps you understand the structure and function of cells, their growth and development, and how they come together to form complex life-forms.

>> **Anatomy:** When you understand how organisms function at the level of the cell, you can then begin to understand how humans (and animals) are constructed. Understanding anatomy gives you the blueprint of a species. Anatomical study ranges from the structure of the very small (cells and tissues) to the very large (the hip-bone-connected-to-the-thigh-bone kind of info).

TIP

If you want to learn how to train someone to increase muscle growth or bone strength, you really need to know how the muscles and bones are constructed.

>> **Physiology:** With a firm understanding of cellular processes (biology) and how the body is put together (anatomy), you can start to examine how cells, tissues, and organs work together in a living body. *Physiology* examines the functions of the living tissues of the body. Whereas anatomy teaches you how the heart is constructed, physiology shows you how the heart works in relation to the lungs and the muscles and reveals its purpose throughout the body. By studying human physiology, you begin to see that the different structures of the body are designed for specific functions that, altogether, keep the entire body functioning while at rest

>> **Chemistry:** Humans are made of matter and require energy to live. Because the body is constructed of atoms, and energy is exchanged through the interaction of various atoms, molecules, and enzymes, you need a basic understanding of chemistry. This knowledge helps you understand what goes on in the body during exercise. After you know the basics of chemistry, you can then focus more closely on the chemistry of the human body.

>> **Biochemistry:** Biochemistry gives you a more in-depth understanding about how the body makes energy from the food eaten and how it uses that energy to keep the cells alive.

>> **Physics:** Bodies are always in motion, even when they seem to be sitting still. Therefore, understanding matter in motion — the realm of *physics* — is essential to the study of exercise science. Physics helps you understand the relationship between energy and force, levers (like joints!), center of gravity, and acceleration.

>> **Psychology:** You can't fully understand exercise and movement unless you also understand the brain and human behavior! Not only do you need to know the anatomy and basic physiology of the functioning areas of the brain, but you also must understand that people learn new things, how people handle stress, and how people prepare themselves mentally for peak performance. Psychology also delves into how emotions influence the body and behaviors.

Getting serious: Focusing on the fields specific to exercise science

Sometimes, the hardest part of starting a career in exercise science is deciding which field to focus on! Your interest may gravitate toward the microscopic: the actions of cells and organ systems and how they function during exercise. Or, maybe you prefer to focus on the way the body performs during exercise and generates forces, or how the body heals through physical training. Maybe you want to blend exercise and nutrition as a means of preventing disease There is a field for all interests within the study of exercise science. We cover some of the primary fields in the following sections.

Biomechanics

Exercise and movement involve forces, levers, balance, and acceleration. Starting with a foundation in mathematics and physics, *biomechanics* studies the mechanics of exercise and physical movement. Exercise can be as simple as lifting a weight or as complex as walking (gait) or doing a high jump. Biomechanics uses technologies that can measure forces (through *force platforms*) and the activation of muscles (through *electromyography*), and it often uses video to analyze all the aspects of body exercise. (Part 3 delves deeply into the biomechanics of exercise.)

Exercise physiology

Exercise physiology is all about the body in motion. As a field, exercise physiology is often associated with a job in a clinical setting (like cardiac rehabilitation) or sports medicine (working with athletes). Understanding how the systems of the body (for example, muscular or cardiovascular) behave during exercise and how they adapt because of exercise training is a major part of exercise physiology. (For detailed information on exercise physiology, head to Part 2).

TIP

Exercise is used as a tool to change the body, as well as to better understand how the body functions. For this reason, exercise physiology is a key component of the many careers and fields that use exercise as a way to improve the body. (You can discover a number of these fields in Chapter 18.)

Fitness and wellness

Cardiovascular disease and cancer are the leading killers of men and women in America. Research has shown a strong link between these conditions and physical inactivity and poor nutrition. Chapter 2 introduces today's view of exercise as a key therapy for health and well-being.

Exercise is Medicine (www.exerciseismedicine.org) is an initiative across the medical and exercise science disciplines. It takes advantage of modern medicine while using exercise to build the foundation of fitness that can lead to many years of health. Fitness and wellness professionals, along with doctors, use exercise and physical activity as part of a comprehensive approach to reduce the incidence of cancer, heart disease, and many other common health challenges. Exercise, body fat reduction, and dietary improvements go a long way toward putting people on a path to health. (Chapter 17 delves into the link between physical inactivity and health problems related to obesity.)

Graduate-level health professions

Having a strong background in exercise science means that you have the knowledge of how exercise can change the systems of the body. You also gain hands-on skills in assessment of the body — things like measuring fitness, body composition, and blood pressure and performing a bunch of cool tests for both athletes and those with chronic diseases. These skill sets are what graduate programs in athletic training, physical therapy, occupational therapy, physician assistant, public health, and more advanced exercise physiology studies are looking for. Exercise science is an excellent degree for a range of bachelor's degree-level careers, as well as a way to be competitively prepared for graduate degree programs in the health professions.

Rehabilitation therapy

Injuries can happen for a variety of reasons: perhaps from a exercise that isn't performed correctly (you lift something wrong, for example), an accident (you fall on an arm), or some underlying health issue (a problem exists with your heart or lungs, for example).

Understanding how the body heals and the interaction between exercise and the healing process is an area of study that spans a number of career fields. These fields often combine medical knowledge with exercise physiology, biomechanics, and even sports psychology. Studies for this field may focus on cardiac rehabilitation, physical therapy, respiratory therapy, occupational therapy, physician assistant studies, athletic training and therapeutic recreation. (Parts 2 and 3 help contribute knowledge to rehabilitation of the body.)

Sports and exercise psychology

After the body has been trained for an activity, the mind becomes the most important aspect of performance. Mood, behavior, and confidence all influence performance, for better or for worse. This area of study seeks to answer questions like, "How do athletes control the stress of a competition and still do their best?" and "How can an athlete be 'in the zone' one day and then perform terribly the next?"

What about people trying to get beyond failed new year's resolutions and make changes to their lifestyle that result in long lasting, consistent health behaviors? Changing a lifestyle that resulted in obesity and heart disease into one that can maintain nutrition and exercise behaviors can be rewarding for an exercise psychologist. Sports and exercise psychology studies human behavior and the mind and applies that knowledge to determine how best to train athletes to get the most out of their performance. If this is an area you find interesting, check out *Sports Psychology For Dummies* by Leif Smith and Todd Kays (John Wiley & Sons, Inc.)

Strength and conditioning

Athletes' bodies can perform at their best only if they've been properly conditioned for the activity. Because exercise requires conditioning the muscular and cardiovascular systems, as well as training the body to hold off fatigue, studying strength and conditioning gives you a deep understanding of how exercise changes the body. You also learn how to apply training principles that are specifically designed to improve performance in a sport. Careers in strength and conditioning range from working with populations trying to condition for fitness to high-level athletes seeking peak performance through strength and conditioning. Parts 2 and 3 cover aspects of conditioning related not only to the muscles (like Chapter 3) but also to the other systems of the body that are essential for peak performance. Part 4 provides more specific guidance on creating a conditioning program.

Understanding the Many Systems That Make Up the Human Body

Single-cell organisms have it so easy! Everything they need is contained in one cell. All their biological processes (eating, generating energy, moving, "thinking," and reproducing) have to be carried out within their single cell, and their range of interactions with the environment is quite limited. Human bodies, on the other hand, are able to adapt and interact with each other and the environment. To function at such a high level, the human body is *much* more complicated. Structurally, it has multiple levels (cells, tissues, organs, and organ systems) that build on each other and that must all function in a coordinated way to maintain the health of the organism — you.

As a student of exercise science, you're introduced to the following systems. Exercise science helps you understand how these systems interact and change as a result of exercise and physical activity.

The brain and nervous system

The brain and the neurons that make up the brain function together as a central processing center where all the information about your body and your environment can be interpreted. The other systems of your body communicate with each other through the nervous system, enabling you to see, hear, move, and interact with your surroundings. This system constantly adjusts and adapts to exercise and your environment. To find out about the nervous system, head to Chapter 7. Chapter 6 explores how your body adapts to different environments.

The circulatory system

Humans need continual sustenance to survive, and the circulatory system is the primary highway over which nutrients like *glucose* (the sugar your body uses for energy), fatty acids, oxygen, and hormones travel. The arteries transfer nutrient-rich blood to your tissues, and thin capillaries create easy access to the tissues. Your veins help guide the nutrient-depleted blood back to the heart and lungs for a refresher. The circulatory system changes its flow during times of stress or exercise. Chapter 5 covers the key functions of the circulatory system related to oxygen and nutrient transfer.

The cardiorespiratory system

To keep a constant flow of oxygen and nutrients coming to your tissue and to keep waste moving out, the body needs a pump and a fueling station. Fortunately, it has both: the heart and the lungs. The heart keeps blood moving, and the lungs serve as the station where oxygen-depleted blood fills up again. Every time a *ventricle* (a chamber in the heart) contracts, its dual chambers either push blood to the lungs to pick up more oxygen (right ventricle) or push oxygen-rich blood to the entire body (left ventricle). Exercise can help train this pump to do more work, push more blood, and get you in shape.

The skeletal system

The human body is about 70 percent water, and most of the tissue in it is made up of some pretty soft stuff. Without a frame to mount the soft, squishy bits on, we'd all be big blobs of humanity! The skeletal system provides a rigid framework that allows you to move about and see the world. Strong bones, constructed with plenty of calcium, mean a strong frame. Functioning joints enable you to move with little effort. When this system begins to weaken (and lose calcium), mobility really drops. You can read about the skeletal system and joints in Chapter 9. In Chapter 10, you can learn about the high-tech methods we have for measuring motion.

The muscular system

Exercise wouldn't be possible without something to produce force. In the body, those "force producers" are your muscles. Muscles provide the horsepower you need to move your body and interact with your world. They're also very adaptable. If you make them do a lot of work, they grow stronger. If you let them sit around and do nothing, they shrink! Strong muscles play a role in good health and quality of life. Head to Chapters 3 and 11 to find out about exercise in general and the muscular system in particular; turn to Chapter 10 to delve into motion analysis.

Energy, metabolism, and nutrition

Humans are hybrid vehicles in a sense that we may only run on a chemical called *adenosine triphosphate* (ATP), but we have systems in our body that can take carbohydrate, fat, and protein and turn them into ATP. The faster we can make the systems run, the more "fit" we are! Chapter 4 explains how we keep the metabolic engine running.

The systems don't run if we can't continually provide our bodies with key nutrients (carbohydrate, fat, and protein), as well as other important nutrients (water, vitamins, and minerals). In Chapter 15, you see how diet can help performance and find some guidelines to get you moving in the right direction.

The endocrine system

Although the brain can control many of the functions of the body through the nervous system, other controls require chemical stimuli. Glucose, for example, can't get into the cells unless the pancreas secretes insulin to help create a pathway into the cells. The endocrine system involves a number of organs and glands that secrete chemicals that bind to receptors both inside and outside cells to essentially open and close cell doors, either letting in or blocking out these chemicals. Sometimes, the release of hormones can cause a fast response (insulin helping to drop blood glucose levels, for example); other times, the release of hormones may cause changes that occur slowly over time (thyroid hormones can slowly make changes in your resting metabolic rate, for example).

TIP

Check out *Anatomy & Physiology For Dummies*, 3rd Edition, by Erin Odya and Maggie Norris, or *Biology For Dummies*, 3rd Edition, by René Fester Kratz (both published by John Wiley & Sons, Inc.), for complete discussions on the endocrine system and the role of hormones.

Examining Exercise from Many Angles

Chances are, when you hear the term *exercise,* you have your own idea of what it means and how people use it in their lives. But you can think about exercise and the connections between it and the world in more ways than you probably imagine. In the following sections, we outline the many ways exercise can be examined.

Studying the science of human performance

When you throw a ball, clear a hurdle, or balance on a beam, you probably focus on the result (were you successful?) or the "feel" of the exercise (the power of your release, for example, or the steadiness of your stance). *Biomechanists* study these aspects of exercise, using the tools of physics and math.

Exercise physiologists examine the energy systems and fuels used during exercise, and how exercise can be used to enhance human performance during athletics and rigorous work situations. focus on these aspects of performance and training.

Both of these careers are focused on answering questions like the following:

>> **How is exercise or any movement impacted by changes in the center of gravity?** Does changing the position of the arms and legs, for example, impact how someone jumps over a high-jump bar or executes a gymnastic move?

>> **What forces and velocities exist in vertical, horizontal, and rotational dimensions?** By knowing the forces, you may change how a spin and rotation are completed in a high-dive maneuver.

>> **How is balance maintained and lost?** Do older people fall because their muscles are too weak to handle a change in direction, or is it due to a delay in the muscle's ability to generate the required force?

>> **How can changes in speed, load, and training volumes affect performance?** In athletics, even a 1 percent improvement can mean taking first place in an event. Exercise scientists look for that improvement by training energy systems, muscles, and the nervous system.

>> **What kind of training is best to condition the athlete, help them train specifically for their activity, and keep them from getting worn out?** For example, can someone run faster simply by changing their running technique? What about tapering activity before a big event to get the most out of a performance? How can they prevent overtraining and a loss in performance?

>> **How can the principles of exercise be used to prevent injury?** Are there ways to land from a jump that can reduce forces on the knee and prevent someone from tearing a ligament? How soon can rehabilitation of muscle and ligaments begin? The goal is to get the athlete back in action quickly and safely.

TIP

Check out *Biomechanics For Dummies,* by Steve McCaw (published by John Wiley & Sons, Inc.) for more on this subject.

Focusing on the health-enhancement aspects of exercise

The human body is meant to move. A body at rest begins to *atrophy* (wither away) and lose muscle mass, bone density, and even heart size. Exercise can be a tool to help the body's systems function at a more optimal level. In fact, regular exercise can produce the following beneficial results:

>> Reduced blood pressure and a stronger heart

>> Increased bone density

>> Improved blood cholesterol levels

>> A stronger immune system

>> Reduced incidence of cancer and heart disease

>> Reduced stress, anxiety, and depression

If exercise is medicine, how do you "prescribe" exercise? Obviously, there are wide-ranging differences among people, including goals, present physical condition, initial fitness level, and underlying health condition. But there are guidelines and principles to set people on the right path. Part 4 is all about improving fitness and performance. Depending on individual goals (weight management, better eating, strength, aerobic fitness), the exercise program can be adjusted to suit needs.

Using exercise as a tool for rehabilitation

Although exercise can serve to prevent a number of chronic health conditions, it's also a key factor during the recovery from a range of health issues that people deal with every day:

>> Cardiac rehabilitation uses exercise to condition patients after heart surgery or heart attack.

>> Cancer patients use exercise to build strength and boost the immune system.

>> Exercises can help provide blood glucose control for people with diabetes.

>> Physical therapy is used for a range of bone, joint, and muscle injuries; arthritis; and stroke recovery.

>> Exercise therapy is used as treatment alongside medical treatments for autism, neuromuscular diseases, and stress management.

In many cases, exercise reverses the years of decline due to a lack of movement and the resulting health conditions that come with physical neglect.

Determining Whether Exercise Science Is the Field for You

Because exercise is an inherent part of life, exercise science is an inherently important field! Exercise science techniques and areas of study are used by medical professionals, athletic departments, sports organizations, corporations, and fitness and wellness industries to enhance performance, improve health, overcome mobility challenges, and more — all by changing the way people move.

To help you determine whether this field is the right one for you, ask yourself these questions:

» **Do I enjoy exercise?** Many people who enter the field of exercise science are avid exercisers, athletes, or people who just like the science of exercise and the idea of living a life of holistic health alongside modern medicine. In many cases, the best professionals are those who "practice what they preach" and are able to lead their clients by example. If you've always enjoyed exercise and improving your health, exercise science may be for you!

» **Do I like helping people?** In almost all the fields within exercise science, you use techniques to analyze and improve the physical function or health of other individuals. As a result, you're in the people business! If you like helping others, especially helping others improve themselves, exercise science may be a good fit for you. Your day may be filled with activity and not much time behind a desk, and your interpersonal skills will be a big plus as you work with people from all walks of life and in all different conditions.

» **Do I want to know about the science behind the exercise?** If you just like activity but you aren't interested in or don't enjoy learning about the science behind the exercise, you may struggle in this field because exercise science is based in anatomy, biology, physiology, psychology, physics, and so on. Conversely, if you like the sciences and can't wait to apply them to human exercise, then you're in for a real treat because, as an exercise science student, you'll be immersed in all of them!

» **Do I want to use exercise as a way to help improve the human condition?** Exercise, physical activity, and movement are tools to change the human body. Exercise scientists use these tools to help individuals heal or improve their condition. Exercise is medicine, and exercise science shows you how to use it effectively to help the individual.

REMEMBER Exercise science provides the foundation for a wide range of careers that use exercise and rehabilitative therapies to help improve the body. As you build your knowledge of the systems of the body and begin to recognize all the ways exercise science can be applied, you'll see the endless possibilities. Chapter 18 outlines ten careers for the budding exercise scientist. Take a gander — and good luck in your studies!

Chapter **2**

Better than a Pill: Exercise Is Medicine

Many people see exercise as a sport or activity done for fun. It may be something they did when they were younger, had time, and were full of energy. But our bodies are made for motion! In fact, not moving is like not eating — we can't live without movement. Exercise helps to maintain the physiologic systems of the body, like the heart, circulatory system, muscular system, and more. Exercise is also an important treatment for living a long and healthy life.

In this chapter, we cover the important benefits of exercise for promoting a longer and healthier life. We introduce the concept of health span as an important quality-of-life marker, and how exercise can add years of good health to a longer life. We also cover the impact exercise has on many common chronic diseases of today. Exercise can be the most important medicine to hold these conditions at bay.

Getting People to Value Physical Activity

Launched in 2007, *Exercise Is Medicine* (EIM) is a collaboration between the American College of Sports Medicine (the world's largest sports medicine organization) and the American Medical Association. The goal is to bring together the medical community with exercise science professionals to include and promote physical activity as part of assessing patients and prescribing treatments that work. Like medication, exercise should be prescribed, with the appropriate frequency, intensity, time, and type of exercise (known as FITT) in order to achieve the desired result. EIM is a big undertaking — most people don't really recognize the huge impact exercise can have on preventing chronic diseases and helping to improve (and even extend) their years of healthy living.

The goals of EIM are as follows:

>> Assessing physical activity for each patient when they visit their doctor

>> Providing exercise-related information and some exercise program planning information

>> Referring the patient to a trained exercise science professional for more in-depth assessment and prescription

The EIM initiative isn't limited to the United States. More than 40 countries are participating. People are getting the message that physical activity and exercise can be life-changing. To learn more about EIM, head to www.exerciseismedicine.org.

In this section, we introduce the concept of exercise, physical activity, and how it can impact chronic diseases.

Use it or lose it: The importance of staying active

Our bodies are built to move! In fact, our bodies adapt to movement by becoming stronger, faster, and more aerobically fit. Add good nutrition to the mix, and our bodies can operate at peak capacity well into middle age. Sadly, our bodies can also move in the opposite direction if we don't move. A body will not stay fit and function well if it doesn't move.

Believe it or not, aging is not the biggest contributor to a decrease in fitness — instead, it's simply being inactive.

TIP

In the United States, 80 percent of adults do not get enough aerobic exercise.

WARNING

PHYSICAL ACTIVITY VERSUS EXERCISE: WHAT'S THE DIFFERENCE?

You've probably heard the terms *physical activity* and *exercise* bandied about, but you may not be clear on what they mean. (Most people aren't, so if you're a little fuzzy on this subject, you're not alone!)

Physical activity is the broader of the two terms. It refers to any movement that uses large muscle groups, is done repeatedly (like mowing the lawn), and results in calories burned.

Exercise is a more specific term and a type of physical activity. It refers to planned activity with a goal to improve or maintain fitness, increase strength, or achieve some other type of fitness outcome. When you're mowing the lawn, you're not exercising, but when you go for a run, you are.

Knowing how intense physical activity should be

Exercise prescriptions or plans for training involve things like the type of exercise, how long it's done, how often it's done, and how intense it is. Often, the intensity is hardest to understand and prescribe. Some people think that the intensity must be high in order to be effective, but the required exercise intensity varies depending on your goals.

One common value that you may see on the treadmill display while you exercise is the MET, which stands for *metabolic equivalent*. Think of MET like the cost of doing movement. What is the cost of sitting still and just resting? That's 1 MET. Vacuuming? 3 METs (three times the energy and oxygen use compared to rest). Using METs allows you to add an intensity "price tag" to various activities. You can also sort activity into light, moderate, and vigorous intensity. Light intensity is any activity that is between 1.6 and 2.9 METs, moderate is 3.0 to 5.9 METs, and vigorous is 6.0 METs or higher. Table 2-1 gives an overview of some activities and their associated MET values.

TIP

To find the MET values of a range of activities, go to the Compendium of Physical Activities website at https://pacompendium.com for the complete list.

SITTING IS THE NEW SMOKING: GET MOVING TO FIGHT OFF DISEASE!

With modern conveniences, jobs using computers, and leisure-time activities that don't involve movement (like watching TV, reading, or playing cards), sitting has become a big contributor to major chronic diseases, like heart disease, cancer, and obesity. In fact, a person's risk of dying goes up based on the number of hours per day they sit. If you sit four to six hours per day, you have a 30 percent increased risk of death; sitting more than eight hours per day leads to a 60 percent increased risk of death compared to people who simply keep their bodies moving through normal daily activity.

Outcomes of sitting that contribute to this increased risk are a lower level of fitness, increased rates of obesity, increased inflammation of blood vessels, increase in blood clots, loss of insulin sensitivity, muscle loss . . . and the list keeps going! These effects contribute to the acceleration of chronic diseases like heart disease, diabetes, osteoporosis, and cancer. Sitting does a lot of damage to bodies.

TABLE 2-1   ## Physical Activities by MET Value

Aerobic Intensity Level	Activity	MET Value
Light	Getting ready for bed	2.3
Light	General gardening	2.0
Light	Washing dishes	2.0
Moderate	Walking for pleasure	3.5
Moderate	Salsa dancing with a partner	4.8
Moderate	Water aerobics/calisthenics	5.5
Vigorous	Playing basketball	7.5
Vigorous	Running 5.0 to 5.2 miles per hour (12 minutes per mile)	8.5
Vigorous	Playing racquetball	10.0

Recommended amounts of physical activity

Using the MET ranges for moderate and vigorous activity, here are the weekly aerobic exercise guidelines for adults in the United States:

150 minutes of moderate intensity aerobic activity or 75 minutes of vigorous intensity aerobic activity

A WORD FROM HIPPOCRATES: THE FATHER OF WESTERN MEDICINE

Hippocrates (460–370 BCE) followed in the footsteps of his teacher, Herodicus, by placing a tremendous emphasis on the health benefits of diet, exercise, and overall fitness. In fact, a quote attributed to Hippocrates is something most exercise scientists and fitness/wellness specialists would be proud to put on the back of their business cards today:

> If we could give every individual the right amount of nourishment and exercise, not too little and not too much, we would have found the safest way to health.

Not bad insight for a guy living a couple thousand years ago.

These are minimum amounts. The more you do, the better!

The level you choose may be related to your starting level of fitness, but the goal is to accumulate! Exercise volume is not just the intensity of exercise but also time. The metabolic equivalent (MET) minute is an indicator of the intensity and duration of activity (exercise volume). If you go for a 20-minute jog at 6 METs, that's 120 MET minutes. If you walk at 3 METS for 60 minutes, that's 180 MET minutes. A good goal is 450 to 900 MET minutes per week. So, choose the intensity (METS) and duration that best fits the MET minute goal.

Movement Matters: Physical Activity and Disease

The main causes of death are heart disease and cancer, but other contributing diseases, like obesity and diabetes, are heavy hitters as well. What happens when all causes of death are put together and associated with levels of physical activity? The picture is clear: Movement matters!

The recommended amount of aerobic activity is 150 minutes of moderate exercise per week. In Figure 2-1, you can see what happens to a person's risk of dying from any cause — look how much risk drops! When you get past about 450 minutes of moderate exercise per week, the risk level stays about the same.

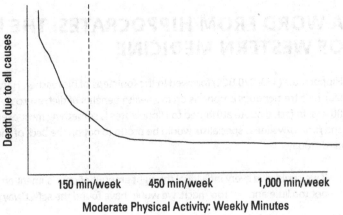

© John Wiley & Sons, Inc.

FIGURE 2-1:
Amount of physical activity and death from all causes.

Many chronic diseases occur as a result of behaviors across time. Inactivity, overweight, and poor diet all can contribute to the development of disease. The good news is that these same conditions can be improved by using physical activity or exercise, dropping body fat, and improving nutrition.

This section covers the use of exercise as a treatment that can improve chronic disease conditions and other health risks that lead to disease.

Treating diabetes using exercise

Type 2 diabetes is a form of diabetes in which the body is still making insulin to help control blood glucose, but the insulin receptor is not able to recognize the insulin, so glucose struggles to get into the cells, leaving the body with elevated blood glucose. High glucose is very damaging to the blood vessels, organs, and brain, and it accelerates the progression of many other diseases, including heart disease. The cause of diabetes is linked to obesity and physical inactivity, which inflame the tissue and prevent insulin from connecting to the insulin receptors.

Type 2 diabetes has reached epidemic levels in the United States. Currently, around 12 percent of Americans have diabetes, and many more have not yet been diagnosed.

The good news? Obesity and physical inactivity can be addressed through lifestyle intervention. If we can get people to become more active and reduce their body fat, they may regain normal blood glucose control. Current medications to treat diabetes are not cures — they only try to manage the elevated blood glucose. Losing weight and increasing activity is the only intervention that can reset the body's control of glucose and reduce the risk of other diseases impacted by diabetes.

METABOLIC SYNDROME: MULTIPLE WHAMMIES AGAINST HEALTH

Often, ailments come in multiples — for example, obesity, high blood pressure, and diabetes. As one organ struggles against a disease or condition, others are affected as well. In the human body, obesity can really get in the way of normal metabolic function. For some people, obesity is accompanied by a number of other problems, such as elevated cholesterol, elevated blood pressure, and diabetes. This grouping of disorders is known as metabolic syndrome, and it affects millions of Americans. The first line of intervention? Reduce body fat and increase physical activity. This prescription can start treating all the parts of metabolic syndrome.

Type 1 diabetes (often referred to as *juvenile diabetes*) is an autoimmune disease often diagnosed in children or young adults. People with type 1 diabetes lack insulin and must take insulin shots or be fitted with an insulin pump that provides doses of insulin. Physical activity is a very effective tool to help maintain safe blood glucose levels in people with type 1 diabetes, too.

Insulin is a hormonal trigger of sorts that binds to receptors on the cell membranes. This binding starts a series of steps that allows a protein known as *glucose transporter type 4* (GLUT4) to enter the cell membranes and create a pathway to pull glucose into the cell. Two things can trigger GLUT4: insulin and exercise. So, in a sense, exercise is almost like an insulin shot. People who take insulin can also factor exercise into their daily plan to help lower their blood glucose. This can mean fewer insulin shots and better blood glucose control. Exercise will also improve their tissue sensitivity to insulin, so even their doses of insulin may be reduced with regular exercise, which can help them maintain a stable body weight.

The bottom line: Exercise is a very important part of treating diabetes! It must be incorporated into any diabetes treatment plan in order to achieve the best possible outcome.

Using exercise to treat cancer

Cancer is an insidious disease that can attack many different areas of the body, from the organs to tissue to blood and bone. The mechanism of how cancer begins are not fully understood, but inflammation can play a role.

According to the U.S. Centers for Disease Control and Prevention (CDC), physical activity is closely linked to reduced cancer rates. In fact, for cancers such as bladder, breast, colon, endometrial, esophageal, kidney, and stomach, cancer rates are reduced by 10 percent to 20 percent in physically active people. Being physically active seems to help fight off the formation of new tumors and slow the rate of growth of others.

The protective effect of physical activity and exercise extends even to those who have already been diagnosed with cancer. Cancer patients who are physically active have seen up to a 40 percent reduction in death from any cause! Additionally, chemotherapy patients who exercise have lowered incidences of *chemotoxicity* (chemical damaging of cell DNA and inflammatory effects of the drug on healthy tissue and nerve damage), as well as better tolerance of the treatment. Exercise can serve as a shield to harden the patient to the rigors of chemotherapy treatment. Some exercise scientists have specific certification for working with cancer patients — for this population, patient safety and appropriate exercise take some additional care.

Surviving heart disease with physical activity

Heart disease, which affects the heart, heart rhythm, blood vessels, and heart valves, and may even include the lungs, is the leading killer in the United States, leading to around 700,000 deaths each year. About one in every five deaths is caused by heart disease.

Heart disease is also referred to as coronary artery disease, because this is where the disease begins. Damage to the inner lining of the blood vessels, maybe from chronic inflammation or high blood pressure, starts this process. The damage happens everywhere in the body, but when it happens in the small coronary arteries, blood flow and oxygen delivery to the heart are reduced. Wherever the arteries suffer damage, plaque (composed of cholesterol) begins to build up. Obesity (which increases inflammation), high blood pressure (which damages artery walls), and elevated cholesterol levels all serve to accelerate the buildup of this plaque, a process known as *atherosclerosis*. Add to that risk factors like smoking and physical inactivity, and blood clots can form, creating a possible lodging of a clot in a narrowed artery leading to a *myocardial infarction* (heart attack), where blood flow through an artery is blocked. When blood flow is blocked, the tissue will die within an hour if it cannot be restored.

Regular physical activity and exercise can help reduce the risk of heart disease by impacting many of the risk factors that contribute to the disease, as well as the condition of the heart itself. Risk factors that can be impacted include the following:

- >> **Obesity:** Consistent exercise, along with a healthy diet (such as a Mediterranean diet), will help reduce body fat, lower inflammation, and ease the load on the heart.

- >> **Hypertension (high blood pressure):** Regular moderate exercise can lower blood pressure values by at least 10 mmHg. Coupled with loss of body fat, blood pressure can be lowered a lot, reducing damage to the arteries.

- >> **Low-density lipoprotein (LDL) cholesterol:** LDL cholesterol can be lowered with a combination of fat loss and diet intervention with reduced saturated fat intake. This can slow the depositing of plaque in the arteries.

The heart muscle itself can be strengthened and the size of the ventricular chamber can be enlarged, so each heartbeat pushes more blood (known as a higher *stroke volume*). Additionally, the cardiac muscle can gain more coronary artery branches, like a tree developing a root system to grab more nutrients. Additional arteries will help deliver oxygen and may save the person's life if an artery is blocked. Even in patients who've already survived a heart attack, exercise can strengthen the heart and bring their fitness back to levels where they can live full and healthy lives.

Slowing Your Grow: Exercise and Health Span

Consider this scenario: You're going to live to be 100 years old! Yay! However, at around age 75, you'll have your first heart attack, suffer nerve damage associated with diabetes, and be so deconditioned and sick that you're mostly confined to your home. Does that sound like a nice 25 years? Nope.

Most people think of life in terms of *lifespan* (the number of years a person lives). But what if you instead considered the *quality* of the years that you have to enjoy living? *Health span* represents the years of life that a person spends in good health, free from the chronic diseases and disabilities of aging. Whether people know the term or not, what most people want is a longer health span, not just a longer lifespan.

Physical activity and exercise are essential parts of an extended health span. In the United States, the current expected lifespan from birth is around 79 years, while health span is only 63 years. The graph in Figure 2-2 shows a hypothetical comparison of two individuals, one (represented by the solid line) who was physically active, ate a healthy diet, and lived to be 100 years old, and another (represented by the dotted line) who was inactive, obese, and suffered from diabetes starting around age 40. Both lived to be 100, but notice the years of good health as shown by a higher continued health score enjoyed by one and the slow decline in health of the other.

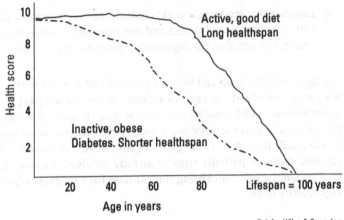

FIGURE 2-2:
Health scores
across a lifetime.

© John Wiley & Sons, Inc.

Staying younger longer

The concept of health span means that you can maintain a healthy body for a larger portion of your lifespan, due to the positive effects of consistent exercise. Research is showing that a combination of both aerobic activity and resistance training can improve function across a range of body systems:

>> **Muscle:** Resistance training that uses loads that are heavy enough to stress the muscle (which is more than 60 percent of the heaviest load you can lift once) and are lifted until you can't continue will help grow and maintain the muscle power fibers that are so important for balance and daily activity. Older, inactive individuals lose these fibers, as well as muscle mass in general, but muscle mass can be maintained into the golden years with exercise.

>> **Heart:** Meeting the recommended amounts of physical activity can help maintain aerobic fitness (measured by *VO2 max*, or the maximum rate of oxygen the body can use during exercise), grow additional blood vessels on the heart and in muscle to better deliver oxygen, and provide a reserve of fitness that can handle daily activity. It can also help you weather illness without huge declines in function.

>> **Immune system:** When you're young, flu season may be an inconvenience, but when you're older and unfit, it may be a real challenge to your immune system. Exercise can strengthen the immune system and help fight the inevitable illnesses that hit as people age. When COVID-19 was at its worst, people who were obese and inactive, had diabetes, and high blood pressure were most at risk. Their compromised immune systems made COVID-19 too much to handle.

>> **Bone:** Bone loss and *osteoporosis* (a disease that weakens the bones) occur when the breakdown of bone is faster than building new bone. The lack of a stimulus to the bone, like the stress and strain of walking or weightlifting, can lead to a fast decline in bone mass, especially in women after menopause. But aerobic exercise and weightlifting can help keep bones strong and prevent fracture.

Mending your brain

The part of aging that's scary for many individuals is the decline in brain function. Neurological diseases such as Alzheimer's disease, dementia, and Parkinson's disease impact millions of older adults, reducing quality of life and leading to an early death. Can the brain be healed? Yes, to some extent. Exercise has been shown to improve brain function. Studies using exercise in older adults have shown improvements in cognitive function, improved motor coordination, improved learning and memory, and increased brain volume.

Exercise causes adaptations that help improve brain function, such as lengthening *dendrites* (the extensions of nerve cells), which can help improve the interconnections across the neurons and improve communication across the brain. Exercise also increases a molecule called *brain-derived neurotrophic factor* (BDNF), which is key to adaptations in the brain to improve cognitive function.

The ability of the brain to adapt and improve function, even in older individuals, is termed *neuroplasticity*, and exercise is a key factor in enhancing this ability. Both moderate and higher-intensity exercise induce the changes, so older folks don't have to work that hard to see positive effects. Consistency is the key to training both the body and the mind.

2

Powering the Body: Exercise Physiology

Find out how muscles make movement possible and how you can train them.

Uncover how the body produces energy from fat, carbohydrates, and protein, as well as short-term, high-intensity energy sources.

See how the heart, lungs, and blood vessels work together to deliver oxygen to tissue to help power movement.

Examine how the environment you move within affects your body during exercise and how you can adapt to your environment so that your performance isn't hurt.

IN THIS CHAPTER

» Grasping the principles of how muscles contract and force is generated

» Looking at different muscle fiber types and structures

» Seeing how muscles work together

» Understanding muscle reflexes

» Building muscle strength

Chapter **3**

Let's Move, Baby! The Muscles

N early every aspect of your life involves movement. Even as you sit and read this book, you're using your muscles: You're sitting in a chair or lying down, holding the book or an e-reader, turning the pages or scrolling, moving your eyes across the page, and so on. Movement can be fairly simple, as in the reading example, or it can be quite complex. To support movement, your body depends not only on your bone structure but also on your muscles. Without muscles, you can't move!

The effect muscles have on movement is determined by muscular makeup. How much force is generated, the amount of joint motion, joint stability, and muscle action differ across muscles, based on their structure.

In this chapter, we explore the different types of muscles, how they're organized into different types of fibers, and how you can use these different fibers to, for example, run fast or run for long periods of time. We also examine the factors that cause muscle fatigue. The variety in your muscles helps you perform a wide range of movements.

The Foundations of Muscle Movement: The Science behind Contraction

If you want to turn on a light, you have to flip the switch to send electricity to the light bulb. If you want to "turn on" a muscle — that is, make the muscle contract — you need to flip a switch in the brain. This "switch" is an action potential that originates in the brain from the motor control centers. As we explain in Chapter 7, various parts of the brain send signals down the spinal cord to initiate movement and cause the muscle to contract. These signals are one part of the story of movement. The actual mechanics of muscle contraction are the other part of the story. Any movement at a joint requires that the muscles connected on each side of the joint shorten.

"How is that even possible?" you ask. "And wouldn't the entire muscle shortening produce a *lot* of force? What if you wanted only a little bit of force? How is that controlled?" Read on for the answers. As you'll see, many factors influence how a muscle behaves.

REMEMBER

A muscle contraction is a very complex piece of work. It involves nerves, different types of fibers, and different types of attachments, and it can span multiple joints. All these factors are significant contributors to the muscular system.

Uncovering the structure of the muscle

A muscle is really many muscles woven together. It's made up of many smaller units of muscle fiber, and each unit of muscle fiber is itself made up of components that, when all are working as they should, make movement possible. Figure 3-1 shows the structures of the muscle as you go to the smaller units. Refer to this image as you read the next few sections.

Bundling up: Myofibrils

As Figure 3-1 shows, bundles of long fibers, called *myofibrils,* are grouped together to form a muscle. Each myofibril is made up of smaller, individual units of contracting tissue stacked end to end. The smallest unit that makes up the myofibril (and the one that does the contracting) is called a *sarcomere.* You can read more about the sarcomere and its role in contraction in "The sarcomere and its parts: Shortening to produce force," later in this chapter.

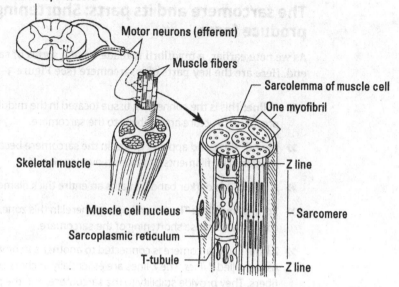

Cross-section of spinal cord

Motor neurons (efferent)

Muscle fibers

Sarcolemma of muscle cell

One myofibril

Skeletal muscle

Z line

Muscle cell nucleus

Sarcomere

Sarcoplasmic reticulum

T-tubule

Z line

Illustration by Kathryn Born, MA

FIGURE 3-1:
The anatomy
of skeletal
muscle tissue.

Releasing calcium: T-tubules and the sarcoplasmic reticulum

One ion that's very important for making a muscle contract is calcium. Although calcium is bound up in bone, it's also found in a system of storage vesicles, called the *sarcoplasmic reticulum*, within the muscle. Calcium can be released from this location and spread throughout a muscle via the *T-tubules* (fluid-filled tubes that sit within the muscle, distributing calcium). All it needs is a stimulus, which it gets by way of the motor unit.

The motor unit: Connecting the nerve and the muscle

In the locations where the nerve actually reaches the muscle, the nerve doesn't just plug into the entire muscle. Instead, each motor nerve connects to only a certain number of muscle fibers. One nerve may connect to 100 fibers, for example, or it may connect to 1,000. This nerve-fiber connection is called a *motor unit*. These connections give your brain some control over just how many of those fibers contract.

The sarcomere and its parts: Shortening to produce force

As we note earlier, a myofibril is made up of a series of sarcomeres stacked end to end. Here are the key parts of a sarcomere (see Figure 3-2):

» **M line:** This is the connecting tissue located in the middle of the sarcomere, providing structure and stability to the sarcomere.

» **I band:** This band appears lighter in the sarcomere because it contains only the thin actin filaments. No myosin overlaps it.

» **A band:** This darker band contains an entire thick filament (myosin).

» **Zone of overlap:** The action happens here! In this zone, actin and myosin connect and cause shortening of the sarcomere.

» **Z line:** Each sarcomere is connected to another sarcomere by rigid connective tissue called *Z lines*. The Z lines are essentially anchors that connect protein fibers. They provide stability to the sarcomere, and the pulling of myosin on actin moves the Z lines closer together during muscle contraction.

» **Actin:** Connected to the Z lines are thin protein filaments called *actin*. Actin has a twisted appearance, similar to what you'd get if you twisted a pearl necklace. It's a fiber that, when activated by a strong pull, can pull the Z lines closer together.

» **Myosin filaments:** Between the actin are thicker looking sets of protein filaments that have small "arms" coming out from them. These thick filaments, called *myosin filaments,* do the pulling. Think of the myosin as a rowboat in the water, and the arms as the paddles that do the pulling.

» **Titin:** Holding myosin in place and keeping it connected to everything is a large, springlike protein called *titin.* Titin, working a bit like a rubber band, helps give muscle an elastic property.

Binding sites for muscle contraction

During a contraction, the sarcomere has to shorten, which happens when the myosin heads grab onto the actin at the binding sites and give them a pull. When a muscle is at rest (that is, not contracting), it can't grab onto the binding sites because the sites are covered. Uncovering the sites involves two proteins:

» **Tropomyosin:** *Tropomyosin* is a long filament protein that lays on top of the binding sites on the actin. When tropomyosin covers the binding sites, the muscle is at rest.

>> **Troponin:** Troponin is a globlike protein that actually moves tropomyosin out of the way, if it has the right incentive, so that the binding site is exposed, a process we outline in the next section.

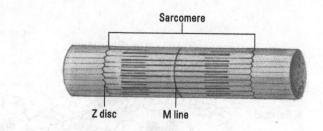

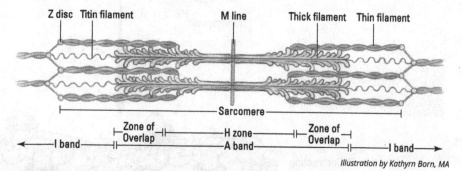

FIGURE 3-2:
The sarcomere.

Illustration by Kathyrn Born, MA

Filaments sliding past each other: Producing muscular force

Because you can't really see the motions within the sarcomere as it shortens, researchers have come up with a theory that explains what happens when the muscle contracts. Here is the step-by-step sequence of what makes the sarcomere shorten:

1. **The brain sends an electrical stimulus down the spinal cord and out to the motor units.**

2. **The motor units spread the signal to the fibers they're connected to, activating the release of calcium from the sarcoplasmic reticulum.**

3. **The calcium binds to the protein troponin, causing troponin to change its shape.**

4. **Troponin's shape change moves the tropomyosin out of the way so that the binding sites become available.**

   Figure 3-3 shows this sequence of tropomyosin movement and calcium binding.

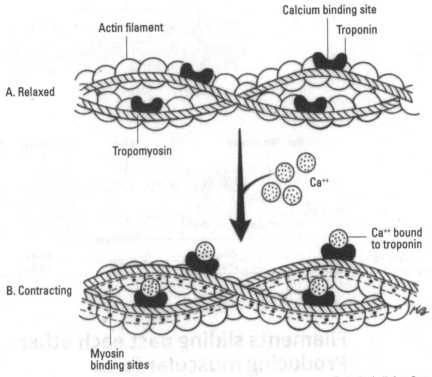

FIGURE 3-3:
Calcium activates
the contraction
sequence.

Illustration by Kathryn Born, MA

5. **The myosin heads attach to sites on the actin, connecting the filaments.**

TIP

   In an earlier analogy, we say that the myosin is like a rowboat and the heads are the boat's oars. This step is akin to the boat putting its oars in the water.

6. **The myosin heads rotate and pull the actin on both sides of the sarcomere toward the center.**

   This action shortens the sarcomere and produces force.

7. **As long as there is energy to power the process and stimuli to keep it going, the myosin heads continue to rotate, releasing, grabbing, and pulling the next site and the next.**

   At this point, the oars of the rowboat are in full swing.

TIP

To visualize this process, put both your hands in front of you, palms facing you, with your fingertips just slightly overlapping. This represents your sarcomere at rest. Now move your fingers inward, fingers sliding past each other. This represents a sarcomere contracting. As the filaments slide past each other and the sarcomere shortens, force is produced.

The Tortoise and the Hare: Fast- and Slow-Twitch Fibers

Some movement activities require endurance, whereas others require a lot of force to be generated over a short period of time. Fortunately, differences in motor units — both in terms of how the nerve functions and the chemistry and action of the muscle fibers — make both types of movement possible.

Muscle fibers are generally divided into two primary groups: slow-twitch and fast-twitch, although an intermediate category also exists. *Twitch* is a reference to the speed and frequency of the neural signal passing along the motor unit.

TIP

The fiber type you're born with may determine your best sport. Fast- and slow-twitch muscle fibers are not interchangeable by nerve type, but there are some variation possibilities within the muscle itself. However, what you're born with will, to an extent, explain a lot about the type of activity in which you excel. Born with a lot of slow-twitch? The 100-meter sprint may not be the event for you, but you may make a great marathon runner! Lots of fast-twitch? Chances are, power sports are great for you. Of course, most people have a combination of slow- and fast-twitch muscle fibers, enabling us to perform a wide range of sport activities. If you examined the best athletes in power sports or endurance sports, you would see a genetic advantage of a higher percentage of either fast-twitch (power) or slow-twitch (endurance) muscle fibers.

Not too strong, but keeps on keeping on: The slow-twitch muscle fiber

Think of slow-twitch muscle fibers like a tortoise: They're not particularly fast, but they do keep on going. Slow-twitch motor units have some common characteristics, outlined in Table 3-1.

TABLE 3-1   ## Common Characteristics of Slow-Twitch Muscles

Nerve Characteristics	Muscle Fiber Characteristics
The nerve is small and reaches a threshold for firing with a small stimulus from the brain.	Slow-twitch muscles have large numbers of mitochondria.
The frequency of the nerve twitch is slow, and the magnitude of the twitch is low.	They're aerobic fibers, capable of making adenosine triphosphate (ATP) by using aerobic metabolism (see Chapter 4). They also use fats, carbohydrates, and lactic acid as a fuel source.
The nerve connects to only a few fibers (maybe 100 to 500 fibers per nerve), making it handy for fine motor control.	They have large amounts of *myoglobin*, an iron-containing protein that transports oxygen through the muscle tissue and gives the fibers a darker, reddish pigment. (Slow-twitch fibers are sometimes called *red fibers*. If you're familiar with turkey, the slow-twitch muscles would be the dark meat!)
	Slow-twitch muscle fibers are relatively smaller and weaker than their fast-twitch counterparts.

REMEMBER

Slow-twitch muscles come in handy for any activity in which endurance is essential. Some muscles have a higher proportion of slow-twitch fibers. For example, the soleus muscle, which is in the lower leg and is important for standing, has a high proportion of slow-twitch fibers. In addition, because the nerve connects only to a few fibers, slow-twitch motor units are usually associated with fine motor skills (like writing, typing, or blinking). The average person may have 50 percent slow-twitch muscle in their vastus lateralis, whereas a marathon runner may be 95 percent slow-twitch muscle.

USING SLOW TWITCH MUSCLES TO COOL DOWN!

TIP

Although slow-twitch muscle fibers run on the by-products of fat and glucose metabolism, they have a unique enzyme that also allows them to use lactic acid as a fuel. Lactic acid is the end product of anaerobic breakdown of glucose, so it's elevated after a bout of very high-intensity exercise, like the 400-meter sprint. The enzyme converts lactic acid back to pyruvic acid, which can then be taken up by the mitochondria. As the slow-twitch fibers are activated, they use the lactic acid as a source of fuel, which helps clear away the lactic acid quickly. You can use this behavior to cool down.

Suppose you're engaged in an intense activity, like running very hard for three to five minutes. During this activity, you build up a lot of lactic acid. What can you do immediately afterward to recover? Activate your slow-twitch fibers by lightly jogging or walking. As you cool down with the light activity, you're clearing away the lactic acid much more quickly than you would if you just stood there with your hands on your knees!

Big, strong, fast . . . and quickly tired: The fast-twitch fiber

Fast-twitch fibers, also called *fast-twitch A fibers*, are like the hare: fast! These fibers are built for speed and for generating a lot of force. The downside is that they tend to fatigue quickly. Fast-twitch fibers and their associated nerves differ from slow-twitch in a number of ways. Table 3-2 outlines their characteristics.

TABLE 3-2   ## Common Characteristics of Fast Twitch Muscles

Nerve Characteristics	Muscle Fiber Characteristics
The nerve is large and takes a higher level of stimulus to reach a threshold for firing. For light activities, the motor unit is generally not active.	Fast-twitch fibers produce their energy by using anaerobic metabolism (see Chapter 4). They don't use much oxygen.
The frequency of the nerve twitch is fast, and magnitude is large.	Anaerobic fibers produce ATP quickly, so fast-twitch fibers can produce more force than slow-twitch fibers.
The nerve connects to many fibers (thousands of fibers per nerve). When the motor does reach a firing threshold, a lot of fibers are activated, and a lot of force is generated.	Anaerobic fibers produce more lactic acid, meaning they fatigue quickly.
	The fibers are large and respond more to strength training.

Fast-twitch X, or intermediate, fibers

One slightly different version of the classic fast-twitch fiber is the *intermediate fiber* (also called *fast-twitch X* or *fast-twitch B*). Although these fibers are still fast twitch, their chemistry is a little different. These fibers have some of the aerobic ATP producing mitochondria, so they can get energy both from aerobic and anaerobic metabolism.

FAST-TWITCH A VERSUS X: LOOKING AT TRAINING'S EFFECT ON YOUR MUSCLES' BEHAVIOR

Can jogging slow down your sprint speed? Maybe. Bodies are very sensitive to training and adapt to the type of training they receive. In the case of muscle fibers, the fast-twitch X fibers may adapt to one type of training at the expense of adaptions to another.

(continued)

(continued)

Fast-twitch X fibers can be trained so that they function more similarly to aerobic fibers or more similarly to anaerobic fibers. If you do a lot of endurance training, you'll improve your endurance, but you may lose some sprint speed. If you do a lot of sprint training, you can improve your sprint speed but lose some of your endurance. If you're a really serious athlete, consider blending your training to include a range of intensity so that all the muscle fibers can adapt and gain performance.

Working in Unison: How the Muscle Behaves

Muscles are much more than simple pieces of flesh that merely contract and relax. In this section, we investigate the properties that help define muscle function. How reactive a muscle is, how much it can stretch, and whether it returns to its normal length are all considerations that affect or dictate muscle function.

Looking at a muscle's response

Muscles produce the force needed for any type of movement, whether it be swatting a bug or running a marathon. Obviously, each action is unique and has particular demands. The force that a muscle or group of muscles can produce is dependent on its behavioral properties, outlined in the following list:

» **Extensibility:** *Extensibility* refers to the muscle's ability to be stretched or lengthened beyond its normal resting length. A good example of extensibility is how the *quadriceps* (the muscle in the front of the upper leg) stretch when the hamstrings are contracted to bend the knees.

» **Elasticity:** Whereas *extensibility* refers to the ability of a muscle to be stretched, *elasticity* refers to a muscle's ability to be stretched or elongated and then to return to its normal resting length afterward. When a muscle is stretched, it returns to its normal length unless an injury occurs from being stretched too far; in this case, the muscle is strained and the muscle fibers are torn.

» **Irritability:** In this context, *irritability* doesn't mean getting angry; instead, it refers to the muscle's ability to respond to stimuli. Also known as *excitability*, irritability describes the reactivity of a muscle and may dictate the timing and amount of stimulus needed for a contraction.

» **Contractility:** In all cases, the muscles must generate tension to create movements. The ability to create tension is referred to as the muscle's *contractility*. The amount of tension or how hard a muscle contracts depends on the muscle's length, its timing, which motor units get innervated, and the position of the joint.

Noting muscles' organizational structure

You may have heard that form follows function — a maxim that definitely holds true when it comes to your muscles. Muscles have a distinct organizational pattern and are connected to the bones in ways that enhance your mobility while simultaneously giving you strength. Read on to discover how muscle organization is key to movement.

The architecture of the muscle fiber

The architecture of your muscles — that is, their size and shape — differs from body part to body part and helps to dictate their function. Some muscles enable a large range of motion, and others have less extensive range of motion but provide support and stability.

Muscles are typically broken up into two structural categories (see Figure 3-4):

>> **Parallel:** Muscles with parallel architecture have fibers that run in a parallel fashion along the length of the muscle. This fiber orientation is more conducive to large ranges of motion. The shapes that have a parallel arrangement are fusiform, triangular, flat, and strap.

>> **Pennate:** In pennate muscle architecture, the fibers are oriented at an angle into their tendons. Because of the larger number of muscle fibers that are attached to the tendon, pennate muscles are able to generate more force. In this category, muscles can be *unipennate* (attaching to one side of the tendon), *bipennate* (attaching to both sides of the tendon), or *multipennate* (attaching to the tendon in multiple locations), depending on the number of tendons and how the muscle fibers attach to them.

Origin, insertion, and lights . . . camera . . . action!

What the muscle attaches to is also a key component of the movement it creates when tension is developed. When you think about the muscle attachments, you need to know the difference between the origin, insertion, and action:

>> The *origin* of a muscle is typically the less movable portion of the attachment. Another way to think of the origin is that it is the more *proximal* (near the center of the body) attachment site of the muscle.

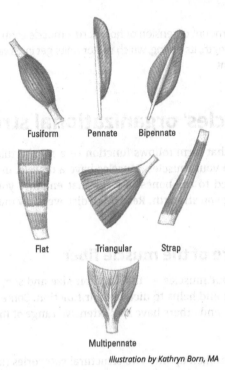

Fusiform   Pennate   Bipennate

Flat   Triangular   Strap

Multipennate

FIGURE 3-4:
Pennate and
parallel muscles.

Illustration by Kathryn Born, MA

>> The *insertion* of a muscle is typically the more movable portion of the attach-
ment and also the more *distal* (away from the center of the body) attachment
of the muscle.

>> The *action* is simply the movement that is created in the joint when tension is
created. What kind of action the muscle is capable of depends on the location
of each of these attachments.

Two things dictate a muscle's function: where the muscles attach and at what
angles they attach. Consider the knee, for example. A number of muscles attach to
the *patella* (knee cap), and each attaches at a different angle. Some pull the patella
up, and others pull it to the outside or inside. If all these muscles work together, the
result is a coordinated upward movement of the patella when the knee is extended
and a coordinated downward movement when the knee is flexed. The angle of pull,
coupled with the amount of force from the muscles, dictates the muscles' effects on
many of the joints. Figure 3-5 illustrates the different angles of pull.

REMEMBER

Typically, muscles generate more than one action. Often, the types of actions that
a particular muscle contributes to depend on the body's position at the time. For
example, your *pectoralis major* (chest muscle) contributes to both horizontal
adduction (when the arm is parallel with the ground) and internal rotation
(regardless of arm position).

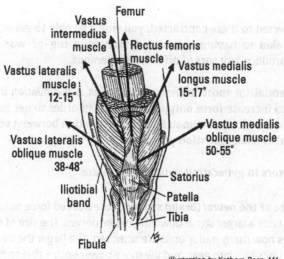

FIGURE 3-5:
The angles of pull.

Femur

Vastus
intermedius
muscle

Rectus femoris
muscle

Vastus medialis
longus muscle
15-17°

Vastus lateralis
muscle
12-15°

Vastus medialis
oblique muscle
50-55°

Vastus lateralis
oblique muscle
38-48°

Satorius

Iliotibial
band

Patella

Tibia

Fibula

Illustration by Kathryn Born, MA

Two-joint and multi-joint muscles

Most muscles span only a single joint and, as a result, provide a standard action with each contraction. For example, the hip flexor attaches at the iliacus of the pelvis and the femur of the thigh; when it contracts, the hip flexes. However, some muscles span two or more joints, and their function is slightly more complex.

>> **A two-joint muscle:** Take the *biceps brachii* (long head), for instance; this muscle originates off the scapula and inserts on the radius in the lower arm. Based on its attachment sites, it primarily supports either elbow flexion or shoulder flexion and is considered a *bi-articular muscle* (that is, a two-joint muscle).

>> **A multi-joint muscle:** An example of a multi-joint muscle is the *erector spinae,* the muscle group that extends along your spinal column and spans multiple joints. When this muscle contracts, the action involves multiple segments of the vertebrae. During contraction, your back is pulled upright, and you stand up straight.

Because muscles often span more than just one joint, their function is largely dictated by the body's position when they contract. For instance, when you're bent all the way over, the erector spinae literally pulls you up (each vertebrae is involved), but when you're already up, it holds you there, keeping you upright.

Pulling harder and harder: Gradation of muscle force

As we explain earlier in this chapter, a motor unit is a single nerve and the few muscle fibers that it connects to. If only one nerve is stimulated and only the few

fibers connected to it are contracted, you won't be able to generate much force —
a scenario akin to having only one person on a tug-of-war team: not strong
enough to produce any sort of effective movement.

REMEMBER

What's essential for most movement activities is a *gradation in strength* (that is,
the ability to increase force output as needed) in order to get just enough muscle
involved to do the job.) Fortunately, the coordination between your brain and your
muscles makes such gradation possible.

The key factors in generating muscular force are

>> **The size of the *neural* (brain) signal:** As the desired force output rises, the
brain sends a larger signal down the motor nerves. The size of the signal
dictates how many motor units are activated. The larger the signal, the more
motor units kick into gear, and the more power you're able to generate.

>> **How strong the signal has to be for the motor units to fire:** Smaller motor
units require less of a signal before they reach a threshold to fire. These
smaller units are the first ones activated. Slow-twitch motor units have the
lowest threshold for recruitment, so they're used first. Activities such as
walking, writing, standing, lifting a light weight, and so on probably use more
slow-twitch fibers!

A muscle fiber never "sort of" contracts. It either contracts or it doesn't. Each
motor unit has a threshold stimulus point. When the signal from the brain is
less than the threshold, the motor unit doesn't contract. If the signal exceeds
the threshold, then all the fibers associated with the motor unit contract. This
all-or-nothing behavior of muscle contraction allows the size of the signal
from the brain to control how many fibers are activated and gives your
body excellent control of how much force you generate.

To generate more force, your body recruits more and more slow-twitch fibers and
then starts recruiting fast-twitch fibers. As the neural signal grows, more slow
twitch motor units are recruited. Just as if you were adding people to a tug-of-war
team, the force generation increases. At some point, the neural signal becomes
great enough that larger, fast-twitch motor units are recruited as well. Usually,
fast-twitch A fibers are recruited first, followed by fast-twitch X. Figure 3-6
shows the sequence of recruitment as the amount of required force increases.

REMEMBER

Motor units are recruited in increasing amounts, based on the size of the neural
signal. Slow-twitch fibers are recruited first, followed by fast-twitch.

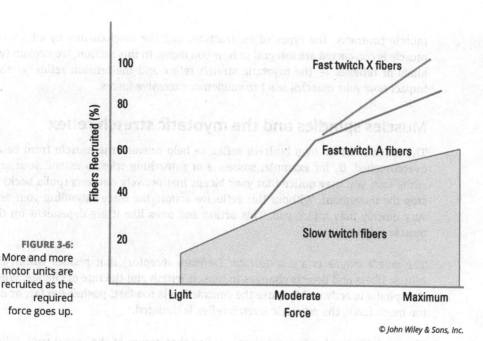

© John Wiley & Sons, Inc.

FIGURE 3-6:
More and more motor units are recruited as the required force goes up.

The chart shows:
- Fast twitch X fibers
- Fast twitch A fibers
- Slow twitch fibers

Fibers Recruited (%): 20, 40, 60, 80, 100

Force: Light, Moderate, Maximum

Acting on Instinct: Hardwired Muscle Reflexes

In any system, some decisions simply don't really need a lot of consideration (hence, the term *no-brainer*). When it comes to movement, some sensory signals are directly linked to a motor response without first going to the brain. If you touch a hot stove, for example, do you really want your nervous system to take the time to send a signal to your brain and your brain to take the time to register the signal as pain and then take more time to send a signal to move your hand from the burning surface? Probably not!

Instead, some movements are *reflexive* — they don't require thought. Of course, not all reflexes are of the "yank your hand from a burning stove" variety. Some simply control how your muscles respond to different kinds of forces or stimuli. Reflexes are important to movement because they speed reactions and provide safety.

Developing tension

Tension and how it's created are at the core of muscle function. Although a contraction leads to movement, not all contractions are the same. How fast the muscle contracts, the types of contraction, and the mechanisms by which the muscle is contracted are integral to how you move. In this section, we explain two kinds of reflexes — the myotatic stretch reflex and the tension reflex — that impact how your muscles react to sudden or excessive forces.

Muscles spindles and the myotatic stretch reflex

The muscle has its own built-in reflex to help prevent the muscle from being overstretched. If, for example, someone or something tries to extend your arm really fast, you may notice that your biceps instinctively *contracts* (pulls back) to stop the movement. Without this reflexive action, the force extending your arm very quickly may injure you. This action and ones like it are dependent on the muscle spindle.

The *muscle spindle* is a *proprioceptor* (sensory receptor) that resides within the muscle fibers and detects changes in muscle length and the rate of change. When the spindle is activated because the contraction is too fast, pushes too far, or has too much force, the myotatic stretch reflex is initiated.

The *myotatic stretch reflex* is a simple reflex that occurs at the spinal cord. When triggered, this reflex contracts the muscle being stretched, called the *agonist* (refer to Chapter 9). As the agonist contracts, the original force, velocity, and range of motion decrease, ultimately protecting the muscle from injury. If you try to kick a ball and miss, for example, the stretch reflex recognizes your blunder and stops you from going too far, preventing you from hurting yourself.

The Golgi tendon and the tension reflex

The last thing you want to happen when you're lifting something heavy or otherwise exerting yourself is to have your muscle pull so hard that the tendon actually pulls away from the bone it's attached to (see Chapter 9 for more on how the muscle and tendon attach to the bone to create movement). Fortunately, your body has a way to stop the muscle from hurting itself: the Golgi tendon organ.

The *Golgi tendon organ* (GTO) is a proprioceptor that is located where the muscle attaches to the tendon. It responds to tension development, much as a spider senses movement on its web. The GTO has a threshold of tension that it considers "too much." When the tension exceeds that amount, the organ sends a signal to the spinal cord and then immediately to the muscle, inhibiting further contraction. Essentially, it turns down the muscle spindle to prevent or minimize additional contraction and keep a lid on any additional tension development. (You can read more about the GTO in Chapter 9.)

You can manipulate how the GTO works to attain your training goals:

>> **Using it to stretch out your muscles:** When you perform a static stretch (refer to Chapter 9) and hold the stretch for a long period, you put tension on the tendon. What you may notice after about 30 seconds is that the muscle starts to relax. This is the Golgi tendon doing its job. It senses the tension you put on the muscle and then reflexively causes a reduction in muscle tension. So, hold the stretch and watch the muscle relax!

>> **Training it to increase strength:** One interesting aspect of the Golgi tendon is that you can actually change its tension threshold. With repeated bouts of exercise, the threshold moves to a higher amount, meaning that you can generate more tension (you become stronger!) using muscle you already have.

But watch out: Highly trained athletes have pushed the threshold so high that they put themselves at risk of tearing the tendon from the bone, but this is unusual and often link to a sudden, significant strain on the muscle or a rapid rise in strength without time for the tendon attachment to adapt and strengthen.

Shortening, lengthening, or not: Types of contractions

Most people equate muscle contraction with movement. Although this is often the case, it isn't always. If you've ever held the door open for someone or simply tried to balance on one foot, you know that some activities require that your muscles fire even though your joints don't move.

Comparing dynamic and static contractions

Muscles act in both a static and dynamic way, providing support for and leading the way for movement. *Static muscle activity* results when a muscle or group of muscles contracts, but the joint doesn't move or moves only minimally. Typically, the purpose of a static contraction is to provide support for the joint or to minimize movement produced by an external force. This type of contraction is considered *isometric*, because the joint doesn't move.

In *dynamic contractions*, the joint and its related body part moves. Dynamic contractions make various types of movement possible, and they occur to control motion from various internal and external influences. *Isotonic contractions*, in which the joint moves, are the most common types of dynamic muscle activity. Isotonic contractions are broken up into either concentric or eccentric components, explained in the next section.

Considering concentric and eccentric contractions

When you think about a muscle contracting, you probably picture a muscle shortening and causing the movement. However, dynamic movement is more complex than that and is dependent on several muscles and/or muscle groups communicating with one another.

When one muscle shortens as it contracts, another muscle lengthens. Each — either lengthening or shortening — is a particular type of contraction:

>> A **concentric contraction** occurs when a muscle shortens during activation.

>> An **eccentric contraction** results when a muscle lengthens during activation. The job of an eccentrically firing muscle is often to resist the motion of another muscle or to control how the joint moves.

REMEMBER

Movement involves a collection of muscles firing both concentrically and eccentrically. Think of the concentric contractions as the movement producers and the eccentric ones as the movement stoppers. Eccentric contractions are also more often employed to control the movement. A good example of controlling a movement is that of hand-eye coordination. If you reach out to grab a door knob and have only concentric muscle firing, you'll reach out toward the knob and strike the door. Nothing — that is, no eccentric contraction — will fire to slow your movement down as you reach the knob or enable you to perform this action in a controlled fashion.

TIP

Understanding the importance of concentric and eccentric contractions is easier if you remember that a muscle is never totally relaxed. Consider what goes on with your arm when you lift a dumbbell. Your biceps contracts and shortens as you flex your elbow. Simultaneously, your triceps contracts to control the amount and velocity of the flexion, but it does so as it lengthens.

Recognizing the different ways muscles work

When muscles contract, they typically do so by applying tension to the sites of attachment and, as a result, create movement. Depending on the factors like fiber architecture, behavioral properties, and types of contractions, all covered in earlier sections, the way the muscles work may also differ (see Figure 3-7):

>> **Agonists and assistors:** The acting muscle responsible for creating a given movement is the agonist. Although any muscle that contributes to the

movement is considered an agonist, some muscles have a greater impact on the movement than others. The muscles with the greatest impact are called simply the *agonists* or *primary movers.* Those that contribute to the movement in smaller ways are referred to as *assistors.* For example, elbow flexion is accomplished when the *biceps brachii* (short and long heads), brachialis, and brachioradialis all contract; however, the biceps brachii is considered the agonist or primary mover, and the others are considered assistors.

>> **Antagonist:** The muscle that contributes directly opposite to the movement that's occurring is referred to as the *antagonist.* Typically, these muscles are located on the side of the joint opposite the agonists, and they cooperate with the agonists by relaxing during the movement.

REMEMBER

The act of the antagonist relaxing or decreasing its gradation (refer to the earlier section "Pulling harder and harder: Gradation of muscle force") during the primary movement is usually an eccentric contraction. However, the key thing to remember is that the antagonist is the muscle that, when contracting concentrically (that is, shortening), provides the opposite motion. When it contracts eccentrically (decreases in gradation), it helps to control the motion and allows the movement that the agonist is trying to accomplish.

>> **Stabilizer:** For a movement to occur, the muscles must act to *fixate* (stabilize) the area so that the limb can exert the force needed to create movement. The muscles that act in this manner are the *stabilizers.* Your *core* (the abdominal muscles) is a good example. When you kick a soccer ball, for example, your core contracts and creates a firm point of support that enables the hip to move and strike the ball. If you don't have good abdominal support, you can strike the ball with only minimal force.

>> **Neutralizer:** *Neutralizers* are the muscles responsible for controlling the influence that internal or external forces may have on the desired movement. Not all muscles that attach to a joint contribute in a way that facilitates the movement; some may actually impede the movement. Therefore, you need muscles around the joint that play a neutralizing role, counteracting muscles that fire in a way that would derail the intended action. Neutralizers also minimize the effect of external forces that can alter the intended movement and potentially cause injury.

REMEMBER

Any muscle can play any of these roles, which are essential to allowing and supporting muscle function. With every movement, an agonist is necessary to create the movement, the antagonist is necessary to help control the motion and allow it to happen, and other muscles are necessary to control the internal and external forces and to create a solid base of support for the movement. In the next two sections, we explain two factors that dictate how muscles work: the length of a muscle and speed of movement.

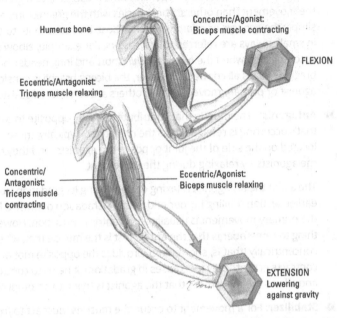

Agonist/Antagonist

Concentric/Agonist:
Biceps muscle contracting

Humerus bone

FLEXION

Eccentric/Antagonist:
Triceps muscle relaxing

Concentric/
Antagonist:
Triceps muscle
contracting

Eccentric/Agonist:
Biceps muscle relaxing

EXTENSION
Lowering
against gravity

FIGURE 3-7:
The relationship
between agonist
and antagonist
muscles.

Illustration by Kathryn Born, MA

Examining the length-tension relationship

A muscle's length influences its force. The *length–tension relationship* explains how much force a muscle can create, given the muscle's length.

A muscle's optimal position for tension development is at approximately 120 percent to 130 percent of its resting length. *Translation:* If your muscle is stretched slightly beyond its normal resting position, it can produce more force. Conversely, when the length of the muscle is less than its normal resting length, how much force it can produce goes down because it has no more room to shorten.

TIP

Have you ever tried to jump up and touch a basketball hoop? If so, you undoubt-edly squatted and then exploded up to touch it. This example shows how the length–tension relationship helps produce force — in this case, jumping higher. Heck, go ahead and stand up from reading this book and try to jump, first, without bending down first and then with bending. Which stance allowed you to go higher?

As you do activities on a regular basis, you begin to identify ways to make the tasks easier. Many of the changes you make relate to the length-tension relation-ship. You alter how much you twist or bend or reach for something, trying to make it easier. Pretty cool, isn't it?

Thinking about the force-velocity relationship

The *velocity* (speed) at which a muscle contracts has a direct impact on the amount of force it can produce. More velocity produces less force; less velocity produces more force.

When the muscle is concentrically contracting (that is, shortening) and you attempt to move a relatively light object, you can do so easily and at a pretty high velocity. Think about throwing a baseball: The ball is light, and you can throw it really fast. Yet, as the object you're trying to move becomes heavier, you're less able to move it as fast. Throwing a shot put, for example, is much more difficult than throwing a baseball, and you can't move it as fast because it's heavier.

REMEMBER

When the resistance grows, movement becomes more and more difficult, as the concentric contraction turns isometric and then progresses to eccentric. Here's what happens:

1. **As the object continues to get heavier, you begin to transition from a concentric contraction, in which the muscle shortens, to an isometric one, at which point no movement is possible.**

   If you've ever been stuck in the middle of a dumbbell curl, you've experienced firsthand what an isometric contraction is!

2. **You transition to a eccentric contraction, the point at which the resistance is greater than the force being produced by the muscle, and the muscle begins to lengthen while it contracts.**

   An eccentric contraction has the ability to create a large amount of force, more than is typically seen with a concentric action. Also, although the resistance is significant enough to warrant an eccentric contraction, as the velocity increases, you start to see a significant increase in how much force the muscle produces.

REMEMBER

Bottom line: Fast concentric contractions can't generate much muscular force, whereas fast eccentric contractions can create more muscular force.

Transitioning between forces: The electromechanical delay

During your normal daily activities, your muscles fire both concentrically and eccentrically, so it's only logical to imagine that a transition occurs between each. The *electromechanical delay* is that transition, and it represents the time it takes for a muscle to go from acting eccentrically to acting concentrically. This phenomenon is often referred to as the *stretch shortening cycle* or the *amortization time*.

Consider what happens when you squat down and then jump. As you squat, your quadriceps muscles lengthen (stretch), representing an eccentric contraction. As you go to jump, they fire concentrically (shorten) to boost you up. The period of time between the end of the eccentric contraction to the beginning of the concentric contraction is the electromechanical delay.

The delay needs to be a relatively quick one to ensure that the energy and elastic properties created during the eccentric portion of the activity aren't lost and actually end up enhancing the concentric portion. If you bend down and sit there for a few moments before you jump, you lose the benefits that the stretch or stored energy has on the activity. Similarly, if the delay is really short, then the muscle isn't able to stretch to its maximal point of force production.

An additional concern with delays that are too long is that the joint is moved into a larger range of motion and injury may result — a situation that occurs in throwers. Research has shown that people who experience shoulder injuries actually have muscles with longer electromechanical delays. Their shoulders are forced to rotate farther than normal, often resulting in additional joint injury.

Plyometric training is a very common training technique in which a muscle is placed under a sudden stretch followed by a forceful contraction. Typically, a load is lowered quickly to induce the stretch, and then lifted as quickly as possible. This type of training for the lower body often involves successive landing-jumping cycles or bounding, sometimes for distance and other times for height. By moving in this way, the athlete is able to take advantage of the stretch-shortening cycle to maximize the force production within the muscles. The result? Higher jumpers and faster runners.

Training Muscles to Work

Muscles are in a fairly constant state of change. If they aren't being used at all (as happens, for example, if you're on bed rest), they begin to *atrophy* (grow smaller and weaker). However, if you train the muscles, they can adapt, get stronger and faster, and even change the chemistry within them. "Use it or lose it" is a pretty accurate statement, and in this section, we explain how you can train muscles to do more work.

Gaining the way you train: Specificity of training

Does being stronger make you faster? Although strength is certainly an important part of training for speed, your neuromuscular system is finicky. If you want to train for speed, you need to do speed training! As simple as this concept is, many people violate the *specificity of training* principle that says your training should be specific to the desired task. For example, some people think — incorrectly — that swinging a heavy baseball bat gives them a faster bat swing or that being able to squat a heavy weight enables them to perform a higher vertical jump. These kinds of violations of the specificity of training principle happen all too frequently.

In this section, we explain the key principles of training specificity.

Training improvements are specific to the muscle fibers used

If you run a number of miles per week at a modest intensity, your slow-twitch muscle fibers will be the primary fibers recruited for the activity (refer to the earlier section "The Tortoise and the Hare: Fast- and Slow-Twitch Fibers"). So, what happens during the big race when you need that big kick at the end to run at a higher intensity? Because you haven't trained for the additional fast-twitch fiber recruitment needed for that kick, your kick will be tiny, and those who've trained more specifically for that moment will pass you by.

TIP

To avoid this scenario, incorporate additional training into your schedule that involves running at a higher intensity! Practice the kick to train your body to recruit the fast-twitch fibers when needed. Then, when the moment arrives, those fibers are ready for action.

Improvements occur at the speed of training and all slower speeds

Slow-speed strength training may help make a muscle strong, but it doesn't give it speed. If you want speed, you need to train the nervous system and muscles to function at speed. Improvements in speed training occur only at the fastest speed you train at. Training at faster speeds also improves your slower speeds, but you can never train slow and hope to be faster. So, match at least some of your training to the speed of the activity!

Changing the load changes your speed

As we explain in the section "Thinking about the force-velocity relationship," earlier in this chapter, force and velocity are related to each other. A light load can be moved quickly, whereas a heavy load is moved more slowly. If you want to swing a baseball bat fast, guess what happens if you pick up a heavier bat? Your swing is slower! Keep training with it, and you get better . . . at swinging a bat slowly. Your bat speed won't improve; in fact, you may actually slow down your speed. Yikes! The lesson? Use loads for training that are very similar to those in your sport.

Adaptations are specific to the joint angle and body position used in training

Functional movements need to be trained, and training needs to replicate as closely as possible the movements you want. If you alter the angles and body positions during training, you'll see those results when you perform the movements in competition. A good coach can help you learn the proper movements. Then it's up to you to train accurately!

You need to train the chemistry of the muscle

As we state earlier, fast-twitch and slow-twitch muscle fibers differ in their chemistry. Slow-twitch fibers are built for aerobic activity, and their enzymes are geared for aerobic energy production. Likewise, fast-twitch fibers have anaerobic enzymes for ATP production. To train for more enzymes (and faster energy production), you need to train those fibers!

Fast-twitch X (or intermediate) fibers can be trained for both anaerobic and aerobic energy production if you vary your training. Be sure to train for the type of adaptation you want to see in those fibers.

Making more muscle and gaining strength

Having more muscle mass has many advantages: Activities of daily living are easier, sport activities are possible, and injuries are less frequent. In addition, muscle burns calories, and stronger muscles lead to stronger bones. Muscle mass becomes even more important as people get older and start to think about things like osteoporosis and playing with their grandkids.

Fortunately, you can develop muscle through training. Muscle grows as a result of stress and damage — which sounds pretty traumatic, but don't worry: The stress is not that great, and surprisingly little effort is required to gain strength.

TIP

In fact, making muscle is a bit like making a callous. If you've ever played a guitar, you know that pressing the strings against the fretboard is a bit painful at first. But with time, nice callouses develop on the fingertips, and playing becomes both easier and less painful.

Many different ways exist to give muscles enough work to grow and adapt. However, a few basic rules apply in all cases of strength training. Follow these rules (outlined in the next sections) to help in your training.

Rule 1: You must lift heavy enough

Weight training is not like aerobic training. Going for a walk is an excellent way to condition your heart and circulatory system. Your muscles, however, need more than that! Because stress and damage cause a muscle to grow (refer to the preceding section), you need to actually cause structural stress to your muscle. If you use loads that your muscles can lift with no stress, you won't see improved strength. The trick is to push your muscles beyond their comfort zone to cause enough stress without injuring the muscle.

REMEMBER

How much is the right amount? Loading is often based on the *one repetition max* (1RM), the load a person can lift just one time. To find this (often after a two-week period of initial training to get past initial muscle soreness), have the client start by lifting a load that feels relatively light a few times, after a rest; add load and lift again. The goal is to work to a point of load that the client can lift only one time. That's their 1RM. As a general rule, training loads need to be at least 60 percent of the 1RM. For example, if you can lift 100 pounds one time only, your exercise weight should be about 60 pounds. Any lighter and the muscle easily lifts the load, and you don't achieve the necessary damage that makes adaptation and growth possible.

WARNING

Use caution when testing the 1RM. Someone who's new to lifting won't be ready to lift their heaviest load. Give them some time to learn to lift smoothly, ad make some initial adaptations, and get past initial muscle soreness from even light loads.

TIP

Eccentric contractions (when the muscle lengthens while contracting; refer to the earlier section "Considering concentric and eccentric contractions") seem to cause the most damage to the muscle during weight lifting. That's good! In fact, you should emphasize the eccentric contractions. So, don't just lift the weight and then drop it: Lower it in a controlled manner to work the muscle during that eccentric phase.

Rule 2: You must lift to fatigue

Lifting a single load, even one that's heavy enough to damage the muscle, doesn't result in *all* your muscles being stressed initially, because the initial lift only needed a portion of the muscle fibers to do the task. In fact, any load that can be lifted more than once is a *submaximal load* (any load less than your 1RM).

When lifting submaximal loads, on repetition 1, you may need only a fraction of your muscle. As those fibers become fatigued, your body calls up more fibers to help carry the load. This process — the used fibers getting tired and the body tapping other muscle fibers as reinforcement — continues with each repetition until all the muscle fibers are involved *and fatigued.* Only at this point, when all your muscle fibers are fatigued, have you worked the muscle, so don't stop early!

Rule 3: Growth happens during the recovery, so eat and rest

Muscles grow during the recovery time between workouts. The point? Recovery is very important to ensure muscle growth. Here are some things you can do to make the most of the recovery time:

>> **Eat enough carbohydrates.** You need energy to fuel the growth. Carbohydrates should make up 50 percent to 60 percent of your diet to fuel the growth of new muscle tissue.

>> **Include an adequate amount of protein in your diet.** Protein helps form the contractile filaments and connective tissue that make up the muscle. You should have between 0.4 and 0.6 grams of protein per pound (g/lb) of body weight. For example, at 0.5 g/lb, a 180-pound person needs 90 grams of protein per day.

>> **Sleep!** During restful sleep, the hormones of muscle growth (growth hormone and testosterone) are highest. If you don't get enough rest, these hormones won't be as elevated.

>> **Base your length of recovery time on the intensity of the training, and take a break between workouts.** The harder the work, the more recovery you need. You can do light work, like gardening, daily with little rest time needed. However, lifting a heavy load, like say 75 percent of your 1RM, causes stress and strain on the muscle and stimulates repair and growth. You can't train a given muscle daily because it needs the recovery time to actually adapt. The more overload you give muscle, the more recovery needed. Usually 24 to 48 hours is enough. Recovery may vary depending on the intensity of the exercise, the condition of the individual, and their age (recovery may take longer for older adults). If you see your loads dropping with each exercise bout, you may need more recovery.

Rule 4: Progressively increase the load as the muscle adapts

Adaptation is great; however, after a muscle has adapted to a load, continuing to train the same way results in a lack of progress. For this reason, you want to engage in *progressive resistance training*, in which you progressively increase the loads as the muscle adapts. One way to track your progress is by the number of repetitions completed. If, for example, you choose a weight that is 60 percent of your 1RM, your muscles should reach fatigue after about 15 to 20 repetitions. If you've adapted enough so you can lift the weight 23 times, it's time to add more load!

TIP

The amount of the increase varies and depends on the size of the muscle. Should you increase five pounds, ten pounds, or more? Rather than think in pounds, consider increasing by a percent of load. Doing so keeps the increase standardized across the different muscle groups. A 10 percent increase in load should be adequate to provide a nice progression in load. This may be tricky for smaller muscles (for example, if you need a 10 percent increase on a 20-pound weight, you'll have trouble finding a 22-pound dumbbell). Use some judgment and perhaps monitor the number of repetitions completed with the new load to determine if it's appropriate.

Seeing how your body adapts to strength training

Strength training doesn't affect just the muscle fibers; it affects the brain and nervous system as well. Nervous system adaptations can happen very quickly, whereas growing muscle tissue takes a bit more time.

Nervous system adaptations

The nervous system adapts quickly to strength training and can result in a substantial increase in strength without any actual change in the size of the muscle fibers. The following neurological adaptations result in substantially increased strength within the first four to eight weeks of training:

» **Increased recruitment of available muscle fibers:** Untrained individuals can't access all the fibers they have for contraction. However, within just a few weeks of strength training, the body is able to recruit more muscle fibers for action. In other words, you can use more of what you always had!

» **Increased frequency of activation:** The brain sends signals for contraction to the muscle in pulses. Any increase in pulse frequency means that the muscles receive these signals more often. Because strength training increases the motor neuron firing rate, the muscle fibers spend more time contracting rather than relaxing.

» **Increased motor unit synchronization:** Just as in tug-of-war, you get the most force if everyone pulls together. Untrained motor units (refer to the earlier section "The motor unit: Connecting the nerve and the muscle") tend to have an unorganized firing rate: Some units fire while others don't. Strength training coordinates (or increases the synchronized action of) the motor units so that the fibers are all pulling at the same time.

>> **Increased threshold for Golgi tendon activation:** The Golgi tendon, covered in the earlier section "The Golgi tendon and the tension reflex," is designed to inhibit additional muscle contraction when too much tension is detected. However, strength training changes this threshold for activation so more force is required to invoke the reflex. In other words, the muscle can generate more force before it gets inhibited. **_Translation:_** You're stronger!

These adaptations benefit anyone who experiences them, but they greatly improve the quality of life for people who suffer debilitating weakness. Think of how a little added strength can help someone walk up stairs or get out of a chair!

Muscle tissue adaptations

Actual changes in muscle tissue due to strength training take a bit longer than neurological changes. However, by 8 to 12 weeks, you should start seeing the following changes in muscle tissue if you follow the strength training rules outlined in "Making more muscle and gaining strength," earlier in this chapter:

>> *Hypertrophy* **(increased muscle size):** The increase in size is seen in both the slow-twitch and fast-twitch fibers. However, the fast-twitch fibers seem much more responsive to strength training and grow the most.

>> **Increase in contractile proteins:** Actin and myosin interaction is the foundation of muscle contraction (refer to the earlier section "The sarcomere and its parts: Shortening to produce force"). Having more actin and myosin means having more pulling power and a stronger muscle. Strength training increases the number of these proteins.

>> **Increase in fast-twitch X to fast-twitch A fiber transition:** Strength training is an anaerobic activity. As a result, when you engage in this type of training, the fast-twitch X fibers become more like the high-power fast-twitch A fibers. Yes, this training may reduce your endurance capacity, but you gain strength!

Recognizing Sources of Muscle Fatigue

Sometimes, the fastest person isn't the one who wins the race; it's the person who doesn't get tired as quickly. Fatigue is a limiting factor in many activities. You try to push yourself as hard as you can, and you try to hang on as long as you can before fatigue grabs hold of you. Depending on the activity, fatigue may come to the muscle in a variety of forms, which we explain in this section.

Running out of gas

As we explain in Chapter 4, the muscle gets its supply of ATP (energy) by metabolizing fuels. Running out of these fuels means fast fatigue:

>> **Creatine phosphate:** This fuel is stored in the muscle for only about ten seconds of high-intensity work. When it runs out, the muscle fatigues!

>> **Glycogen:** Glycogen is stored in the liver and muscle. You have about 2,000 calories' worth, which is enough for about a 20-mile run. When that fuel runs out, the muscle can't keep going!

Suffering from bad (lactic) acid

Lactic acid interferes with muscle contraction. Sarcomeres contract when calcium binds to the protein troponin, which helps open a binding site for the myosin to grab (refer to the earlier section "The Foundations of Muscle Movement: The Science behind Contraction"). Unfortunately, lactic acid (and the acidic hydrogen ion [H^+] that makes up part of it) competes with the calcium for the troponin binding site. As a result, the H^+ ion from the lactic acid prevents the calcium from binding to the troponin. Without calcium binding to troponin, muscle contraction is blocked. As acid levels increase during activity, more muscle contractions get blocked, and you start to fatigue.

TIP

You can recognize the fatigue that results from lactic acid as it happens. As you exercise and your muscle fibers begin to build up lactic acid, blocking contraction, you may notice that your running stride becomes "choppy" or your pedal rate starts to vary. What's happening is that the non-fatigued muscles are trying to help out with the movements, and your body uses different muscle activation strategies to do the same work. This situation can slow you down and also make your movements less precise.

More bad (lactic) acid: Slowing nerve conduction

Normally, electrical signals move quickly along the axons of the nerve, skipping from node to node like a stone across water (Chapter 7) has more on the nervous system). However, when H^+ ions from lactic acid build up, the signals slow down. If you're trying to coordinate a movement, as you do when you run, jump, or shoot a basketball, for example, you may notice that the sequence of your movements starts getting thrown off a bit. The reason is that the signals just don't quite get to the muscle in time, resulting in fatigue and reduced performance.

Getting the message from your brain to stop

One last cause of fatigue can be your own brain. Lactic acid and the resulting acidity (H^+ ions) can cause you to feel tired and in pain — and even nauseous — and can cause you simply to stop. Because motor activity is linked to sensory information (refer to Chapter 7), physiologic pain can result in a reduced motor output to the muscles. A reduced output from the central nervous system results in less effort (like less load lifted or slower running speed) and, therefore, fatigue.

WARNING

Athletes have been trained to push well beyond the normal limits at which most of the rest of us would fatigue, even to the point of injury. To some degree, this is a good thing, but it can be taken to extremes. Pushing beyond what you used to think was fatigue may get you to perform better (like finishing that last mile of the race). Pushing to the point of weakness and leading to injury (like a runner collapsing from exhaustion during a marathon) can mean you won't finish the race. The trick is to understand the limits of your body's performance.

Chapter **4**

Keeping the Big Wheel Turning: Exercise Metabolism

Your body runs on one fuel source: adenosine triphosphate (ATP). But because you can store only a small amount of ATP, as soon as you begin to use it up, you need to create more. Fortunately, you can make more ATP using energy systems in the muscles with fuels such as carbohydrates and fats.

Some of these systems kick in fast and furious, providing an almost instant supply of ATP; others provide energy at a slower rate. Some get depleted quickly; others can go forever. Some sport activities and movements use one system more than the others.

In this chapter, we explain how your body's ATP systems work and note which activities use one system more than another.

Introducing The ATP-PC Energy System: Give Me Energy Now!

Your life depends on the energy you get when you break chemical bonds, specifically the bonds holding together a molecule called ATP. Adenosine is connected to three phosphates by high-energy bonds. These bonds hold the energy that drives all the biological actions in your body. To produce energy, you just need to get the bonds to break!

Breaking (chemical) bonds

An essential component that drives chemical reactions is a *catalyst*. In the human body, these catalysts are *enzymes*. It takes a reaction with water and the help of a special enzyme — ATPase — to liberate energy from ATP. After the energy is liberated (along with a phosphate being lost), you end up with *adenosine diphosphate* (ADP). (The *di* part of *diphosphate* means "two.")

When ADP is present, other energy systems turn on to replenish ATP. Here's what's happening:

$$ATP + H_2O \rightarrow ADP + P_i = \text{energy liberated}$$

$$ADP + P_i \text{ (from another energy system)} = ATP \text{ replenished}$$

Where is ATP stored? Well, if it's used for movement, where do you think you'd put it? In the muscle! But strangely, muscle stores only enough ATP for about two seconds of work. That's like having $5 in the bank — certainly not enough to pay the bills. Fortunately, your body has a way to produce the ongoing energy you need.

Replenishing energy as you use energy: The air compressor analogy

To understand how the human body's energy system works, think of an air compressor. An air compressor is a big tank that holds air that you can use to fill tires or run machinery. Attached to this tank is a small motor that compresses air and a gauge that shows the amount of air pressure in the tank.

Now, imagine that the tank is full of compressed air and the motor is turned off. How can you make the compressor turn on? Simple: You use some air! When you use air, the pressure in the tank drops, and that drop in pressure signals the motor to turn on to compress more air.

Your body's energy system follows essentially the same principle. You have only two seconds of ATP stored in your body, but when you use it, you turn on your body's energy systems to start making ATP!

Three primary systems provide ATP:

>> **Phosphocreatine (ATP-PC):** This system provides an immediate boost of energy that lasts only a few seconds.

>> **Anaerobic glycolysis:** This system provides energy for activities lasting longer than a few seconds (closer to five minutes) but that still need a lot of ATP quickly.

>> **Oxidative (aerobic) system:** This system provides energy for activities that don't need ATP at very high rates but need the ATP to last for a very long time without fatigue (like your entire life!).

REMEMBER

As you can see, the systems that make ATP provide energy at different rates. The moment you start to move, you use your small stores of ATP and turn on *all* the systems that make ATP. Because your metabolism always needs ATP, you're always making it and always using it! As a result, you can get energy for long walks or high jumps without having to shift gears. The energy will be there for you! The following sections explain these three energy systems in detail.

Phosphocreatine: An immediate source of ATP

If the high-energy bond of ATP is broken for activity, that energy needs to be replaced if you want to continue moving. One way your body replaces the used energy *fast* is to "steal" it from another substance. *Phosphocreatine* is the most immediate source of energy to remake ATP (see Figure 4-1). Phosphocreatine is stored within your muscle, and you have enough for about ten seconds of all out, high-intensity exercise.

TIP

To better understand how the phosphocreatine system works, imagine that you have $100 in your pocket and a friend who replenishes your money as you spend it. You spend $10 on lunch, for example, and immediately, your friend hands you $10. You spend another $50 on some clothes. Immediately, your friend gives you $50! Wow! As long as your friend doesn't go broke, you can keep spending! But when the friend goes broke, you're both out of luck. If you're running a 100-meter sprint, you'll deplete your stores of phosphocreatine. Because phosphocreatine stores last only 8 to 10 seconds, as you run that race, you're using ATP as fast as possible, with ATP replenishment coming from phosphocreatine. As soon as those stored are depleted, you can't produce ATP fast enough, and you'll slow down. So, in this intense exercise case, fatigue is happening due to a depletion of phospho-creatine stores.

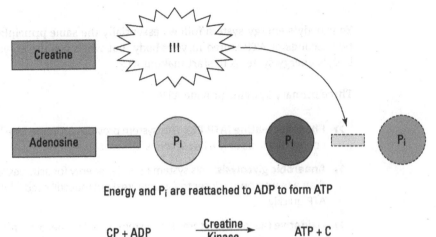

Energy and P$_i$ are reattached to ADP to form ATP

$$CP + ADP \xrightarrow[\text{Kinase}]{\text{Creatine}} ATP + C$$

FIGURE 4-1:
How
phosphocreatine
remakes ATP.

© John Wiley & Sons, Inc.

REMEMBER

High-intensity activities that last under ten seconds — activities like the sprinting for 100 meters, high-jumping, running to first base in baseball, swinging a bat or golf club, or lifting a very heavy weight (one that you can lift maybe only five times) — all get their ATP mostly from phosphocreatine.

CREATINE LOADING: EFFECTIVE AID OR EXPENSIVE URINE?

Because phosphocreatine is so important for high-intensity exercise, athletes want to store as much of it as possible. The human body can create some of the components, like creatine, from amino acids. However, some research has shown that supplementing the diet with creatine may also provide positive effects. In laboratory testing, creatine supplementation showed positive improvements in high-intensity exercise performance (producing a better effort at weight training, for example, or leading to increased strength and longer efforts at sprint cycling, resulting in improved sprint time).

The benefits seem to vary: Some subjects responded to the supplementation; others didn't. Side effects appear to be minimal (nausea and possibly cramping). In addition, the addition of creatine to the cells pulls water with it, causing some water weight gain — an effect that may be beneficial for those needing to cool themselves with sweat but not great for those who need speed (the added weight can slow them down). So, the jury is still out on the effectiveness of creatine supplementation.

Anaerobic glycolysis: Fast energy with a price

Wouldn't it be nice to be able to generate enough ATP to run hard for longer than the ten-second burst of phosphocreatine? Well, you do have a system of ATP production that works very quickly to give you ATP. Using the glucose (the simplest form of carbohydrate) in your body, you can produce a lot of ATP pretty fast (not as fast as the phosphocreatine system can produce ATP, but still plenty fast). However, this ATP production method has a side effect of sorts: It leads to fatigue.

ATP supplies are used up within two seconds of exercise. This loss of ATP immediately turns on the system within the cell that can use glucose to provide energy to form more ATP. The chemical reactions that accomplish this take place within the cell.

YOUR STARTER FUEL: GLUCOSE AND GLYCOGEN

Because humans run on ATP, you'd think that we should just eat ATP. Not possible! Instead, the energy for ATP is tied up in other molecules. One is the monosaccharide or simple sugar glucose. Your body has the necessary enzymes to rearrange a molecule of glucose so the energy within the molecular bonds can be used to remake ATP. How sweet is that?

Many versions of sugars exist, as do other chains of glucose like starches, but the simplest is *glucose*, the primary component of starches, or carbohydrates, like pasta, grains, and rice. Glucose is a 6-carbon molecule that serves as an essential fuel to help energy systems in our body produce ATP.

REMEMBER

Although you carry a small amount of glucose in your blood, you actually store glucose in the muscle and liver in the form of *glycogen*. Think of glycogen as a glucose snowball — a multitude of glucose units connected together. Your body has about 2,000 calories of glycogen — enough to run about 20 miles.

GETTING GLUCOSE INTO THE CELL

Because glycogen is kept in two locations (the muscle and liver), the process of getting glucose ready for ATP production varies, depending on the location of the glycogen:

>> **From the liver:** Glycogen is broken apart into individual glucose units (in *glycogenolysis*). This glucose is dumped into the blood so that it can be transported to the muscle or to other cells that need it. (This is why we have blood glucose.) From there, the glucose gets into the cell by way of special proteins that act like gateways (think of the revolving doors at a fancy hotel).

GLYCOGEN SUPERCOMPENSATION: CARB-LOADING FOR PERFORMANCE

Having as much glycogen as possible stored in the liver and muscles before any big activity or event (a marathon, the Tour de France, and so on) is clearly advantageous. Normally, you store glycogen after a workout, using a glycogen-making enzyme called *glycogen synthase,* along with carbohydrates in the diet. Briefly storing more glycogen than normal is possible, however. The recipe for *loading,* or *supercompensating,* is very simple:

1. **Reduce your training volume and intensity.**

   Known as a *taper,* this action reduces your use of glycogen. Filling the gas tank is easier if you aren't using as much gas, right?

2. **Increase your dietary intake of carbohydrates.**

   Maybe bump it up to 60 percent to 70 percent of your diet. The enzymes for glycogen synthesis store the extra carbs as glycogen.

3. **A day or two before the big event, reduce your training even further and increase your carbs to at least 70 percent.**

   Doing so drives maximal glycogen supercompensation.

The result? You have extra stores of glycogen, you feel rested, and you probably can run faster and longer than you ever did during training. See Chapter 15 for more sports nutrition information.

REMEMBER

ATP is required for glucose to get into cells, so you actually use energy to start the process of creating ATP. The end result is a glucose molecule with a phosphate attached (called *glucose 6-phosphate*) — just what you need to start making some ATP quickly inside the cell.

>> **From the muscle:** Location is everything! Because some glycogen already exists in the muscle, you simply need an enzyme to break the glycogen snowball apart and grab a floating phosphate. The result? A glucose 6-phosphate that didn't cost you any ATP.

Cooking up ATP, oxygen-free: Anaerobic glycolysis

The cell is a bit of a soup, full of nutrients and enzymes. Chemical reactions can take place quickly in this environment and help produce ATP at a very fast rate. Because oxygen isn't used, the process of breaking down glucose is *anaerobic* (without oxygen).

Two primary steps are involved with anaerobic glycolysis. The first step requires an investment of energy, but the second step doubles your energy. If you want to make money, you have to spend a little, and that's what happens here (see Figure 4-2):

1. **Invest energy and prime the pump.**

   In this first phase, glucose is taken into the cell and "trapped," by attaching a phosphate and converting glucose into glucose 6-phosphate. Capturing and trapping the glucose takes energy (ATP) and an enzyme. Later, another phosphate is added and another ATP used. This process gets the molecules in a position to produce ATP by converting it to fructose 6-phosphate.

2. **Produce double the energy.**

   In this phase, the molecule splits in two, and each one goes through a series of reactions, starting from glucose 3-phosphate (G3P), to 1–3 biphosphoglycerate (1–3 BPG), to 3 phosphoglycerate (3-PG), during which you generate two ATP. After water removal, phosphoenolpyruvate (PEP) is converted to a strong acid, *pyruvic acid,* and two more ATP are generated. You just doubled your money — you went from 2 ATP to 4 ATP — and you have a net gain of energy!

   The reason you can get one more ATP is because muscle glycogen doesn't take energy to trap the glucose, so one less ATP is invested!

REMEMBER

This outcome almost seems too good to be true: fast energy, double your energy . . . so what's the catch? The end result of glycolysis, pyruvic acid (or *pyruvate*) is a strong acid that very quickly causes fatigue.

One way to slow the acid buildup is to convert the pyruvate to a less-acidic acid — *lactic acid.* An enzyme (lactate dehydrogenase, or LDH) converts pyruvic acid into lactic acid:

Pyruvic acid ———— Enzyme (LDH) ———— Lactic acid

Unfortunately, lactic acid can be just as bad, as we explain in the next section.

THE METABOLIC DOWNSIDE: LACTIC ACID AND FATIGUE

The unfortunate side effect of anaerobic glycolysis is the accumulation of lactic acid. Your body doesn't respond well to acid. Proteins begin to break down, and cells can die. To prevent too much acid from building up, a number of fatigue-related changes take place when lactic acid accumulates from exercise. These changes are designed to slow you down and prevent damage.

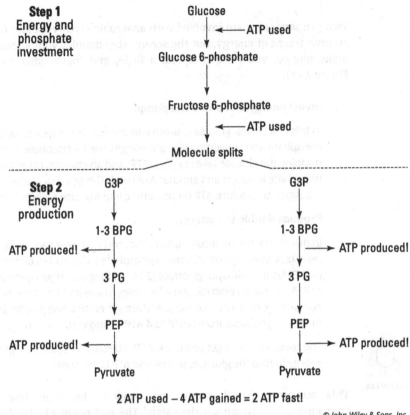

Step 1
Energy and
phosphate
investment

Glucose
←— ATP used
Glucose 6-phosphate

Fructose 6-phosphate
←— ATP used

Molecule splits

Step 2
Energy
production

G3P

1-3 BPG

ATP produced! ←

3 PG

PEP

ATP produced! ←

Pyruvate

G3P

1-3 BPG

→ ATP produced!

3 PG

PEP

→ ATP produced!

Pyruvate

2 ATP used – 4 ATP gained = 2 ATP fast!

© John Wiley & Sons, Inc.

FIGURE 4-2:
Producing ATP,
using anaerobic
glycolysis.

REMEMBER

When we talk about acid in this context, we're really talking about a particular ion. Think of the unit of acidity, pH (which stands for the *power of hydrogen*). The hydrogen ion (H^+) is what makes acid, well, acid. The concept can be confusing sometimes, because a higher concentration of H^+, or more acidity, is reflected by a lower pH value. So, the accumulation of lactic acid really means the accumulation of hydrogen ions and a drop in pH.

UNDERSTANDING HOW H⁺ CAUSES FATIGUE

Following is a step-by-step description of how H^+ can cause fatigue (see Figure 4-3 for an illustration of this process):

1. **Hydrogen ions block muscle contraction.**

   H^+ ions compete with another ion, calcium (Ca^{++}), for the affection of a protein (troponin). Calcium normally binds to troponin in the muscle to cause muscle contraction. As H^+ builds up, it competes with Ca^{++} for troponin binding and starts to block contraction. The result? Less force produced and fatigue.

2. Hydrogen ions slow nerve signals to the muscle.

Normally, nerve signals can skip along a nerve like a stone across water. H^+ in the cell slows down the skipping. As a result, you can't get a coordinated signal to the muscles. Uncoordinated signals interfere with motor skills. Your running strides are altered, and you experience more fatigue.

3. Hydrogen ions block an enzyme necessary for anaerobic glycolysis.

Early in the anaerobic glycolysis process of making ATP, a particular enzyme, *phosphofructokinase,* is very sensitive to H^+. When H^+ levels rise, phosphofructo-kinase slows its ability to help run glycolysis! When this happens, you can't make more lactic acid. Of course, you can't make more ATP either. Result? Even more fatigue.

4. Hydrogen ions cause pain.

You may have felt the pain of lactic acid in your muscles when you worked hard. And when the pain was high, you reduced your effort (which means a reduced motor stimulus leaving your brain); that's also fatigue.

REMEMBER

Lactic acid causes fatigue at the brain (called *central fatigue*), as well as at various locations around the muscle and cell (known as *peripheral fatigue*). Head to Chapter 7 for a more in-depth discussion of the brain's role in movement.

RECOVERY FROM EXERCISE: GETTING RID OF LACTIC ACID

Because lactic acid is such a major player in fatigue (and fatigue means poor performance), getting rid of lactic acid fast is desirable if you want to get back in action quickly. Here are some suggestions:

>> **Breathe it off.** Thank goodness for chemistry! Blood contains a substance called *bicarbonate* (HCO_3^-). When you breathe, the HCO_3^- in your blood can combine with the nasty H^+ to form a weaker, and less nasty, acid called *carbonic acid.*

$$H^+ + HCO_3^- \;\text{---}\; H_2CO_3$$

Can you see two substances in there? Well, when blood passes through the lungs, it's converted into carbon dioxide and water:

$$H_2CO_3 \;\text{---}\; H_2O + CO_2$$

The extra CO_2 makes you breathe harder. You've probably found yourself breathing hard when you've pushed the intensity a bit too much. Maybe it's because lactic acid is building up!

Source of fatigue # 1

Lactic acid interferes with muscle contraction

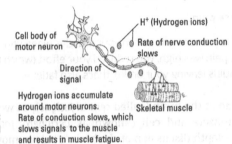

Calcium binding site

Troponin

Tropomyosin

Ca^{2+}

H^+

H^+

H^+ (Hydrogen ion)

Ca^{++} (Calcium)

Hydrogen ions from lactic acid
compete with calcium for binding sites.
This blocks muscle contractions.

Source of fatigue # 2

H^+ (Hydrogen ions)

Cell body of
motor neuron

Rate of nerve conduction
slows

Direction of
signal

Hydrogen ions accumulate
around motor neurons.
Rate of conduction slows, which
slows signals to the muscle
and results in muscle fatigue.

Skeletal muscle

FIGURE 4-3:
How lactic acid
causes fatigue.

Source of fatigue # 3

Depleting stores of glycogen

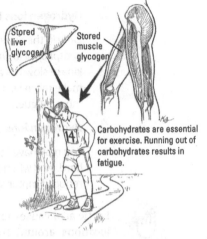

Stored
liver
glycogen

Stored
muscle
glycogen

Carbohydrates are essential
for exercise. Running out of
carbohydrates results in
fatigue.

Illustration by Kathryn Born, MA

TIP

>> **Use your muscles.** As you'll see when you study muscles, muscle fibers favor either fast or slow ATP production. Aerobic fibers, known as *slow-twitch* muscle fibers, are unique. They actually use lactic acid just like glucose and produce ATP! Slow-twitch fibers are used mostly during light exercise. So, when the big sprint is over and all that lactic acid has built up, what should you do? Walk! Light jog! If you use your slow-twitch fibers, you'll get rid of the lactic acid more quickly. Even during exercise, slow-twitch fibers can use lactic acid. So lactic acid is not all bad, depending on the situation.

The Oxidative (Aerobic) System: It Just Keeps Going and Going

Mitochondria are nature's batteries. These organelles contain enzymes that can rearrange molecules through a number of steps to ultimately create ATP. The reason mitochondria are so good at producing ATP is because, as long as they have a source of fuel and oxygen available, the only waste they produce is carbon dioxide and water, which you can breathe out.

Mitochondria (see Figure 4-4) are located in the cell. From a standpoint of exercise, you'll find that they may be more numerous in some areas than in others. As Chapter 3 explains, different muscle fibers have different characteristics. Some are aerobic muscle fibers and have a lot of mitochondria; others are anaerobic fibers and have few mitochondria.

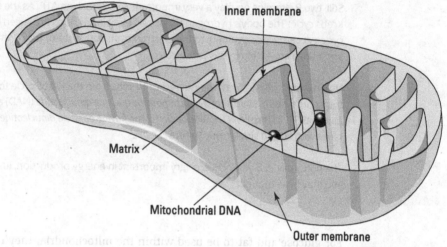

FIGURE 4-4:
A mitochondrion.

In the mitochondria, chemical reactions occur that take fat and glucose and produce H^+ ions. These ions create the power to make the ATP that feeds your muscles.

Mitochondria produce ATP much like a battery produces energy. To understand these chemical reactions, picture a battery. A battery has a positive and a negative charge at either end. The flow of electrons across this electrical gradient is what runs your radio. Inside the battery, positive charges are created, usually using an acid that produces hydrogen (H^+) ions. The foods we eat (fats, carbohydrates, and even proteins) all contain H^+ ions. Our energy systems can gather these ions to make ATP.

Aerobic metabolism: Making ATP with glucose, fat, and protein

You can make energy from the foods you eat. This process, called *aerobic metabolism*, involves a series of complex chemical reactions — too complex for the purposes of this book. However, you may find it useful to take a step-by-step look at the basics behind the creation of ATP from the nutrients in foods.

B VITAMINS: THE ENERGY VITAMINS?

You may have heard that B vitamins are the "energy vitamins," a phrase that may lead you to think that, just by consuming these vitamins, you'll have energy. Unfortunately, that isn't the case. You get energy through the aerobic and anaerobic systems.

Still, two B vitamins do play a very important role in making ATP. As the section "The Krebs cycle: The body's hydrogen producer" explains, H^+ ions produced by the Krebs cycle get carried, or shuttled, to the electron transport system. Two B vitamins — niacin and riboflavin — help in this process.

Niacin and riboflavin form the carriers of H^+ ions from the Krebs cycle to the electron transport system. Niacin forms *nicotinamide adenine dinucleotide* (NAD) and can combine with H^+ to form NADH. Riboflavin forms *flavine adenine dinucleotide* (FAD) and combines with H^+ in a similar way to form FADH.

The bottom line: B vitamins are very important in energy production, just not the way you may have thought.

For glucose and fat to be used within the mitochondria, they're rearranged into various molecules that can "plug into" the aerobic metabolic pathway and act much like kindling does to feed a fire. The "fire" of ATP production in the mitochondria is a sequence of molecular rearrangements, and glucose, fat, and protein serve as the starting point.

Using glucose and fat to make ATP

As the earlier section "Cooking up ATP, oxygen-free: Anaerobic glycolysis" explains, glucose can be broken down to two pyruvic acid molecules through the process of glycolysis. Pyruvate is a 3-carbon molecule that can be converted into a key molecule that the mitochondria can use to make energy when oxygen is present. That molecule is a 2-carbon unit called *acetyl coenzyme A* (CoA). The left-over carbon is lost when carbon dioxide (CO_2) is formed.

$$2 \text{ pyruvate} \text{ ———— } 2 \text{ acetyl CoA} + 2 \text{ } CO_2 \text{ (produced as waste)}$$

Fat is a very long chain of carbon, hydrogen, and oxygen. Fats can be brought to the mitochondria, and from there, a number of 2-carbon acetyl CoA units can be created in a process called *beta-oxidation* (in this context, *beta* refers to the number 2). Think of a fat like a long chain of sausage links, with each individual link being a 2-carbon beta unit.

REMEMBER

Both carbohydrates and fats can be broken down into acetyl CoA molecules, which are the primary entry points into the Krebs cycle. In this way, both glucose and fat can undergo aerobic metabolism. You can read about the Krebs cycle in the later section "The Krebs cycle: The body's hydrogen producer."

Using protein for ATP

Protein isn't a big contributor to ATP production. In fact, under normal conditions (like eating enough food every day), you may get only about 5 percent to 10 percent of your energy from protein. Instead, protein is used to make things: muscle, enzymes, and antibodies — pretty important stuff! Muscle is the greatest storage location for protein, so anything that steals protein results in the loss of muscle mass.

Protein can be used for energy in two ways:

>> **As components within the Krebs cycle:** The big wheel of the H^+ ion producer needs a number of molecules to keep things going. Protein can be broken down into its building blocks (called *amino acids*), which can then be used within the Krebs cycle (after the liver takes out the nitrogen, that is).

>> **As energy after being converted into glucose:** If carbohydrates are low in the body, the liver can convert protein into glucose in a process called *gluconeogenesis* (think "glucose-new-make"). Although using protein in this way can save you when you don't have any carbs, it uses up your muscle, so it's not a good idea in the long run.

The Krebs cycle: The body's hydrogen producer

For your "battery" to run, it has to produce H^+ ions. Fortunately, that's what the Krebs cycle does. The Krebs cycle is a series of chemical reactions that rearrange molecules and release H^+ ions.

As Figure 4-5 shows, enzymes are needed for each reaction. For example, the starting molecule, acetyl CoA, is rearranged to form citrate, then isocitrate, then alpha-ketoglutarate. At that rearrangement, an H^+ ion is released and carried onward for ATP generation. The process continues with additional rearrangements (succinyl CoA → succinate, and so on).

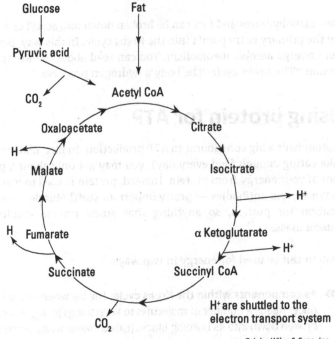

FIGURE 4-5:
The Krebs cycle:
The body's
hydrogen-
producing
machine.

Glucose

Fat

Pyruvic acid

CO_2

Acetyl CoA

Oxaloacetate

Citrate

H

Malate

Isocitrate

H^+

H *Fumarate*

α Ketoglutarate

H^+

Succinate

Succinyl CoA

CO_2

H^+ are shuttled to the
electron transport system

© *John Wiley & Sons, Inc.*

CO_2 is released during "turns" of the cycle as a waste product, and H^+ ions that are released are carried or shuttled onto the location for energy production (the electron transport system). As long as the big wheel keeps on turning, H^+ can be produced through the molecular rearrangements.

The electron transport system: Running the battery

The electron transport system (ETS) can be thought of as the guts of a battery; it uses the supply of H^+ to produce ATP. Located on the inner mitochondrial membrane, it's responsible for using the energy from the H^+ ions that are produced by the Krebs cycle to drive ATP production. Just like a battery gets its juice by having an electrical gradient, the ETS creates a chemical (H^+) gradient across the inner mitochondrial membrane. This is where the energy for ATP production comes from.

Figure 4-6 illustrates this process. Electrons are removed from H+ and passed down a series of reactions (almost like water running over a dam). The energy created by this cascade of electrons is what generates ATP. At the end of the sequence, H+ remains and must be eliminated or neutralized.

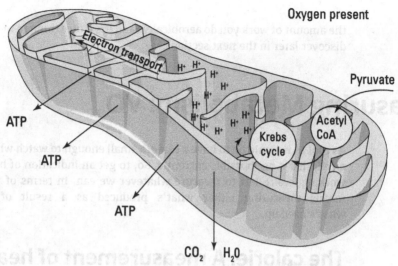

Oxygen present

Electron transport

H^+ H^+

H^+

H^+

H^+

H^+

H^+ H^+

H^+

H^+

H^+

Pyruvate

Acetyl CoA

ATP

ATP

Krebs cycle

ATP

CO_2 H_2O

© John Wiley & Sons, Inc.

FIGURE 4-6:
The electron transport system — using H^+ to make ATP.

Here's how the process works: Electrons from the hydrogen ions that have been obtained by way of the Krebs cycle are passed along a chain of reactions passing from the inner membrane of the mitochondria to the outer membrane. This transfer creates an energy gradient that provides the energy needed to remake ATP. A key component is the enzyme ATPase, which uses the energy from the flow of H+ to reconnect the phosphate to ADP, thus forming ATP. The H+ ions that are left over need to be removed.

Can you think of anything that combines well with H+ to form a neutral substance? See the next section for the answer!

Water under the bridge: Understanding oxygen's role

Now you may be thinking, "But H^+ ions cause fatigue! I don't want H^+ accumulating in my mitochondria!" Ah, well, this is where oxygen plays its part in the story.

When you combine H^+ and oxygen, you get water:

$$2H^+ + O = H_2O$$

Water is as neutral a substance as it gets. As long as oxygen is available, the H^+ is neutralized. *Translation:* The oxygen acts as a buffer, eliminating the H^+ ions and assisting with ATP production. If you want to make a lot of ATP, you need to get a lot of oxygen into the mitochondria. Therefore, oxygen use is related directly to the amount of work you do aerobically (and it's a nice thing to measure, which you discover later in the next section).

Measuring Metabolism: VO$_2$

As cool as it would be to have a camera small enough to watch what goes on inside a cell, that's not possible currently. So, to get an indication of how hard cells are working, we're left to measure whatever we can. In terms of metabolism, that means measuring either what's produced as a result of metabolism or what's used up.

The calorie: A measurement of heat

Your system runs on ATP. The chemical energy from ATP breakdown is used to make your muscles move and to perform all other actions. But did you know that only about 20 percent of the ATP energy goes to your muscle? What happens to the other 80 percent? It produces heat! That's why shivering keeps you warm and why you need to sweat when you exercise. One way to determine work intensity and calories burned is to measure the amount of heat produced during exercise.

WHY NO CARBS MEANS MUSCLE LOSS

Glucose is essential to burn fat. Fat and glucose both enter into the Krebs cycle (that big wheel of H$^+$ producers, explained in "The Krebs cycle: The body's hydrogen producer," later in this chapter) at the same point, as acetyl CoA. However, glucose also contributes to other parts of the cycle. Without glucose, that big wheel won't keep on turning.

Without glucose, fat continues to accumulate in the form of acetyl CoA but can't get through the Krebs cycle. The body responds by letting the liver convert the acetyl CoA to an acid called a *ketone*. Ketones slow the metabolic rate, reduce appetite, and build up levels of acid in the blood (and your body does not like acid). Left unchecked, ketosis can lead a person with diabetes into a coma.

In healthy people, restricting carbs (as you do in a low-carb diet) also brings on ketosis. However, instead of just messing with their fat metabolism, they also start losing muscle mass. Here's why: Protein can be used for ATP production within the Krebs cycle, *and* the liver can turn protein into glucose! If you deprive your body of glucose, it responds by depriving you of your muscle mass, a situation that slows metabolic rate even more and makes it hard to lose body fat. So, eat your carbs!

In the early days of measuring heat, exercisers were placed inside a sealed chamber surrounded by water; oxygen was fed into the chamber, and carbon dioxide was removed. As the person exercised, researchers measured the change in water temperature. A *calorie* was defined as the amount of heat it took to raise 1 milliliter (or 1 gram) of water 1 degree centigrade. Because raising 1 milliliter 1 degree takes a pretty small amount of heat, the standard is to deal in numbers a thousand times bigger. So a *kilocalorie* (heat needed to raise 1 *liter* of water 1 degree centigrade) is what people usually mean when they talk about calories.

Measuring the volume of oxygen consumed

Measuring the heat produced during exercise is difficult. Fortunately, oxygen, which is used to make ATP, can also be measured. As a result, it has become a primary variable when determining both work intensity and calories burned.

Oxygen concentrations in air can be used to measure heat. The air around you is about 21 percent oxygen. Now, take a breath and then exhale. The concentration of oxygen in the air you just exhaled is only about 16 percent oxygen. Where did the rest of the oxygen go? You used it in the mitochondria to make ATP!

By measuring how much air you are moving each minute (breathing in and out), you can then determine the *volume of oxygen* (VO_2) you use each minute. VO_2 is usually measured in liters used per minute (L/min). At rest, VO_2 may be as low as 0.25 L/min; during peak exercise, it may be as high as 6.0 L/min.

If you worked as hard as you can, perhaps running faster and faster on a treadmill until you fatigued, eventually you'd hit the peak of your ability to use oxygen to make ATP. This is known as the *maximal oxygen uptake*, or VO_2 *max*.

Because the use of oxygen is directly related to physical work, measuring VO_2 is the primary tool to assess how hard the work is. VO_2 is directly linked to ATP productions and heat produced (calories); therefore, if you know VO_2, you can estimate calories burned. For every liter of oxygen consumed, about 5 kilocalories are burned. So, the equation is

$$\text{calories burned} = VO_2 \text{ L/min} \times 5$$

Exercise physiologists use this equation to determine how many calories various activities burn.

Comparing fitness levels: VO$_2$ and body weight

Suppose you have a 200-pound man and a 120-pound woman. Each can lift 150 pounds. Who's stronger? Trick question? Maybe.

On the one hand, both have the same strength (each can lift 150 pounds). But based on size, the woman is stronger. Factoring strength based on body weight seems like a better way to compare.

Likewise, if two individuals can use, say, 4 liters of oxygen per minute during peak exercise, you may think they have the same level of fitness. However, you really need to factor in body size to determine oxygen use relative to body weight.

REMEMBER

TIP

When you want to compare the fitness levels of individuals, you need to determine VO$_2$ according to body weight. Follow these steps:

1. **Convert each person's weight into metric units.**

   To convert pounds into kilograms, take the weight in pounds and divide it by 2.2.

2. **Covert L/min to mL/min by multiplying the L/min value by 1,000.**

3. **Adjust for body weight.**

   Divide the mL/min value by the weight in kilograms. This calculation gives you the milliliters of oxygen used per kilogram of body weight each minute, a unit represented as mL/kg/min.

4. **Compare the VO$_2$ max to determine who is more fit.**

   As Table 4-1 shows, the higher the VO$_2$ max number, the more fit the individual.

TABLE 4-1 **Fitness Categories Based on VO$_2$ Max (in mL/kg/min)**

	Low Fitness	Average Fitness	High Fitness
Men	Less than 45	46 to 55	56 or more
Women	Less than 40	41 to 49	50 or more

Say you're comparing a man who weighs 180 pounds and a woman who weighs 135 pounds. Both have a VO_2 max of 4.0 L/min, and you want to determine who is more fit. Table 4-2 shows the comparison, using the preceding steps.

TABLE 4-2   **Comparing VO_2 Max: An Example**

	Man	Woman
Weight converted from pounds to kilograms	180 pounds ÷ 2.2 = 81.8 kg	135 pounds ÷ 2.2 = 61.4 kg
VO2 max converted from L/min to mL/min	4.0 L/min × 1,000 = 4,000 mL/min	4.0 L/min × 1,000 = 4,000 mL/min
mL/min adjusted for body weight	4,000 ÷ 81.8 = 48.9 mL/kg/min	4,000 ÷ 61.4 = 65.1 mL/kg/min
Conclusion	His VO_2 max is 48.9 milliliters of oxygen used per kilogram body weight each minute. The man's fitness level is average.	Her VO_2 max is 65.1 milliliters of oxygen used per kilogram body weight each minute. The woman's fitness level is in the highest fitness category!

TIP

By using this method of displaying VO_2 max, you can compare people of different sizes and make tables of fitness norms (so you can compete against your friends or at least see whether you have a decent level of fitness!).

Measuring metabolism during exercise

Technology has advanced to the point where it's now possible to measure the concentration of oxygen and carbon dioxide in every breath taken. All you have to do is capture the air and redirect it to an analyzer, like the one shown in Figure 4-7.

REMEMBER

Just as items in a store cost a certain amount of money, exercise and work intensity cost a certain amount of oxygen to make ATP.

Here are some basic principles of VO_2 related to work:

>> If work intensity goes up, VO_2 goes up.

>> Whoever has a higher VO_2 max can do more work.

>> Work that uses a lot of muscle mass uses more oxygen (VO_2) and, therefore, burns more calories.

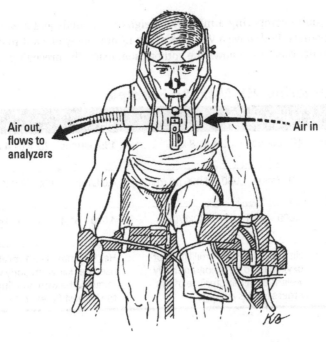

Air out, flows to analyzers ← ---- ← ---- Air in

FIGURE 4-7:
Measuring VO₂ by analyzing the concentration of gas in your breath.

Illustration by Kathryn Born, MA

Given this information, which activity do you think burns more calories: sit-ups or walking? You've probably heard that if you want to lose fat around the belly, you should do sit-ups. But how much work does a sit-up entail versus walking? Sit-ups use a small amount of muscle mass (abdominals and hip flexor muscles) and walking uses a much larger amount of muscle mass (legs, hips, and arms) in order to carry and move the entire body. So it "costs" more ATP and more oxygen, and it burns more calories to walk than it does to perform a sit-up. In fact, walking up an incline can use even more muscle and burn even more calories. One key to caloric expenditure is to involve a lot of muscle.

TIP

Other activities that use a lot of muscle and, therefore, use a lot of calories include biking, cross-country skiing, dancing, hiking, jogging, rowing, swimming, and walking up a hill (which uses even more leg muscles than regular walking).

Measuring changes in metabolism: The anaerobic threshold

In earlier sections, we explain how both aerobic and anaerobic systems make ATP. The aerobic systems, using fat, carbohydrates, and oxygen can keep making

ATP. However, these systems work only at low to moderate work intensity; when you go beyond that, you have to start also using the anaerobic system. But anaerobic metabolism has a key downside: lactic acid, which leads to fatigue. As a person moves from easy to heavy work, a transition in metabolism occurs that shows up as a big increase in lactic acid in the blood. This sudden increase in acid represents the *anaerobic threshold* (AT).

Think about what happens at low-, moderate-, and high-intensity exercise. At low intensity,

>> **Aerobic (slow-twitch) muscle fibers are doing most of the work.** These fibers don't produce lactic acid. In fact, they can even use lactic acid for energy!

>> **Aerobic metabolism (the Krebs cycle) is producing most of the ATP.** With oxygen available, only water and carbon dioxide are produced.

>> **Fat and carbohydrates are both being used for energy.**

At moderate intensity,

>> **The work is getting harder, and oxygen delivery to the muscle can't quite keep pace with the exercise intensity.**

>> **Fast-twitch (anaerobic) muscles are starting to be used in addition to slow-twitch muscles.** Fast-twitch fibers make lactic acid, so lactic acid starts to accumulate.

>> **Fat is used less as a fuel percentage, but overall fat use is near its peak due to the added intensity.** If you're fit enough to work at this intensity for more than 20 minutes, this may be a more ideal intensity for exercise and fat use.

At high intensity,

>> **All your muscle fibers are being used, and lots of lactic acid is produced.**

>> **Fat metabolism is reduced, and glucose becomes the primary fuel source because you can get ATP fast from both aerobic and anaerobic glucose metabolism.**

>> **With anaerobic metabolism kicked into high gear, lots of lactic acid is produced.**

REMEMBER

Because lactic acid is related to fatigue, the point where lactic acid increases is a key index of how hard you can work before fatigue (see Figure 4-8). For this reason, athletes tend to race at an intensity just below their anaerobic threshold.

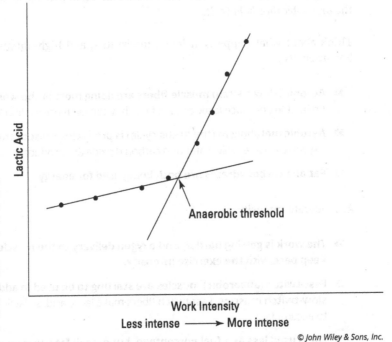

FIGURE 4-8:
The anaerobic threshold — the point where lactic acid begins to accumulate, leading to fatigue. Regression lines are drawn through data to help identify the breakpoint.

Anaerobic threshold

Work Intensity

Less intense ⟶ More intense

© John Wiley & Sons, Inc.

TECHNICAL STUFF

Measuring lactic acid (which you do by taking a blood sample) is not the only way to measure the anaerobic threshold. As we note earlier, lactic acid can be converted to CO_2 and then breathed off (ventilation). Researchers can actually measure either CO_2 production or even changes in ventilation to identify the threshold — tactics that are easier than poking a finger to get a blood sample!

THAT'S ONE SMART TREADMILL!

As we explain in this chapter, for every 1 liter of oxygen used, about 5 kilocalories are burned. By knowing VO_2, you can estimate the number of calories burned. Researchers have established prediction equations for walking, running, cycling, and stepping that can estimate the VO_2 cost of work intensity. These equations are built into exercise equipment software. All the equipment needs is the workload and your body weight to determine how many calories you burn.

Here's an example: Julie is walking on a treadmill at 3.5 mph (93.8 meters/min). She weighs 125 pounds (56.8 kg). The equation for VO_2 estimation in mL/kg/min for level walking is

$$VO_2 \text{ mL/kg/min} = (\text{speed in meters/min} \times 0.1) + 3.5$$

Plugging in Julie's numbers, you get

$$VO_2 \text{ mL/kg/min} = (93.8 \times 0.1) + 3.5 = 9.4 + 3.5 = 12.9$$

Next, you convert VO_2 to L/min by multiplying Julie's VO_2 mL/kg/min by weight in kilograms and then dividing the result by 1,000:

$$12.9 \text{ mL/kg/min} \times 56.8 \text{ kg} = 732.7 \text{ mL/min} \div 1,000 = 0.733 \text{ L/min}$$

Finally, to get the kilocalories, you multiply VO_2 L/min by 5 (every L/min of oxygen used burns 5 kilocalories):

$$\text{kilocalories} = 0.733 \text{ L/min} \times 5 = 3.7 \text{ kilocalories per minute}$$

If Julie walks for 20 minutes, she burns 74 kilocalories ($3.7 \times 20 = 74$).

By inputting your body weight, exercise machines can give a pretty decent estimate of your calories burned. Pretty handy!

Training for Improved Metabolism: It's the Enzymes!

When it comes to making ATP, you know that you need a starting fuel (phosphocreatine, carbohydrates, or fat) and then a way to transform the molecules to get the energy out of them. So, what magic ingredient transforms the molecules? Enzymes! As we explain earlier, enzymes are the components that drive chemical reactions. What's particularly interesting — and helpful in the context of improving performance — is that you can create more enzymes. How? By training! The key is to tailor your training to the type of enzyme changes you want.

PREDICTING 10K TIME, USING THE ANAEROBIC THRESHOLD

Imagine you just tested an athlete on a treadmill doing a running test. You measured ventilation during the test. Can you predict the running speed of the athlete during a 10K race? You betcha. Take a look at the following illustration.

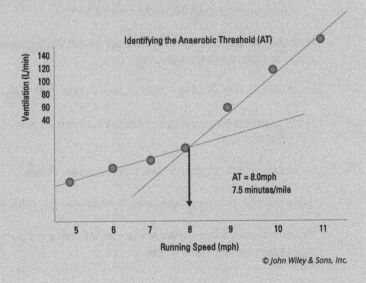

© John Wiley & Sons, Inc.

Notice that, at 8 mph, the ventilation suddenly increases at a higher rate. That's the point at which lactic acid is accumulating, carbon dioxide is accumulating, and ventilation is increasing.

Running at 8 mph, your runner is running at a 7.5 minute-per-mile pace (60 min/hour ÷ 8 miles/hour = 7.5). Because you know that a 10K race is 6.2 miles, you can do the calculation to estimate how long it will take this runner to complete a 10K race:

6.2 miles × 7.5 minutes/mile = 46.5 minutes

So, the 10K time is closely related to the pace at which the anaerobic threshold occurs. You can use these kinds of calculations to track training progress or even to compare runners, because any changes in the anaerobic threshold mean changes in race pace or performance. Useful!

Getting better at what you're doing: Training specificity

They say practice makes perfect. Well, that may be true only if the practice itself is near perfect. Bodies tend to adapt to the exercise conditions they're given. Run slowly, and you improve at running slowly. *Specificity of training* means that improvements in training are specific to what you're doing and includes things like the speed of movement, the load lifted, the intensity of the exercise, the angle or position of the limbs, the environment . . . you get the idea. Improvement in training is very finicky!

REMEMBER

Energy systems are simply a combination of chemical reactions. They start with a molecule (phosphocreatine, glucose, or fat) and use enzymes to help the reactions take place. The more enzymes you have, the faster you make ATP, and the way to get more enzymes is to train in ways that use particular enzymes.

Training the ATP-phosphocreatine system

The phosphocreatine system (explained earlier, in "Phosphocreatine: An immediate source of ATP") provides the energy for the highest intensity of activity. You only have up to about ten seconds of phosphocreatine stored. A training regimen for improving this system includes the following characteristics:

>> High-intensity exercise intervals of five to ten seconds in length.

>> Short rest bouts between intervals. (Don't worry, no lactic acid was made during this activity.)

>> Activities that use the same muscle you would use for competition because improvements are specific to the muscle used.

By following such a regimen, you should see the following training improvements:

>> Phosphocreatine breaking down at a faster rate

>> Some increase in phosphocreatine storage (although diet influences this, too)

>> Improvement in all-out effort because you make energy faster

Training the anaerobic glycolytic system

The anaerobic glycolytic system (see "Anaerobic glycolysis: Fast energy with a price") uses glucose as its primary fuel. It's useful for high-intensity activity that lasts longer than ten seconds and that can last as long as five minutes. The side effect of this system is lactic acid.

If you want to improve this system, do the following:

>> Train, using a high-intensity interval activity of between 30 and 60 seconds.

>> Include rest intervals of between one and five minutes of light activity (which gets rid of lactic acid). Then hit it again!

>> Use the muscles you'll use for competition.

TIP

This training regimen uses up glycogen, so you may need a rest day to restore.

Here are the training improvements you should see:

>> Faster ATP production (more enzymes)

>> Faster removal of lactic acid (thank goodness!)

>> Faster speed and quicker recovery — in other words, improved performance

Training the oxidative (aerobic) system

The oxidative system (explained in "The Oxidative (Aerobic) System: It Just Keeps Going and Going") is the ultimate ATP producer, using fats, carbs, and even proteins to make ATP. The aerobic system can be trained a number of ways, depending on what you're trying to achieve:

>> If you're in lousy shape to begin with, you can improve your aerobic fitness by exercising lightly as few as two times per week.

>> If you want to train the aerobic system, engage in moderate-intensity exercise, which is a great because it uses mainly the aerobic system to make ATP.

>> If you want to improve the aerobic system, engage in high-intensity training. You may even see improvements in the aerobic system while working on the glycolytic system. Bonus!

TIP

Use large muscle groups so that you maximize the use of the aerobic system. Activities like walking, jogging, swimming, hiking, biking, and rowing are ideal.

You should see the following training improvements:

>> More enzymes, producing more ATP

>> Less lactic acid at the same running speed

>> Improved ability to get oxygen into the mitochondria

>> More mitochondria, which is like having a bigger aerobic muscle

>> Improved ability to deliver blood (which carries oxygen) to the muscle

>> A bigger heart, which means a bigger pump to push more blood and more oxygen through your body

REMEMBER

If you want to make energy both during very high-intensity activity and more modest-intensity activity, you need to train specifically for it. Your body is like putty, but you have to do some work to shape it the way you want, both inside and out! For more specifics on training for various activities, see Chapter 11.

Chapter 5

The Body's Engine: The Cardiovascular System

All the contracting muscles, nerve stimuli, and metabolic activity of the body would not take place if the necessary nutrients were not made available. Glucose, fat, protein, and oxygen get transported to the cells through blood flowing to the body's tissues. Wastes, like carbon dioxide, are also removed through blood flow.

The heart is the pump that moves the blood through the blood vessels throughout the body. If this pump is strong, you can do a lot of work. If it weakens, you weaken. In this chapter, we look at how the cardiovascular system works at rest and during exercise.

The Heart's Structure: A Muscle Made to Pump

The heart is designed to be an efficient pump. Its structure and the way it works all serve to move oxygenated blood to all the tissues and organs in your body. Becoming familiar with the different components that make up the heart helps you understand how the heart works and why you can't talk about movement or exercise without a firm knowledge of the heart muscle.

Heart chambers and valves

The heart collects blood and, like a policeman directing traffic, sends it out to two different locations. It has two different types of chambers:

>> **Atria:** The atria are small chambers on the topside of the heart. They collect blood that is returning to the heart via the veins.

>> **Ventricles:** The ventricles are the larger, more muscular chambers on the lower half of the heart. They get their blood from the atria above and later squeeze to pump the blood away from the heart.

Heart valves, which open and close in a coordinated way to help keep the blood moving in one direction, are between the atria and ventricles, as well as between the blood vessels and the heart.

Two halves of the whole

Just as the atria on the top portion and the ventricles on the lower part of the heart have their own purpose, the left and right sides of the heart (each with one atrium and one ventricle) have different functions.

The right side

The right side of the heart is responsible for two things:

>> Collecting all the blood that has been out delivering oxygen to the muscles and tissues. Blood returns to the right-side atrium by way of large veins called *vena cavae* (singular *vena cava*).

>> Pumping the blood out of the right-side ventricle and to the lungs, where it can pick up oxygen.

The left side

The left side of the heart works in the same way as the right side, except for the direction of the blood flow:

>> The left-side atrium collects oxygen-rich blood from the lungs by way of the pulmonary veins. This blood is ready to feed oxygen to the tissues.

>> The left-side ventricle pumps the oxygenated blood out to the entire circulatory system of the body.

TIP

When the left ventricle squeezes blood out, you can feel the wave of blood. Place your fingers on the side of your neck (at your carotid artery) and you can feel the waves go by. This is one way to measure heart rate!

Seeing How the Heart Works

Imagine that you're playing in a swimming pool, and you decide to squirt water with your hands. If you're like most people, you'll cup your hands to make a chamber, fill the chamber with water, and then squeeze down quickly to force the water out of the opening you leave. The heart works in a similar way. It moves blood throughout the body by filling its chambers and then squeezing down to force blood through the cardiovascular system.

Watching the blood flow through the heart

Although the right side of the heart collects oxygen-depleted blood from the body and sends it to the lungs for oxygen, and the left side of the heart collects oxygenated blood from the lungs and sends it out to the body (refer to the earlier section "Two halves of the whole"), their actions occur simultaneously. This is why the heart beats in a nice, coordinated fashion.

Table 5-1 outlines the steps involved in the movement of blood through the heart. You can see this path in Figure 5-1.

TIP

The sounds your heart makes are the product of the valves closing in Steps 3 and 5. In Step 3, when the valves between the atria and the ventricles close to stop the blood from flowing back into the atria, you hear the first heart sound (lub). In Step 5, when the valves in the ventricles close to stop the blood from flowing back into the heart, you hear the second sound (DUP). Because the valves leading from the ventricles to the lungs and body are larger than the valves separating the atria and ventricles, they produce a louder sound when they close: *lub DUP!*

REMEMBER

The term used to denote contraction of the ventricle (Step 4) is *systole* (pronounced *sis*-tol-ee). The term used to denote relaxation of the ventricle (Step 5) is *diastole* (pronounced die-*ASS*-tol-ee).

TABLE 5-1   ## How Blood Moves through the Heart

Step	Right Side of Heart	Left Side of Heart
Step 1	Deoxygenated blood returns to the right atrium, where it collects. This is known as the *venous return.*	Oxygen-rich blood returns to the left atrium from the lungs, where it just picked up a fresh supply of oxygen.
Step 2	The valve separating the right atrium and the right ventricle opens, and two-thirds of the blood flows into the ventricle. The remaining one-third stays in the atrium until the atrial muscle contracts, forcing it out. ***Tip:*** Think of this action as akin to wringing the water out of a sponge: When you take a sponge out of a water bucket, a lot of the water just drips off the sponge, but to get the rest, you have to give the sponge a squeeze.	The valve separating the left atrium and the left ventricle opens, and two-thirds of the blood flows into the ventricle. The remaining one-third stays in the atrium until the atrial muscle contracts, forcing it out.
Step 3	The right ventricle contracts, squeezing down on the blood that's inside, and the pressure builds. The valve between the right atrium and right ventricle closes to keep the blood from going backward. *Lub.* You can hear this sound of the closing with a stethoscope.	The left ventricle contracts, squeezing the blood, and the pressure builds. The valve between the left-side atrium and ventricle closes, keeping the blood from backing into the left atrium. *Lub.* You can hear this sound of the closing with a stethoscope.
Step 4	As the right ventricle squeezes and the pressure builds, the valve holding the blood in the right ventricle opens, and the blood is pushed out to the lungs through the pulmonary artery.	As the left ventricle contracts, the valve holding the blood in the left ventricle opens, and the blood is pushed out to the entire body through the aorta.
Step 5	The heart muscle relaxes. Some of the blood that was pumped out flows backward to the heart and closes the heart valves. *DUP!* You can hear the sound of the closing with a stethoscope.	The heart muscle relaxes. Some of the blood that was pumped out flows backward to the heart and closes the heart valves. *DUP!* You can hear the sound of the closing with a stethoscope.

A NOISY HEART: HEART MURMURS

Normally the sounds you hear during the pumping cycle of the heart are clear and sharp (lup DUP... lup DUP... lup DUP). But, sometimes heart valves get leaky, either because they don't close all the way or because the seals leak. The result is that blood squirts backward through the gap and makes a rumbly sound.

Leaky valves between the atria and ventricles cause a sound like "phyyyth dup... phyyyth dup... phyyyth dup. Heart murmurs can be minor and no worry, or they can be more significant and interfere with the heart's ability to adequately pump blood.

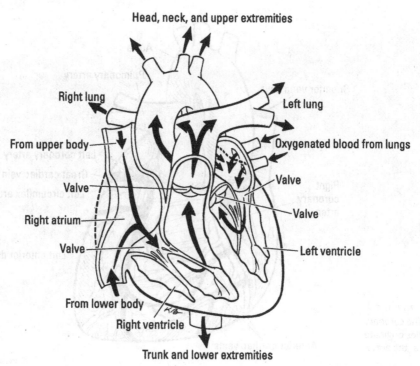

Head, neck, and upper extremities

Right lung

Left lung

From upper body

Oxygenated blood from lungs

Valve

Valve

Right atrium

Valve

Valve

Left ventricle

From lower body

Right ventricle

Trunk and lower extremities

FIGURE 5-1:
The direction of
blood flow
through
the heart.

Illustration by Kathryn Born, MA

Getting blood to the heart

The heart is very generous, sending oxygen-rich blood throughout the body. But what about the heart muscle itself? The heart is pumping and pushing and using quite a bit of oxygen, so it needs a constant supply of oxygen, too. Figure 5-2 shows the coronary arteries (darkened in the image). Notice that they originate in the aorta, just past the valves of the heart.

When the heart is in systole (contraction), the arteries that supply blood to the heart squeeze shut, meaning the heart is doing work but not getting any oxygen. After systole is completed and some blood rushes back toward the heart, the ventricle is in a relaxed state (diastole). During this phase, the blood coming back to the heart enters the coronary arteries, which are located on the aorta just beyond the valves between the aorta and the ventricle (see Figure 5-3).

REMEMBER

The heart uses oxygen during the contraction phase and receives its supply of oxygen during the relaxation phase.

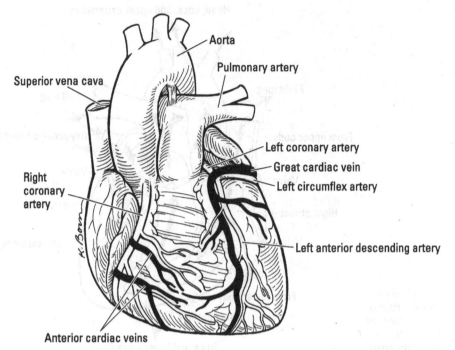

Aorta

Pulmonary artery

Superior vena cava

Left coronary artery

Great cardiac vein

Left circumflex artery

Right
coronary
artery

Left anterior descending artery

FIGURE 5-2:
The coronary
arteries originate
at the aorta.

Anterior cardiac veins

Illustration by Kathryn Born, MA

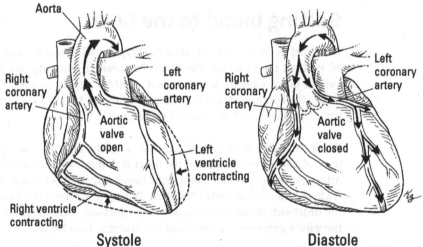

Aorta

Right
coronary
artery

Left
coronary
artery

Left
coronary
artery

Right
coronary
artery

Aortic
valve
open

Aortic
valve
closed

Left
ventricle
contracting

Right ventricle
contracting

Systole

When the ventricles contract,
the walls squeeze the coronary
arteries shut, preventing blood flow.
The blood within the ventricle is
pushed out through the aorta.

Diastole

When the ventricles relax,
suction pulls blood back
toward the heart. The aortic
valve closes, and backward
pressure sends blood into the
coronary arteries.

FIGURE 5-3:
During diastole,
the blood flows
back toward the
heart, providing it
with oxygen.

Illustration by Kathryn Born, MA

Identifying the force behind the heart beat: Blood pressure

If you've ever pumped up an air mattress with a foot pump, you know that you have to push hard enough to overcome the air pressure that is already in the mattress in order to push air into the mattress. The heart functions in a similar manner: It has to generate enough pressure to push blood out into the system of arteries that deliver blood (and oxygen) to the tissues. It uses two primary pressures, systolic and diastolic blood pressure, to accomplish this task (see Figure 5-4):

>> **Systolic pressure:** As we note in the earlier section "Getting blood to the heart," systolic blood pressure is the pressure generated during the ventricle's contraction phase. Imagine that you're holding one end of a long rug and you snap it. You see a wave of rug move away from you. In a similar fashion, when the ventricle contracts, a large wave of blood is sent away from the heart. This wave actually stretches the arteries (they bulge as the wave moves past). Normal values for systolic blood pressure at rest range from 90 to 120 mmHg. (**Note:** Blood pressure is reported in *millimeters of mercury,* abbreviated to *mmHg.*)

TIP

Try feeling this systolic pressure wave yourself. Place the pads of your first two fingers across either your carotid artery (at the neck) or your radial artery (palm side up, thumb side of your wrist). If you get the location right, you can feel the ventricular pulses as they move past.

>> **Diastolic pressure:** Because the vessels are full of blood, pressure already exists in the system. The pressure in the circulatory system during the resting phase is called the *diastolic blood pressure.* Normal values for diastolic blood pressure range from 50 to 80 mmHg.

Setting the pace: What controls heart rate?

A single cardiac cell is a wondrous thing. All by itself, it'll beat in a nice rhythmic fashion. Of course, if all cardiac cells decided to beat at their own pace, the heart would never be able to squeeze in a coordinated movement. Therefore, special heart cells tend to pace the entire heart so that blood moves through in a coordinated fashion.

Introducing the sinoatrial node

Within the atria and ventricles is a specialized tissue that spreads across the chambers. This tissue receives an impulse and quickly spreads it to all the cardiac muscles in the chamber. All it needs is an initial pulse, which comes from one spot in the right atrium: the *sinoatrial node* (or *SA node*).

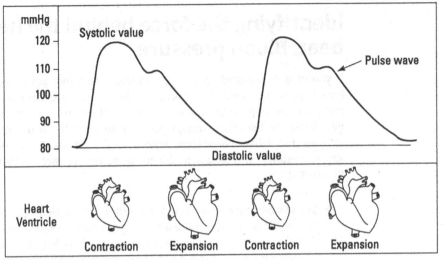

FIGURE 5-4:
The contraction phase generates systolic pressure; the resting phase, diastolic pressure.

© John Wiley & Sons, Inc.

Think of the SA node as the heart's pacemaker. Although all cardiac tissue can contract on its own, the SA node seems to contract faster than all other heart tissue. Because it beats the other tissue to the punch, your heart rate is set according to the rate at which the SA node fires.

UNDER PRESSURE: HYPERTENSION AND HEART DISEASE

Blood vessels are fragile things. They stretch and can handle large loads of blood, but if they stay under pressure for too long, they begin to become damaged. Prolonged systolic pressure over 120 mmHg and/or diastolic pressure over 80 mmHg may cause the arterial walls to begin to scar and fill in. This narrows the arteries and is a key part of atherosclerosis, the leading cause of stroke and heart attacks. Because you can't feel hypertension (high blood pressure), you must have your blood pressure measured to discover whether you have a problem.

Pressure can hurt the heart as well. During systole, if the heart has to push against a lot of pressure (called *afterload*) or if it has a lot of blood returning to it (called *preload*), it must use more oxygen to do more work — a situation that can fatigue the heart and weaken it.

Stimulating and contracting the heart, step-by-step

The sequence of stimulus and contraction is like a carefully choreographed dance that moves blood through the heart (see Figure 5-5):

1. **When the atria have filled with blood and the blood begins to flow to the ventricles, the SA node fires.**

2. **This electrical signal sweeps across the atria, stimulating the atria to contract and push the blood into the ventricles.**

3. **The electrical signal is delayed at a junction between the atria and the ventricles, called the *atrioventricular node* (or *AV node*).**

   The delay at the AV node lasts only about one-tenth of a second, but it gives the atria a moment to do their work. You don't want the ventricles to contract while the atria are contracting. If they did, the blood would go forward and backward.

4. **The electrical signal emerges from the AV node and sweeps across the ventricles through fast conducting tissues (left and right *bundle branches* and *purkinje fibers*), causing an almost immediate stimulation of the ventricle, followed by ventricular contraction.**

5. **The stimulated cells *repolarize* (reset) to their original state.**

   This happens in between heart beats.

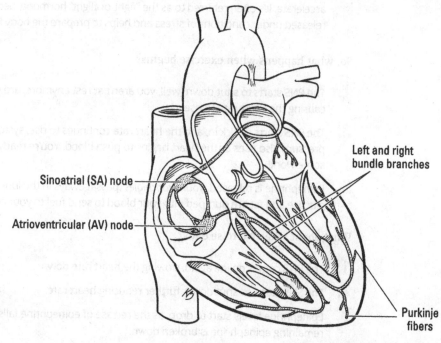

Sinoatrial (SA) node

Atrioventricular (AV) node

Left and right bundle branches

Purkinje fibers

FIGURE 5-5: The sequence of electrical stimulation of the atria and ventricles shown on an electrocardiogram.

Illustration by Kathryn Born, MA

Fast or slow, what makes it go? The nervous system's influence on heart rate

If the SA node were allowed to pace heart rate without any influences, we would all have a resting heart rate of about 90 beats per minute. Is your resting heart rate that high? Probably not. So, something is slowing it down. And something speeds it up when, for example, you start to exercise. That something is actually two things: your nervous system and hormones that can influence heart rate.

Here's what happens during periods of rest and activity:

>> **Your heart rate at rest:** During resting conditions, your body focuses on things like digestion and, well, rest! Under these conditions, the *parasympathetic nervous system* (PNS) is at work. The PNS has nerves that connect to the SA node and cause it to slow down at rest.

>> **Your heart rate when action is required:** When you start to exercise or when you're under stress of some type, your body needs to push blood and oxygen to the muscle. In this case, the *sympathetic nervous system* (SNS) gets to work. The SNS also connects to the SA node, but when it kicks in, heart rate begins to rise in relation to the amount of stimulation. Some heart rates can go as high as 200 beats per minute!

The SNS also stimulates the adrenal gland, which contains a hormone called *epinephrine*. When it's released into the blood, epinephrine causes heart rate to accelerate. It's often referred to as the "fight-or-flight" hormone, because it's released under conditions of stress and helps to prepare the body for doing work.

So, what happens when exercise begins?

1. The PNS starts to shut down (well, you aren't at rest anymore, are you?), causing the heart rate to rise.

2. The SNS starts to kick in, and the heart rate continues to rise; systolic blood pressure also rises as the heart begins to push blood. You're ready for some work!

3. Epinephrine is released, your *bronchioles* (passageways in the lungs) dilate, and glucose and fat are dumped into your blood to send fuel to your cells.

What about when exercise ends?

1. The PNS comes online again, slowing the heart rate down.

2. The SNS starts to shut down, further reducing heart rate.

3. Epinephrine levels start to drop, as the release of epinephrine falls and the remaining epinephrine is broken down.

Key measures of heart function

Because your body depends on the blood and oxygen that your heart pumps out each minute, the strength of your heart muscle is a key measure of exercise ability. Here are a few important components related to heart function:

>> **Stroke volume:** The ventricle chamber holds the blood just before it's pumped out for circulation. The more you can pump, the more blood and oxygen you can deliver. *Stroke volume* refers to the amount of blood that is pumped out of the ventricle with each heartbeat. Usually stroke volume is about 70 milliliters per beat in a resting heart.

>> **Ejection fraction:** Ejection fraction is very similar to stroke volume, but it's a better indicator of heart strength. *Ejection fraction* refers to the percentage of blood that is pumped with each heartbeat. A normal, strong heart can eject about 60 percent of its blood with every beat, whereas a weak heart ejects less than 50 percent.

>> **Rate pressure product (RPP):** RPP is a key indicator of the oxygen demand of the heart muscle. Because the heart needs oxygen to push, how hard it pushes (systolic blood pressure) and how fast it pushes (heart rate) influence oxygen need. The harder and faster the heart pushes, the more oxygen it needs. You use the following formula to calculate RPP:

>> RPP = heart rate × systolic blood pressure

>> **Cardiac output:** The total "horsepower of the heart" is related to how much the heart can pump with each beat, as well as how fast the heart is beating.

REMEMBER

Cardiac output is the total amount of blood that is pumped by the heart each minute. You can calculate it by using this simple equation:

cardiac output = heart rate × stroke volume

Cardiac output is directly related to work intensity. If work intensity goes up, cardiac output goes up.

Delivering Fresh Air to Your Cells

As we explain in Chapter 4, producing energy (adenosine triphosphate, or ATP) requires oxygen to help run chemical reactions in the mitochondria. Although oxygen is certainly available in the atmosphere, how does oxygen get from the atmosphere into your lungs, then into your blood, and finally into your cells? Through a series of steps and biological processes, of course. Read on to discover how pressure, the simple act of breathing, and key biological processes let your body get all the oxygen it needs while also removing carbon dioxide.

Transporting oxygen through the body: The pressure gradient at work

A gas (like air) always moves from an area of higher pressure to an area of lower pressure. Think of a balloon. If you blow it up and let it go without tying off the end, what happens? The air comes rushing out. Why? Because of the difference in pressure between the air inside the balloon and the air outside the balloon! Without this pressure gradient, air and oxygen would not be able to travel through your body.

You may take breathing in and out for granted, but it's an essential part of getting oxygen to your cells. To breathe in and out, your body creates changes in air pressure:

» **Breathing in:** Two sets of muscles help you create a low pressure condition in your lungs. The *diaphragm* is a muscle just beneath your lungs that contracts during *inspiration* (breathing in). By contracting, the diaphragm creates low pressure in the chest, and this low pressure draws air in. The *intercostal muscles* (the muscles between your ribs) can also contract and expand your chest.

Try this: Put your hand just below your chest and above your belly. Now breathe in through your nose (like you're smelling a flower). Do you feel your belly push outward a bit? This is your diaphragm contracting. Now take a big breath and breathe in hard. Feel your entire chest expand? Those are the intercostal muscles at work.

>> **Breathing out:** After breathing in, you can simply relax the muscles you used to pull air in. When you do so, the pressure in your lungs rises and pushes the air back out. Or, you can force the air out by contracting your intercostal muscles, which pulls the chest inward and sends the air out.

Paying attention to partial pressure

Imagine a room full of air. You can't see the air, but molecules of the gases that make up air (oxygen, carbon dioxide, and nitrogen) are bouncing all around in the room. Right now you're sitting at the bottom of a giant ocean of air (the atmosphere) that's pushing down on you. The amount of pressure the atmosphere generates is known as *barometric pressure*. You measure barometric pressure by measuring the height of a column of mercury in millimeters (mmHg). At sea level, air pressure is around 760 mmHg.

Air is composed of three main gases:

Gas	Its Percentage of Air
Oxygen	20.93%
Carbon dioxide	0.04%
Nitrogen	79.03%

Using this information, can you guess how much pressure the oxygen component generates? If 20.93 percent of air is oxygen, it generates 20.93 percent of the pressure. Knowing this, you can do a simple calculation to determine how much of the pressure is generated by the oxygen alone.

To calculate the pressure of the oxygen component, you multiply the air pressure at sea level by the concentration of the gas (well, actually the concentration in decimal form, so divide 20.93 percent by 100 to get 0.2093). The resulting number is called the *partial pressure* because it's only a portion of the total pressure. The partial pressure of oxygen is represented as PO_2. The partial pressure of carbon dioxide is represented as PCO_2.

Here's the calculation for PO_2:

$$PO_2 = 760 \text{ mmHg} \times 0.2093$$

$$PO_2 = 159.1 \text{ mmHg}$$

You use the same method to determine the partial pressure of any gas (like CO_2 or nitrogen).

Each gas moves independently from higher to lower pressure, based on its own partial pressure.

REMEMBER

Tracking the movement of O_2 and CO_2

Aerobic metabolism (refer to Chapter 4) needs oxygen to get to the mitochondria, and then it needs the carbon dioxide to get out of the cells and into the atmosphere. How are these feats accomplished? By creating partial pressure gradients for each gas so that they move from higher to lower pressures. As Table 5-2 shows, the pressure does the pushing! The pressure to move oxygen comes from the atmosphere, and the pressure to move CO_2 comes from the production of CO_2 in the cells.

TABLE 5-2 **Partial Pressure Gradient for Oxygen (PO_2) and Carbon Dioxide (PCO_2)**

Atmosphere		Lung		Blood Moving through the Lung		Cells and Mitochondria
$PO_2 = 159.1$	→	$PO_2 = 104.0$	→	$PO_2 = 40.0$	→	$PO_2 = 2.0$
$PCO_2 = 0.3$	←	$PCO_2 = 40.0$	←	$PCO_2 = 46.0$	←	$PO_2 > 46.0$

Notice in which direction the gases move: The oxygen moves from the atmosphere to the lung to the blood moving through the lung and finally to the cells and mitochondria. The carbon dioxide moves from the cells and mitochondria to the blood moving through the lungs to the lungs and finally back out into the atmosphere. Just what you want!

REMEMBER

Carrying gases in the blood

Gases can exist not only in the atmosphere but also in fluid environments. If you've ever opened a can of soda or poured a glass of champagne, you've observed the gas coming out of a fluid: Think of the bubbles rising in a glass of champagne! Dissolved gases within a fluid establish the partial pressure of the gas in that fluid.

REMEMBER

Unfortunately, the fluid part of blood can't carry enough oxygen to supply your needs. Nor can it help get rid of all the CO_2 that your cells create. To solve this dilemma, the body has a variety of means to transport oxygen and carbon dioxide through the blood. These lifeboats for oxygen and carbon dioxide transport are the keys to your survival.

Transporting oxygen

The primary carrier of oxygen in our blood is *hemoglobin* (Hb), an iron-containing protein within your red blood cells. Hemoglobin is the stuff that gives your blood the red color (it's the iron), and it carries 99 percent of all your oxygen.

Each gram of hemoglobin can carry four oxygen molecules (about 1.3 milliliters of oxygen). The more hemoglobin you have, the more oxygen you can carry in your blood. If you're iron-deficient, your hemoglobin levels drop, and you become *anemic*, a condition that reduces your ability to carry oxygen in the blood.

Figure 5-6 shows hemoglobin picking up oxygen from the lungs and carrying it through the blood and then dumping the oxygen into the tissue. Typically, hemoglobin is saturated with oxygen after leaving the lungs, with 98 percent of hemoglobin bonded to oxygen. Saturation levels drop as the oxygen is deposited in the tissue.

Hemoglobin can be finicky. It can either carry or dump oxygen, which it does depends upon three key conditions:

>> **The partial pressure of oxygen in the vicinity:** If PO_2 is high, as it is in the lungs when the blood moves through, the hemoglobin picks up and carries the oxygen. If PO_2 is low, as it is deep in the muscle tissue and the cells, the hemoglobin lets go of the oxygen and dumps it in the place where it's needed, inside the cell.

>> **Temperature:** Hemoglobin holds on to oxygen more when the temperature is low. During exercise, when the temperature of the tissue rises, hemoglobin dumps its oxygen much faster and, in doing so, makes an exercising muscle happy.

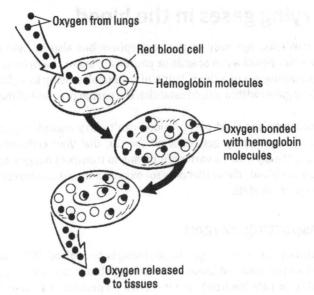

Oxygen from lungs

Red blood cell

Hemoglobin molecules

Oxygen bonded
with hemoglobin
molecules

FIGURE 5-6:
Red blood cells
and the hemoglo-
bin contained in
them pick up,
transport, and
deposit oxygen.

Oxygen released
to tissues

Illustration by Kathryn Born, MA

» **The pH level:** The level of acidity in the blood influences hemoglobin's
carrying capacity. If the pH level is more basic (as it is during rest), hemoglobin
hangs onto the oxygen, but when things get acidic (as they do during exercise), the hemoglobin dumps more oxygen to the tissue.

LOSING RED BLOOD CELLS . . . THROUGH YOUR FEET?

It may sound a bit odd, but runners can lose red blood cells through their feet. Think
about the act of running: foot strike after foot strike. The loads on the feet can easily be
six times your body weight. Now, think of the small blood vessels passing through the
tissue of the feet at the moment of each foot strike. The impact can be strong enough to
actually destroy the red blood cells that are squeezing through the capillaries. Large-
volume running can lower hemoglobin levels and cause anemia. Because running is an
aerobic activity, the reduced oxygen carrying ability can really slow the runner down. For
runners who have high training volumes, getting adequate iron in the diet is essential.

Here's what happens with hemoglobin and oxygen as they move through the body:

>> **At the lung:** In the lung, hemoglobin encounters high PO_2, cooler temperatures, and a nice basic pH. Oxygen from the lung is pushed by a pressure gradient and picked up by hemoglobin. The oxygen-hemoglobin partnership, known as *oxyhemoglobin,* is secure. Off we go!

>> **At the muscle:** Hemoglobin, carried in the blood, arrives at the muscle. Conditions in the muscle (especially if the muscle is exercising) are much different from conditions in the lung: low PO_2, an acidic environment, and a high temperature due to the ATP being used. Under these conditions, hemoglobin dumps its oxygen to the eagerly awaiting muscles (the oxygen-deprived hemoglobin is called *deoxyhemoglobin*), and then it's back to the lung to repeat the process.

Transporting carbon dioxide

Carbon dioxide is the waste product of aerobic metabolism, and your body has to get rid of it! Once again, hemoglobin comes to the rescue! But CO_2 can also be carried in other ways:

>> **Dissolved in the blood:** CO_2 dissolving in blood is just like gas dissolving in a soda! Only about 10 percent of CO_2 is transported in this way.

>> **Bound to hemoglobin:** Instead of latching onto the iron portion of hemoglobin, CO_2 latches onto the protein portion of hemoglobin (together they're called *carbaminohemoglobin*). Twenty percent of CO_2 is carried this way.

>> **Carried in the blood by altering its chemistry:** When PCO_2 is high, the carbon dioxide combines with water (with help from an enzyme in the red blood cell) to form a weak acid, called *carbonic acid:*

$$CO_2 + H_2O = H_2CO_3$$

Carbonic acid immediately breaks into two parts:

● **H+ (hydrogen ion):** H+ is like acid and can actually bind to your good friend hemoglobin and be carried away.

● **HCO_3 (bicarbonate):** Bicarbonate can actually be carried in the blood, so you can hold quite a bit of it. Seventy percent of your CO_2 is carried this way.

AEROBIC PERFORMANCE ENHANCEMENT: DOPING

Red blood cells play a key role in aerobic performance, especially for endurance events, like the marathon, cross-country skiing, or long cycling events. Sometimes, athletes try to gain an advantage by boosting their red blood cell volume to unnaturally high levels. This is known as *blood doping*.

In blood doping, athletes often receive transfusions of red blood cells (often their own, which they have stored in a refrigerator) just before a big event. Because the blood carries more oxygen with more red blood cells, these athletes are able to work harder and perform better for up to 14 weeks after the infusion. Alternatively, a doping athlete can take a manufactured hormone called *erythropoietin* (EPO), which makes the body create more red blood cells. Both of these techniques can be tested for, and each year, athletes are disqualified for their cheating ways.

When the CO_2 reaches the lung, all the processes that have helped carry CO_2 reverse:

1. Dissolved CO_2 diffuses into the lung.

2. Carbaminohemoglobin gives up its CO_2 to the lung.

3. Bicarbonate recombines with H^+, reforms carbonic acid, and the CO_2 then diffuses into the lung.

Extracting oxygen from the blood: a-VO$_2$ difference

If you had a million dollars in a vault but you didn't have the combination, the money really wouldn't help you, would it? Same with oxygen in the blood: Your oxygen-rich blood is great for your muscles to do work, but only if you can extract the oxygen!

Here are the keys steps to get the most oxygen out of the blood (see Figure 5-7):

1. Starting with the artery, the hemoglobin loads up on oxygen.

   Each hemoglobin molecule can carry 1.34 milliliters of oxygen. Hemoglobin values can range from 11 milligrams to 17 milligrams per 100 milliliters of blood. So, for example, if a hemoglobin level is 15, you can carry about 20 milliliters of oxygen ($15 \times 1.34 = 20$) in each 100 milliliters of blood.

2. The blood vessels, and lots of them, irrigate the muscle.

The more blood vessels moving through the muscle, the closer the oxygen gets to the cells — much like irrigating a farm field! (You can read more about the role of the blood vessels in the next section, "Observing Blood Vessels in Action.")

3. The partial pressure gradient draws oxygen from the hemoglobin and pushes it into the tissue.

The more mitochondria available (the mitochondria are organelles that produce ATP by using oxygen), the more oxygen extracted, and the more oxygen extracted, the more work you can do!

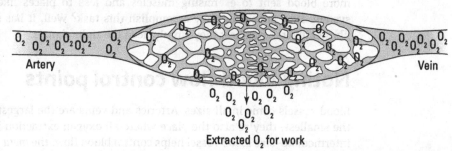

© John Wiley & Sons, Inc.

REMEMBER

If you measure the amount of oxygen present in the arteries (Step 1) and then measure the amount of oxygen left over in the veins after it went through the tissue (Step 3), you can discover how much was extracted. Here is the calculation you use to determine *arterio-venous oxygen difference* (a-VO$_2$ difference):

arterial O$_2$ – venous O$_2$ = amount of O$_2$ extracted

20 ml/dl – 15 ml/dl = 5ml/dl

So, the a-vO$_2$ difference is 5 ml/dl.

REMEMBER

As work intensity and the need for more oxygen increase, the a-vO$_2$ difference increases, meaning that more oxygen is extracted. Unfit people can't extract as much oxygen as fit people. They just don't have the "combination" to unlock all the available oxygen. That's why training is so important!

Observing Blood Vessels in Action

If you have summer water fights, you must learn proper water hose self-defense. If someone is chasing you around with a hose and squirting you with water, what do you do? You kink the hose to immediately stop the water flow. Then, when your friend looks at the nozzle to figure out why the water stopped, you unkink the hose, and they spray themselves! Fun right? In this way, you can control where and when the water flow occurs.

Your body is full of blood vessels that are squirting blood in many directions and to many places. Unfortunately, you don't have enough blood to supply every tissue the maximal amount of blood it may need. Therefore, the body needs a way to divert blood to areas that need it the most. During exercise, for example, you need more blood sent to exercising muscles and less to places like your digestive system. How does your body accomplish this task? Well, it has some of its own "hose kinkers" in place; they simply need the right signals.

Noting blood-flow control points

Blood vessels come in all sizes. Arteries and veins are the largest. Capillaries are the smallest; they're also the place where all oxygen extraction takes place. One intermediate-size blood vessel helps control blood flow: the *meta-arterioles*. When you're thinking about blood-flow control points, you need to be familiar with this blood vessel.

REMEMBER

Meta-arterioles are the vessels that control the flow of blood by either squeezing down or relaxing. They're smaller than arteries but larger than capillaries. Wrapped around the vessels are muscle bands, which squeeze tightly to reduce the amount of blood that can move through a vessel. They don't squeeze shut completely, but they can keep a lot of blood out (or let a lot in).

Factors that open and close blood vessels

The circulatory system is under constant influence from different stimuli to route blood flow to tissues of the body. Depending on which control system is activated, blood vessels may contract to divert blood flow, or they may relax to allow more blood to flow to the tissue. The primary controls are within the nervous system and chemical sensors in the blood vessels.

The nervous system's role in blood-flow control

Nerves are necessary to shift blood. The two primary controls of the nervous system play a very important role in blood-flow control. The PNS is most active at rest, and the SNS is working during stress and exercise:

>> The PNS relaxes blood vessels to areas of digestion, such as the gut, kidneys, pancreas, and even saliva glands. This increases blood flow to the digestive organs. However, blood flow to the skin is reduced.

>> The SNS increases blood flow to the skin (to get rid of heat), dilates arteries going to active muscle (to get more blood and oxygen to the tissue that needs it), and reduces blood flow to areas that are inactive.

These changes, which can happen quickly at the onset of exercise, help to provide more blood to the areas that need it without placing much additional strain on the cardiovascular system. (For more information on the PNS and SNS, refer to the earlier section "Fast or slow, what makes it go? The nervous system's influence on heart rate.")

Chemoreceptors: Sensors that know when you're working

Physical activity produces waste products like lactic acid and CO_2. A lack of oxygen to the tissue also triggers waste due to anaerobic metabolism.

Have you ever had blood briefly shut off to an arm or leg? After you free the limb, you can feel the rush of blood because the arteries are wide open, waiting for blood. The waste products caused those blood vessels to open wide because of a response by chemoreceptors.

Chemoreceptors sense chemical stimuli in the blood. These chemicals include the following:

>> **pH:** The more acidic the area (due to a lot of lactic acid, for example), the more the blood vessels widen (called *vasodilation*).

>> **Temperature:** The higher the temperature, the more vasodilation.

>> **PCO_2:** Chemoreceptors sense the rise in carbon dioxide and cause dilation in order to bring more blood supply to the tissue.

TIP

One reason you want to warm up with some light activity before exercise is because doing so helps you activate the blood-flow control mechanisms that deliver blood and oxygen to the muscles you'll use during the activity.

Noting the Effects of Exercise on the Cardiovascular System

The moment you start exercising, a multitude of changes begin to happen across your body as different systems come online to facilitate the activity. The cardio-vascular system, as the engine of the work, will show rapid and immediate (also called *acute*) adjustments. The type of work being done influences the type of response. Aerobic and strength exercises provide two good examples to help you understand the changes that take place.

Acute adjustments to aerobic exercise

Take a boat out on a lake and push the accelerator. Off you go! Gas is burned, the engine roars, the prop turns, and the nose of the boat rises. After you get up to cruising speed, things level off: The motor stays at a steady roar, and the nose of the boat comes down to water level. Same thing with your body.

When you take off on a run or a ride, your heart kicks in and roars to life, pushing blood through the body, beating faster and stronger. Then after a few minutes, you seem to level off. These responses are the result of what's happening in your cardiovascular system. Take a look at the adjustments that occur.

As the level of aerobic work increases

As the level of aerobic work increases, your body initiates a series of reactions that provide your cells with the oxygen they need to function under the increased workload. Here's what happens:

1. The blood flow per minute, called *cardiac output,* increases.

Cardiac output is increased in a couple of ways — by increasing the heart rate and by increasing the stroke volume:

- *Heart rate increases.* The PNS stops holding back heart rate, and the rate starts to rise. At the same time, the SNS kicks in fast, and heart rate rises even more. The stress hormone epinephrine is released, causing an additional rise in heart rate. The heart rate increases each time the workload increases until it can't go any higher, and you're at your limit!

- *Stroke volume increases.* More blood fills the ventricle, so more blood can be pumped out. The SNS kicks in and causes the heart muscle to beat more forcefully, squeezing out more of the blood it has.

REMEMBER

Stroke volume has limits! Just as you can't squeeze a sponge dry, you can only squeeze so much blood out of a ventricle. Stroke volume hits its highest point usually around 50 percent of a person's peak aerobic fitness, or VO_2 max. (Refer to Chapter 4 for more on aerobic fitness.)

2. Your cardiac output rises and then stabilizes.

Because cardiac output is related to the amount of work you do, it stabilizes within a few minutes and matches blood flow per minute to the demands of the work. Remember that cardiac output is the product of heart rate multiplied by stroke volume, as we explain in the earlier section "Key measures of heart function."

3. The active muscle gets more blood.

Blood vessels to active muscle dilate and bring more blood. The SNS, as well as the waste products of exercise (lactic acid, heat, and CO_2), are causing dilation.

4. Your blood pressure (systolic) rises.

The added force of heart contraction creates a larger pressure wave during the contraction phase (systole). In a normal response, the systolic blood pressure rises with more work.

Diastolic blood pressure, which is the pressure in between heart contractions, shouldn't change much. After all, nothing is different! Just the amount of time at rest changes. (The earlier section "Identifying the force behind the heart beat: Blood pressure" has more on systolic and diastolic pressures.)

5. Respiration (ventilation) rises.

Both the rate of breathing and the volume of each breath increase as work increases. More CO_2 is produced as a waste product, stimulating even more ventilation. Additional movement stimulates mechanical receptors, which also stimulate ventilation. If the work is heavy enough, lactic acid indirectly stimulates ventilation (because lactic acid can be converted to CO_2; refer to Chapter 4 for details).

6. Body temperature rises and sweating begins!

As the heat from energy production rises, blood flow to the skin increases. When body temperature exceeds an internal threshold, the hypothalamus in the brain, which senses body temperature, initiates a sweat response to dissipate the heat. The sweat comes from the water in the cells, the space between the cells, and the blood.

As the boat levels: The steady state

What happens if you just pick one work rate and stay at that work rate for, say, ten minutes? You may notice some adjusting going on the first few minutes, but things start to stabilize in a few minutes.

REMEMBER

The point at which heart rate and oxygen consumption have caught up to the work demand and remain at a stable level is called the *steady state*. At the steady state, heart rate, blood pressure, and most other variables remain stable (as long as you don't change the work rate). You may sense steady state a few minutes into your run, where breathing feels consistent and you can continue at the intensity for an extended period of time.

Here's what happens to your heart rate, your oxygen consumption, and your breathing in the steady state:

>> **Heart rate:** Your heart rate rises to meet the blood-flow demand. This acceleration period often lasts a minute or two because that's generally how long the heart rate takes to catch up to the required work. After it does, your heart rate stays about the same for the rest of the time you spend at that work rate.

>> **VO_2:** Your oxygen consumption shows a similar rise at the beginning of work, but it, too, levels off after it catches up to the work demand.

>> **Ventilation:** Your ventilation rises rapidly at the beginning of work, but it stabilizes after your system has matched the energy demand of the work.

TIP

If you're doing steady-state work, cardiac output must stay the same. But in a hot environment, you sweat a lot! All that heat dissipation means that blood is pushed to the skin to help radiate heat, and blood plasma is lost as you continue to sweat. These changes result in a drop in stroke volume!

Fortunately, the body compensates for the drop in stroke volume by increasing heart rate to maintain a steady cardiac output. This upward rise in heart rate while at a steady state is called *cardiovascular drift*. An easy way to counter cardiovascular drift is to replace fluids to help offset the sweat loss.

Acute adjustments to strength training

Strength training is an anaerobic activity. Most efforts are quite intense and last only about a minute. During strength training, a number of things take place in the cardiovascular system, some of which may seem the opposite of what you may expect!

Strength training requires that many muscles contract. Contracted muscles squeeze down on blood vessels and produce a variety of effects. The magnitude of response depends on how much muscle is being contracted.

During the lift

The following steps outline what happens during the lift:

1. The internal pressure slows the blood returning to the heart.

As the venous return drops, the heart has less blood to pump with each beat.

TIP

Think of it like a big balloon of pressure in the middle of your body that holds blood in the limbs and briefly prevents it from returning to the heart.

2. Blood is pushed out of the blood vessels and into the space between the cells, called the *interstitial space*.

Fluid being pushed into the interstitial space is a condition known as *edema*.

Blood vessels can leak, and when they're under pressure, they can lose some of their plasma into the interstitial space. The plasma shifting to different locations actually results in reduced blood volume. You can often feel this effect. Ever wonder why your biceps feels tight and "pumped" after a lift? The trapped plasma in your interstitial space causes this sensation.

3. Both systolic and diastolic pressures increase.

These can be quite high. Good thing this period is brief.

4. Sensory nerves in the blood vessels sense the rise in pressure.

The receptors that sense the rise in pressure are called *baroreflexes*.

5. Baroreflexes affect the heart and blood vessels in an attempt to counteract the high pressure.

Baroreflexes do the following:

- Reduce heart rate (yes, heart rate goes down during the lift!).

- Generate signals to the blood vessels to dilate.

WARNING

No one wants high blood pressure, but during a weight-lifting bout, it's hard to avoid, at least for a moment. However, you can inadvertently make matters worse by holding your breath. Holding your breath during a lift (called a *valsalva maneuver*) can greatly increase blood pressure, and it can be dangerous, especially for people with heart disease. Instead of holding your breath, breathe out in a smooth, controlled manner during the exertion portion of the lift. Breathe in on the lowering or the easier part of the lift. Doing so helps you maintain normal breathing patterns during exercise and helps minimize blood pressure increases.

After the lift

After the lift, the pressure drops rapidly, and more reflexes kick in:

1. After the lift, when pressure drops quickly, the baroreflex kicks in again and does the opposite of what it did during the lift.

The baroreflex can sense both increases and decreases in blood pressure. After the lift, the following happens:

- The drop in pressure causes an increase in heart rate. You may feel your heart rate take off just after setting the weight down.

- Blood vessels starts to constrict to bring pressure back up. If pressure doesn't increase fast enough, you may even feel a little dizzy!

2. Blood returns to the heart.

The pressure inside the body has been released, and all the blood held back in the limbs now rushes back to the heart.

3. When the blood fills the right atrium, it causes a stretch, which initiates a reflex acceleration of heart rate (known as the *Bainbridge reflex*).

You may feel your heart is beating fast and strong, as it handles the excess blood that's returning to it.

4. Edema sticks around, letting you feel pumped for a while.

For about 30 minutes after the lift, you still have plasma trapped in the interstitial space. Your blood volume will remain a bit lower, at least until the fluid leaks back into the veins (via the lymphatic system).

TIP

You may realize now that, although weight lifting makes the heart rate increase, it's due to reflexes and pressure changes and not aerobic training. So, if you want to do "cardio," don't rely on weight training — do aerobic training!

Making Long-Term Changes to Cardiovascular Performance

A wonderful thing about your cardiovascular system is that it adapts and grows stronger and more efficient if you give it a stimulus (like aerobic training). People who are inactive and out of shape can see huge improvements in their cardiovascular and aerobic abilities. Aerobic fitness comes about due to a number of specific adaptations, which we examine in the following sections.

REMEMBER

To make changes in the cardiovascular and muscular systems, you need a well-balanced conditioning program that includes *both* aerobic and strength training.

Adapting to aerobic exercises

Exercise is a fantastic medicine for the body. By doing aerobic training, you can change many aspects of your cardiovascular system. It's like getting a complete overhaul to a car's engine! Just look at all the changes:

>> **Heart rate:** Your resting heart rate is lower after aerobic training, because of the following factors:

- *The PSN has become more dominant at rest.* Therefore, it slows the heart rate down more at rest than before. In addition, your heart rate comes back down to rest faster after a workout!

- *The size of the heart chamber (ventricle) has grown.* With larger ventricles, fewer heart beats are needed to pump the same amount of blood at rest.

>> **Blood pressure:** In people with high blood pressure, exercise can lower resting blood pressure. In some cases, it may lower blood pressure as much as 10 mmHg! Moderate aerobic exercise seems to exert the best effect.

>> **Stroke volume:** Long-term aerobic training increases stroke volume (that is, more blood can be pumped with each stroke) because it

- Helps to remodel the ventricles, enlarging the ventricles

- Strengthens the heart muscle, enabling it to pump out more blood

>> **Cardiac output:** Your maximal work output increases, partly due to the increase in stroke volume. If you can pump more blood, you can work harder!

REMEMBER

Because cardiac output represents total blood flow and is related to the work you're doing, you only see improvements in cardiac output during very hard work. For more on cardiac output, refer to the earlier section "Key measures of heart function."

>> **Blood vessels:** The density of capillaries in the muscles increases, meaning more oxygen can be delivered to the muscle. Just as making more water lines improves the irrigation of a farm field, aerobic training causes an increase in the irrigation of the muscle!

>> **Oxygen extraction:** Aerobic training helps you use more of the oxygen your blood is bringing you. This adaptation is caused by

- The increase in the size and number of mitochondria, which draw the oxygen from the blood

- The increased availability of the oxygen (because you have so many blood vessels!)

REMEMBER

Consistent aerobic training makes physical changes in the heart, in the blood vessels, and in your ability to use oxygen. All these changes happen at the same time and could never be replicated with a pill or supplement. Exercise is the best medicine for changing your body to become fit and able to do more work!

Adapting to strength training

Strength training is mostly an anaerobic activity, so it doesn't really stress the cardiovascular system much. As a result, strength training doesn't produce many adaptations to the cardiovascular system. Heart rate, stroke volume, cardiac output, oxygen extraction . . . very little change is seen in these variables. Instead, all the adaptations happen to the muscles, the motor nerves, and the brain.

With strength training, your body adapts pretty specifically to the type of exercise you're doing. If you stress your muscles by strength training, then the skeletal muscles adapt. (See Chapter 3 for more information on these adaptations.)

Chapter **6**

Earthlings and the Earth: Adapting to Your Environment

Being a warm-blooded mammal has its advantages. By generating your own internal body heat, you can maintain your metabolic function without having to rely on the external environment. Whether the day is cold or warm, your cells stay happy and functioning. But conditions can arise that make the body either too hot or too cold. Controlling body temperature can become quite difficult in extreme environments, a situation that can impair performance and even result in death.

In addition, as a creature who breathes air, you certainly value the oxygen that conveniently surrounds you, waiting to fill your lungs. However, as you ascend in altitude, the conditions change, and oxygen is not quite so available, a situation that presents problems for high-flying and high-climbing humans.

In this chapter, we explore how the body maintains its temperature under both hot and cold conditions and how it's affected by and acclimatizes to heat and altitude. By the end of this chapter, you'll see how tough the environment can be on your body and the ways that your body can adapt to conditions to continue to perform its best.

Keeping It Just Right: The Basics of Temperature Regulation

The human body is finicky when it comes to temperature. It likes a very narrow range that hovers around 98.6°F (37°C). Too far above or below that point, and cell function begins to decline, and systems don't function. Your body maintains an acceptable temperature through a series of control systems, starting with the hypothalamus in the brain. The hypothalamus signals other mechanism to either warm you up or cool you down.

The hypothalamus: Your internal thermostat

The hypothalamus is an almond-size section of the brain located just above and slightly to the front of the brain stem. One of its key metabolic functions is body temperature regulation.

Blood continually courses through the hypothalamus, where its temperature is monitored. Each person has a hypothalamic thermostat set at a predetermined temperature, or *set point*. That set point is around 98.6°F (37°C). The goal of the hypothalamus is to balance the gain of heat (due to exercise or the environment) with heat loss so that the set point is maintained.

REMEMBER

Body temperature is not the same everywhere on the body. For example, the skin, also called the *shell*, is cooler than the blood, and the blood is cooler than active muscles and organs. The hypothalamus monitors the *core temperature* (the temperature deep within the body). The core temperature is the most important temperature to keep near its set point.

TECHNICAL STUFF

The hypothalamus does more than just regulate body temperature. It controls a range of functions like thirst, blood pressure, hunger, and hormone release. In some cases, the hypothalamus releases chemicals that impact the body directly (like releasing vasopressin to boost blood pressure) or that cause other organs to release their hormones. For example, the hypothalamus may release a hormone that causes the pituitary gland to release growth hormone.

FEELING FEVERISH?

Although your set point is supposed to be maintained at 98.6°F (37°C), it can be modified. Under conditions of illness or infection, your body activates defenses to combat the nasty invaders. One of these self-defense tools is heat! The hypothalamus raises the body's set point, causing a rise in core temperature as high as 104°F (40°C). A high core temperature may fight the illness, but it can also be a danger to your cells if it goes too high, which is why medications may be given to block the flames of a fever.

Pass the heat, please: The core-to-shell model of heat transfer

Hot things like to transfer their heat to cooler things. In order for the heat being generated in the muscle (lots of heat) to leave the body, it must come in contact with cooler and cooler locations. Therefore, the direction of heat movement looks something like this:

Heat in muscle → Cooler blood → Cooler skin → Cooler environment

As we explain in the next section, your body has ways of moving heat away from its core by cooling the shell (skin). Problems can arise, however, when these mechanisms fail or when extreme environmental conditions overwhelm the body.

Some Like It Hot — But Not Your Body!

Hot environments can pose a serious challenge to the body. If you add the heat generated during heavy exercise, you can be hit with a double whammy! Understanding the different ways your body gains heat from the environment can help you plan for the conditions.

Looking at the mechanisms of heat gain

The gain of heat by the body can come from within, or it can be from the external environment. Is the day sunny? Humid? Does the ground give off any heat? If the mechanisms of heat gain are combined, you can be in for a very hot day! Here are the variety of ways you can gain heat:

>> **Heavy exercise:** A large percentage — 80 percent, in fact — of the calories your body burns is lost as heat. The harder you work, the more heat you produce.

>> **Heat from the sun:** A sunny day can add 20 percent more heat load than a cloudy day. The sun heats the skin, making it harder to dispel the heat.

REMEMBER

Heat dissipates by going from higher- to lower-temperature environments, as we explain in the earlier section "Pass the heat, please: The core-to-shell model of heat transfer." If your skin is warmer due to heat from the sun, the internal heat can't dissipate as effectively.

>> **Reflected heat:** Heat can reflect off many surfaces, like asphalt, metals, and water. (Ever run on a black asphalt surface on a sunny day? You may have noticed how hot it is!) The reflected heat is why stadiums can get so hot in the summertime, or why a city street is a lot hotter than a country lane.

>> **Hot air:** A hot day can also warm the skin, making it hard for heat to get from the core to the skin. In this situation, the heat stays trapped inside the body (it's that core-to-shell model of heat transfer principle again).

>> **Covered skin:** For heat to leave the skin, the skin must be exposed. Your clothing traps the hot air near your skin and prevents heat from leaving. Think about how hot it gets, even when you're wearing only a light shirt.

>> **Humid days:** As the next section explains, one way to cool the skin is through sweating. The sweat itself doesn't cool you off; the sweat evaporating off the skin does the trick. Very humid air, however, already has all the water it wants, and it isn't willing to take your stinky sweat! On humid days, you can't cool your skin through evaporation.

TECHNICAL STUFF

Because the environment is such a contributor to heat gain, people try to measure the environmental conditions by using a variety of indexes. One is called the *heat index*. This index, shown in Figure 6-1, calculates a temperature by considering the air temperature and the relative humidity. Unfortunately, this method excludes the heat of the sun.

Temperature (°F)

Relative Humidity (%)	80	82	84	86	88	90	92	94	96	98	100	102	104	106	108	110
40	80	81	83	85	88	91	94	97	101	105	109	114	119	124	130	136
45	80	82	84	87	89	93	96	100	104	109	114	119	124	130	137	
50	81	83	85	88	91	95	99	103	108	113	118	124	131	137		
55	81	84	86	89	93	97	101	106	112	117	124	130	137			
60	82	84	88	91	95	100	105	110	116	123	129	137				
65	82	85	89	93	98	103	108	114	121	128	136					
70	83	86	90	95	100	105	112	119	128	134						
75	84	88	92	97	103	109	116	124	134							
80	84	89	94	100	106	113	121	129								
85	85	90	96	102	110	117	126	135								
90	86	91	98	105	113	122	131									
95	86	93	100	108	117	127										
100	87	95	103	112	121	132										

FIGURE 6-1: The heat index factors together air temperature and humidity.

Courtesy of the National Weather Service

Turning on your personal air conditioner: The body's cooling mechanisms

To cool off, your body has a variety of mechanisms to move heat from your body's core to the shell. Some of these mechanisms work better than others:

>> **Convection:** Hot air molecules can sit just above the skin, keeping the skin hot and preventing it from cooling. With *convection cooling,* air blows on the skin, sweeping away the hot air so the skin can release more heat. If you've ever stood in front of a fan when you're really hot, you know what convective cooling feels like.

>> **Conduction:** When something hot touches something cold, the heat moves to the colder object. In *conductive cooling,* the skin comes in physical contact with a cooler object — a cold towel, cold water, ice cubes, or anything else that can be touched — that transfers the heat away from the skin. Some people may even wear cooling vests, which can go underneath clothing. Ever wonder how firefighters stay cool? Cooling vests!

>> **Radiation:** Infrared rays can warm a fast-food hamburger, and they also can take heat away from the skin. *Remember:* Your blood is warmer than your skin. When the core temperature rises, the hypothalamus signals blood vessels in the skin to open wider, which lets more hot blood move to the skin. When

the hot blood gets near the surface, its heat can radiate away. Another effect of this cooling mechanism is that your skin looks flushed; that's the result of the widened blood vessels. Hopefully, you'll never get warm enough to cook a burger!

>> **Evaporation of sweat:** Water vapor holds far more heat than water itself (think of steam, which is hotter even than the boiling water that produces it). When your core temperature rises above the set point, the hypothalamus triggers sweat glands in the skin to release fluid (sweat) onto the skin. This fluid has been heated by the blood coursing through the skin. When it reaches the surface of the skin, it turns to a vapor (evaporates) and takes the heat with it. Humidity can interfere with sweat evaporation. Just dripping sweat doesn't cool the way sweat evaporation does.

REMEMBER

Sweat evaporation, which does 80 percent of the work in cooling the body, is the most important cooling mechanism your body has. The more skin you have exposed to the environment, the more sweat evaporation can take place (remember how humidity affects evaporation, though). Modern *wicking* clothing helps move water that may otherwise be trapped on the skin to the surface of the clothing, helping to continue to cool the skin even with the skin covered!

Adding insult to injury: Exercising in hot environments

Athletes can't hide from the heat. They often must perform in conditions that would make most of us run inside for some iced tea. If their bodies' cooling mechanisms are working, things may go just fine. However, if the athletes are unaccustomed to the heat or if they can't cool themselves, *hyperthermia* (a rise in body temperature above the set point) is inevitable, a situation that results in a decline in performance and possible serious injury.

When athletes encounter a hot environment for the first time, they notice an immediate effect on performance. Heat reduces their ability to perform well.

Seeing the effects of a hot environment on the body

Exercising in a hot environment produces certain changes in the body:

>> **A faster rate of glycogen (carbohydrate) use:** As carbs are used more quickly, athletes deplete the primary energy source for much of their work. Have you ever heard of the marathon runner that "bonks," "crashes," or "hits the wall" with fatigue during a race in hot weather? They've run out of glycogen! (Chapter 4 has more information on glycogen and exercise metabolism.)

- **Reduced muscle blood flow:** With so much blood going to the skin to help cool the body, less blood is available for the muscles. Less blood flowing to the muscles means less oxygen for the muscles, fewer nutrients, and reduced performance.

- **Increased blood lactic acid:** Because the muscle is starving for oxygen, it relies on anaerobic metabolism to keep going. The resulting lactic acid contributes to *bonking* (the sudden fatigue that comes from either a loss of glycogen stores or a rise in lactic acid) and a very unpleasant feeling in the muscles. (For a detailed explanation of what lactic acid is and how it affects the body during exercise, refer to Chapter 4.)

- **High rate of water and electrolyte loss through sweating:** Sweat evaporation is the body's primary cooling mechanism. In the untrained individual, the sweat contains not only water but also electrolytes (sodium and potassium), which are important for cell function and the transport of nerve signals. They must be maintained within the body.

WARNING

Dehydration reduces performance. Evan a 2 percent loss in body weight due to sweating results in a reduction in performance. You also run the risk of heat injury. To prevent dehydration, you must replace fluids lost as quickly as possible, both during and after the activity.

- **Increased heart rate:** With blood going to the skin for cooling and more fluid being lost due to sweating, a reduction in blood volume occurs. With less blood volume, the heart must beat even faster than usual to push the same amount of blood.

Too hot to handle: Heat injury

Athletes are known to push themselves very hard, sometimes ignoring warning signs of injury. When this happens in a hot environment, the result can be very bad. Even hours after being in the heat, the illness can continue.

WARNING

Heat injury is a leading cause of death among athletes, and the injury has three primary stages of severity, listed here from least to most severe. Action should be taken at the first signs of heat injury:

- **Stage 1 — Heat cramps and dizziness:** During the early stages of heat injury, the cells become dehydrated, and fluid is lost from the blood. The result is a feeling of nausea and dizziness, as well as muscle cramps.

  Treatment: Get the person out of the hot environment! Give them cool fluids as soon as possible, massage the cramps, and have them stretch. If they're dizzy, have them lie down.

DETERMINING HOW MUCH FLUID YOU NEED TO REPLACE

Did you know that 1 liter of fluid weighs 1 kilogram? Additionally, 1 pound of fluid is 16 ounces. To determine how much fluid is lost due to sweating, do the following:

1. **Weigh the person (with minimal clothing) before the activity.**

2. **Weigh the person after the activity.**

3. **Subtract the after-exercising value from the before-exercising value.**

   The difference in weight represents the loss of fluid!

Here's an example using both pounds and kilograms. Before a long run, Taylor weighs 180 pounds (81.8 kilograms). After the run, Taylor weighs 177 pounds (80.5 kilograms). Using pounds and ounces, 180 pounds – 177 pounds = 3 pounds of fluid lost; 3 pounds × 16 ounces = 48 ounces that need to be replaced. Using kilograms and liters, this is 81.8 kilograms – 80.5 kilograms = 1.3 kilograms lost; 1.3 kilograms equals 1.3 liters to replace.

Get Taylor drinking! Remember that Taylor has also lost things like sodium and potassium, so sports drinks may be a nice solution to the problem.

>> **Stage 2 — Heat exhaustion:** If the athlete pushes past cramps and ignores the nausea and dizziness, things can become quite severe. Heat exhaustion causes extreme losses in fluid. Symptoms of heat exhaustion include the following:

- Cold clammy skin, despite a high internal temperature
- Pale complexion
- Collapsing from dizziness or even losing consciousness
- Headache and nausea
- Weak and rapid pulse
- Shallow breathing

WARNING

Treatment: Call 911 immediately. Get the person in a cool environment immediately! Heat exhaustion is very dangerous and needs immediate care by a physician. The person with heat exhaustion may need so much fluid that it must be administered intravenously. The sufferer's sweating mechanism is shutting down due to the loss of so much fluid, and the condition can progress to heat stroke (and death) quickly, so you must act fast! Until emergency responders arrive, cool the sufferer with cold water and, if available, ice.

>> **Stage 3 — Heatstroke:** At this point, the person has collapsed completely and their ability to cool themselves has shut down. Symptoms of heat stroke include

- Very high body temperature (106°F/41.1°C or more)
- Dry skin (sweating has shut down)
- Unresponsiveness
- Labored breathing

WARNING

Treatment: Without immediate treatment, death can occur quickly (often due to things like liver or kidney failure). Call 911 immediately, and, if possible, immerse the sufferer in ice. Your goal is to cool them down fast!

Getting your body to adapt to the heat

TIP

Fortunately, the body is equipped to acclimate to hot environments. It only takes about 10 to 12 days, and the recipe is pretty straightforward:

>> **You must exercise in the hot environment.** Sorry, sitting in a sauna or lying out in the sun doesn't count! Adaptations only occur when you work in the actual environment.

>> **Take it easy and work up intensity.** Whatever the training intensity you're used to, back it off to about 60 percent to 70 percent for three to five days. As your body starts to adapt, you can build up intensity.

>> **Show some skin.** Wear minimal clothing to help your skin cool through sweat evaporation. Clothing should be light, breathable (wicking material), and reflect light. If you normally wear pads (you play football, for example), start without them for a while.

TIP

>> **Take water breaks.** Stay hydrated! Drinking about 8.5 ounces (250 milliliters) of water every 15 minutes helps offset sweat losses.

Within 10 to 12 days, your body will acclimatize. The following changes that occur help cool your body faster and allow better (and safer) performance:

>> **Sweat rate increases.** Your sweat glands put out more sweat, which means more cooling.

>> **Sweating begins earlier.** The sweat mechanism kicks in more quickly, so you don't get too hot before things start to cool.

>> **Sweat is more watery.** The sweat glands reduce the amount of sodium and other substances in the sweat, a combo that helps conserve electrolytes. Watery sweat also evaporates faster, which is cool — literally and metaphorically!

>> **Plasma volume increases.** The kidneys retain more fluid for the blood, and because some of the sweat comes from the blood, this translates into more fluid volume.

>> **Your body uses less glycogen.** Glycogen use drops after acclimatization, which means you don't fatigue as fast. (Glycogen, which is a stored form of glucose in the muscle and liver, is discussed in greater detail in Chapter 4.)

>> **Your skin is cooler.** Due to all the preceding changes, the skin stays cooler, enabling heat to move from the core to the shell more easily.

>> **Your heart rate is reduced.** Because of all the fluid increases and improved cooling, the heart doesn't have to work as hard, and your performance in the hot environment will be similar to your performance in a cooler environment.

When Chillin' Ain't Cool: Exercising in Cold Environments

Humans are capable of surviving in space, so it's not hard to believe that cold environments *can* be conquered. Obviously, standing in Antarctica in your running shorts isn't a wise move, and certainly exercising in cold environments has risks that you must be aware of. But proper clothing and understanding how much heat you generate during the activity can go a long way toward ensuring that you safely handle cold environments.

The chill can kill: Introducing hypothermia and wind chill

When heat loss exceeds the body's ability to generate heat, a condition of hypothermia may develop. In *hypothermia*, the body temperature drops below 95°F (35°C), and a loss of body function results. Causes of hypothermia include

>> Exposing skin to cold air, which rapidly draws heat away

>> Exposing skin to cold water, which dramatically accelerates heat loss

>> Wearing wet, cold clothing, or falling into cold water

WARNING

Being both wet *and* cold rapidly lowers body temperature. If you can't generate heat to offset the drop, you risk hypothermia! Symptoms of hypothermia include the following:

>> **Shivering:** The muscles are being activated to rapidly contract as a way to generate heat.

>> **Fatigue and sleepiness:** These symptoms indicate that the nervous system is beginning to slow down, as are body functions.

>> **Slowing heart rate and breathing:** The central nervous system is slowing its function. If body temperature drops too much, breathing can stop entirely — and so can your heart.

>> **Unconsciousness:** Let's hope you're getting help by this point!

Hypothermia progresses through three stages:

>> **Stage 1 — Mild:** This stage may almost seem like a stress response as the body tries to offset the drop in core temperature. It involves shivering, fast heart rate, and an increased use of glucose.

>> **Stage 2 — Moderate:** Body temperature keeps dropping. The shivering becomes pretty severe as the body forces muscle contractions to generate heat. Coordination of movement becomes slow and error prone, and people in this stage may experience mild confusion. You may notice that the sufferer looks pale and has very cold hands. The reason is that the body is constricting blood vessels to the body's shell as a way to keep the core warm. Lips may even look pale or blue.

WARNING

>> **Stage 3 — Severe:** The body begins to shut down. Heart rate drops very low, respiration falls, and blood pressure drops. Confusion, disorientation, uncoordinated muscles, and weakness mean that the person is probably not in a position to save themselves. Organ failure and death can follow.

TIP

Treat hypothermia before it becomes a problem. If you see someone who is likely suffering from hypothermia, get them dry, wrap them up, and give them heat! Your goal is to warm their core (their chest and trunk) and to get them away from the frigid environment!

Wind chill can become a problem when the combination of air temperature and wind is such that skin freezes quickly if exposed to the elements. You may feel all warm on the inside, but wonder why your fingers are frozen. When air temperature gets down around 10°F (−12°C), it takes only a small breeze to create conditions that can freeze the skin within minutes. Ultimately, how severe the problem is depends on air temperature, how warm you are, the length of exposure, and the wind chill.

Keep the heat: Dressing for the cold

The key for success in cold weather exercise is insulation. You have to cover the skin and provide layers of insulation to keep the heat. Here are some suggestions:

>> **Layer clothing.** Air is an insulator. By layering clothing, you create layers of air, which help hold heat in.

>> **Wear clothing that can wick away moisture.** Wet clothing loses its air pockets of insulation. Newer clothing materials let water escape without losing the air insulation layer. It's worth the extra money for some nicer winter materials, especially if you exercise outdoors often or frequently engage in outdoor, cold-weather activities!

>> **Adjust clothing based on how much heat will be produced during the activity.** A heavy-work, high-heat-producing activity requires less insulation than a light-work, low-heat-producing activity. *Remember:* Dressing too heavy can actually bring on hyperthermia (refer to the earlier section "Adding insult to injury: Exercising in hot environments" for details on this condition)!

Kids lose heat much more quickly than adults do, so keep them well insulated. Older folks also may get colder faster and not generate as much heat, so be sure to wrap them well!

A HAPPY LUNG IS A WARM, MOIST ONE!

Try breathing on a window. See the moisture? Your lungs like to be warm and wet. But cold air sucks the moisture right out of them. Dry and irritated lungs get stiff and narrow and make breathing hard. The result may be *cold air–induced asthma,* a condition that can make breathing very difficult, reduce exercise capacity, and create uncomfortable situations for just about anyone.

So, how can you avoid cold air–induced asthma? One simple treatment is to put a scarf or mask over your mouth while you exercise. Doing so warms the air slightly and keeps more moisture from escaping. Drinking extra water in cold climates can also offset the water lost in the breath.

Live High and Train Low: Exercising at Different Altitudes

Humans are a finicky lot. We can't live in the ocean, don't like the desert much, and are mostly confined to warm climates under 10,000 feet. So, when we do venture outside our comfort zone, the body's ability to do work is immediately impacted. Fortunately, we can adapt (sort of), which helps extend our range of wandering this planet.

REMEMBER

Oxygen is the currency needed for life. Normally, people live within an ocean of air (oxygen, carbon dioxide, and nitrogen). But as you travel higher into the atmosphere, the lower pressure reduces the pressure pushing oxygen into your blood and muscles. With less oxygen to help you do work, your performance suffers (or worse). The following sections have the details.

Revisiting oxygen transport

As we explain in detail in Chapter 5, pressure is the key behind all gas movement. Air always flows from high pressure to low pressure. The highest pressure of oxygen is in the atmosphere; next is your lungs; and then the blood. Oxygen is "pushed" from your lungs into your blood based on a pressure difference, and from there, it's pushed into your muscle cells:

Oxygen in atmosphere → Air in lungs → Blood → Muscle cells

Because humans aren't fish and can't take oxygen from a fluid, we need something to carry the oxygen in our blood. That carrier is *hemoglobin*. Hemoglobin can pick up a bubble of oxygen and transport it to the muscle cells. It contains iron, which bonds to the oxygen and gives you nice, red blood. All the hemoglobin needs to do its job is a nice push (pressure). Refer to Chapter 5 for details on the role hemoglobin plays in transporting oxygen.

REMEMBER

As the pressure of oxygen in the atmosphere drops — as it does at higher altitudes — less oxygen is pushed into the blood, resulting in less oxygen for the hemoglobin to carry.

Each gas that makes up air (oxygen, carbon dioxide, and nitrogen) exerts a pressure independent of other gases. The individual pressure for each gas is known as that gas's *partial pressure*. Here are the partial pressure values of each of these three gases (for details on how to calculate partial pressure, refer to Chapter 5):

>> **Oxygen:** 159 millimeters of mercury (mmHg)

>> **Carbon dioxide:** 0.03 mmHg

>> **Nitrogen:** 600.7 mmHg

Barometric pressure is the pressure exerted by the total of all the gases, and it's 760 mmHg at sea level.

TIP

Partial pressure can be modified, either by changing the concentration of the gas (like adding a bottle of oxygen) or by changing the pressure. So, when you're exercising or climbing at altitude (which drops partial pressure), you can use some supplemental oxygen from a breathing system and increase the partial pressure. Doing so allows mountain climbers to actually climb higher than typically possible — provided they don't run out of their extra oxygen!

When going up brings you down: Altitude and reduced aerobic capacity

Problems caused by low air pressure at high altitudes don't really begin until you get above 5,000 feet, but above that altitude, not enough pressure exists to push oxygen fully into the blood. As a result, less oxygen is available to you for exercise. As you go higher, you experience more pronounced effects:

>> **At 10,000 feet:** Your fitness is about 20 percent lower than at sea level. You run slower and get tired faster. Even a simple walk takes more effort.

>> **At 14,000 feet:** Your aerobic ability is 30 percent weaker. If you're out climbing in Colorado, just hiking up a hill may feel like you're running your hardest. You have to stop periodically just to catch your breath. Your heart rate may be near its max.

>> **At or above 20,000 feet:** At this level, few people function very well unless they're acclimatized. Simply not enough oxygen is being pushed into the blood to enable you to do much work.

REMEMBER

You can avoid the drop in atmospheric pressure as you go up in altitude. Head to the later section "I think I can, I think I can . . . Adapting to high altitudes" for information. Still, due to the loss of oxygen and reduced ability to do work, your training intensity at altitude will be lower than training under 5,000 feet. You won't be working at your peak, so training improvement can be more difficult.

WHY AM I ALIVE IN A JET FLYING AT 40,000 FEET?

Jets fly at very high altitudes and take air into the cabin at that altitude, and people manage just fine, even though a person would normally die at 40,000 feet. What gives? Pressure!

The concentration of oxygen in the air at 40,000 feet is the same as at sea level, but there is so little pressure that the oxygen can't get pushed into the blood. To counter this situation, jets have cabins that are pressurized to the equivalent of an altitude of about 8,000 feet — enough pressure that most people don't have any problems. However, doctors may suggest that people with heart and lung ailments avoid flying for fear of issues that may arise due to the slightly less-than-ideal conditions.

A sick view from the top: Identifying altitude illnesses

Not everyone has difficulty adjusting to changes in altitude, but that doesn't mean that, when you and the family go skiing in Colorado at 10,000 feet, someone isn't at risk for some of the following symptoms of altitude sickness:

>> **Dehydration:** Dehydration is common for two reasons. First, the air is dry higher up, and you lose water simply by breathing. Second, your kidneys release fluid (you hit the bathroom more) as a way to concentrate the blood to carry more oxygen.

>> **Headaches:** Mild headaches are common with dehydration. If your headache gets worse and progresses to significant pain and debilitation, watch out — you may be sensitive to more serious conditions.

>> **Fatigue and insomnia:** These symptoms usually go away within two days as you adjust.

TIP

When arriving at higher altitudes, take a few days to adjust, drink lots of water, and don't exert yourself too much.

In the following sections, we outline some of the more serious conditions that can occur at high altitudes.

High-altitude pulmonary edema

At high altitudes, some people are susceptible to more serious conditions that are life-threatening. These individuals experience changes in their lung tissue that cause fluid to accumulate in the space between the lungs and the blood, blocking oxygen from getting to the blood. Called *high-altitude pulmonary edema*, the condition produces these symptoms:

>> Coughing and flu-like symptoms

>> Difficulty breathing (you gasp for breath)

>> Skin (lips and fingers) that may look blue

>> A tight chest and wheezing, which indicate the lungs have fluid surrounding them

REMEMBER

If these symptoms occur, the single best treatment is to get down from the altitude! Get below 3,000 feet.

High-altitude cerebral edema

WARNING

Whereas high-altitude pulmonary edema is an accumulation of fluid in the lungs, *high-altitude cerebral edema* is the accumulation of fluid in the brain. This condition is often fatal, so take it seriously! If you see these symptoms, get down from the altitude immediately:

>> Nausea and/or vomiting

>> Weakness, confusion, and/or memory loss

>> Severe headache

>> Balance problems

>> Hallucinations

REMEMBER

The preceding symptoms are all signs that your brain function is in trouble. The only treatment that works? *Get down from the altitude!*

I think I can, I think I can . . . Adapting to high altitudes

Given time at high altitudes, your body will acclimatize. How much time depends on just how high you're going. Altitude acclimatization takes longer the higher up you are. Hiking at 10,000 feet, for example, may mean waiting three to four days for acclimatization to occur. When you're climbing at 20,000 feet, you may need a month or more before your body adjusts.

THE DRUG THAT DID MORE THAN HELP ALTITUDE ILLNESS

Researchers in the early 1990s were working on a medication that can dilate blood vessels in the lungs and heart to help reduce fluid around the lungs, as well as deliver more oxygen to the heart. Clinical studies started to show an interesting side effect. Patients reported that they had erectile improvement. Research on the altitude illness treatment was abandoned, and a drug, later called Viagra, was developed. This story goes to show that new discoveries come via unusual pathways!

REMEMBER

So, what changes occur during acclimatization to high altitudes? The key is oxygen. You can't change the atmosphere, so the only way to acclimatize to altitude is to improve your body's ability to load up on oxygen and deliver it to the cells. Key adaptations to altitude include the following:

>> **New blood vessels form.** Yes, your body actually produces new blood vessels to help deliver more oxygen to the muscles so that they don't starve.

>> **Red blood cell production increases.** More red blood cells means more hemoglobin, which in turn means you can carry more oxygen. Even though the push of oxygen is less, you make up for it by having more hemoglobin carrying oxygen. Many hands make light work, the saying goes. This is your body's best adaptation to high altitudes.

>> **Blood vessels dilate.** Wider blood vessels can deliver more oxygen to the tissue and help keep you moving.

Living high and training low: The best of both worlds

So, you want to be the best you can be? Well, then, you need to take advantage of the best that sea level and altitude can give you. We call this the *live high, train low method*, and it lets you use the enhanced oxygen delivery adaptations that occur at high altitudes while you exercise at low altitudes:

>> **Live high:** Achieving the adaptations that enable your blood to carry more oxygen takes time living in a high-altitude environment. Some people even sleep in tents that have reduced pressure or reduced concentrations of oxygen to simulate altitude (that's getting pretty serious).

» **Train low:** Your strongest training happens only when you have the most oxygen available, so you train at lower altitudes. By taking advantage of the adaptations in your blood to carry more oxygen while you train at lower altitudes, you can push your fitness and performance to the max!

This method gives you the best of both worlds. It may not be for everyone (we are *not* suggesting that you commute back and forth between the mountains and sea level!). However, some top aerobic athletes do try to take advantage of the live high, train low method.

3

The Physics of Movement: Basic Biomechanics

Understanding the mechanism of motor control and how the brain communicates with the body for movement.

Identify the kinds of motions, laws of motion, and the types of forces the body generates.

Discover how muscles and joints are oriented, how they keep the body stable, and how to keep joints and muscles flexible.

Analyze movement and functional activities (like making a jump shot), using a systematic approach.

Chapter **7**

Planning Your Movements: Motor Control

Movement is a puzzle. Just walking across the room requires cooperation between muscles that move the legs, arms, and torso, plus balancing that noggin on top. Add to that changes in terrain, environment, and obstacles, and you can see how the brain has to coordinate many functions to execute movement. This is motor control.

Like any good relationship, communication occurs between the information coming to the brain from sensors that monitor what the body is experiencing (like pain, pressure, temperature, body position, and balance) and the information the brain is sending out in movement-related signals (like muscle contractions). These feedback systems help keep your body continually updated so that the movements you execute match the conditions you experience, and this constant communication is the basis of coordinated movement.

In this chapter, we explain how the brain and interconnected nervous system both sense body position and movement and initiate a movement response.

Introducing the Main Player: The Neuron

The primary functional part of the entire nervous system is the *neuron*. Neurons are small by themselves, but linked together, they form the system by which signals are sent and received throughout the body. We all have billions of neurons in our bodies.

Neuron basics: Parts and functions

A neuron looks a bit like a tree with roots (see Figure 7-1). Here are the parts of a neuron and what they do:

» **Dendrites:** The thin, fingerlike sensory nerves that appear on one end of the neuron. Dendrites pick up signals from the *axon terminals* of other nearby nerves.

» **Cell body:** The larger area containing the nucleus of the neuron. The cell body is responsible for keeping the neuron alive and functioning. The *nucleus* contains the genetic information for the neuron.

» **Axon:** The single nerve fiber that carries an electrical signal to the next neuron. Axons are bundled together, forming a nerve, and they can be very long or quite short. For faster conduction speeds, some axons are covered with a fatty coating called a *myelin sheath*. The myelin sheath allows nerve signals to jump along the outside of the nerve, hopping from open space to open space in the sheath (these spaces are called *nodes of Ranvier*), much like a stone skipping across water.

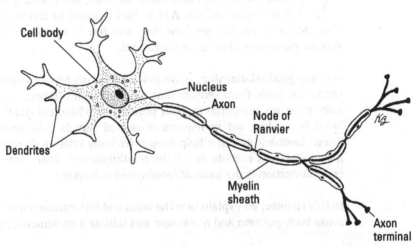

FIGURE 7-1: The parts of a neuron.

Illustration by Kathryn Born, MA

REMEMBER

Neurons form connections to each other, creating branches of interconnections, which allow for information to pass across great distances and from various locations. So, any particular neuron is actually getting inputs from a variety of neurons that are connected to it (at the dendrites). If the inputs are enough, they cause a stimulus in the neuron. If they aren't sufficient to cause a stimulus in the neuron, nothing happens. So, one muscle may get a stimulus to contract, while a nearby muscle does nothing. It all depends on the sum of all the inputs.

REMEMBER

Neurons are not all alike. Some have specific functions within the body. Some like to sense; others like to signal:

>> **Sensory neurons:** Sensory neurons are connected to the sensors of the environment. The sights and sounds around us are picked up by sensing organs (eyes, ears) with the information transferred to sensory neurons in the brain. These brain neurons have dendrites that pick up the sensory information from many inputs and send signals along their axons to the brain. This action is a bit like sitting in a crowded room, listening to conversations and then trying to explain to someone what you're hearing! In that scenario, you're the sensory neuron, picking up the signals (the bits you overhear) and passing them on.

>> **Motor neurons:** As their name implies, motor neurons influence movement. Signals from the brain and spinal cord travel out to the muscles along motor neurons. Motor (muscle) movements are governed by the signals that come down the motor neurons. Contracting muscles, relaxing muscles, and controlling many complex actions that make up a movement. These neurons influence which muscles are activated and which are relaxed when you throw a ball — how hard, which muscles work, which joints move, and which do not. The signals can be excitatory (called *excitatory postsynaptic potentials*) to cause movement or inhibitory (called *inhibitory postsynaptic potentials*) to inhibit movement.

>> **Interneurons:** Interneurons located in the brain or spinal cord form a bridge between sensory and motor neurons. As we explain later, some movements can happen quickly after a sensation. These reflexes are hardwired into the body using interneurons.

Neurotransmitters: The bridge over River Synapse

You may think that a sensory or motor neuron is like one long wire running through your body. Not so! In fact, neurons are more like small noodles, lined up in a row but not actually connected. Not connected? Nope. Which brings up the question, "How do signals get transmitted?" The answer: neurotransmitters!

Neurotransmitters are chemicals located in little sacs at the end of an axon terminal. When the nerve signal reaches these sacs, the sacs move to the edge of the axon and open up, releasing a chemical into the small space (called a *synapse*) between the two neurons. These chemicals float across the synapse and connect to the dendrites, stimulating the nerve to continue the signal. Think of the neurotransmitter as a ferry carrying a wagon across a river.

Different nerves have different neurotransmitters. Neurotransmitters that cause muscles to contract are not the same neurotransmitters that cause some nerves to either excite or inhibit. By having different types of neurotransmitters, the body can organize a variety of signals, instead of having one signal that tries to control everything.

Orders from Above: Motor Control

For movement to occur, the muscles need some coordinated instructions. Fortunately, we all have brains! The brain and the associated nervous system provide the input to the muscles, stimulating them to contract and move.

In the following sections, we give you a tour of the central processing center (the brain) and the bundle of neurons (the spine) that transmit the signals the brain sends to the muscle.

The brain: The central processing center

As the central processing center, the brain receives sensory information (related to body position, balance, visual input, sound, and more) from all areas of the body and sends out information to the body in response. Some key areas of the brain include the following (see Figures 7-2 and 7-3):

>> **Cerebral cortex:** The wrinkled and wavy outer layer of the brain, this area has regions for both sensory information processing as well as motor function. Note the many different areas (limbic, primary visual, secondary visual, posterior parietal, auditory, and so on) within the cortex in Figure 7-2.

>> **Sensory cortex:** Located toward the back (posterior) of the brain, the sensory cortex contains regions of sensory information like vision, taste, pain, temperature, and pressure.

>> **Motor cortex:** The motor cortex is located toward the middle of the brain in the frontal lobe. It's a key area for initiating movement; it also helps coordinate movement (which is nice when you're trying to play darts and not put a hole in the wall).

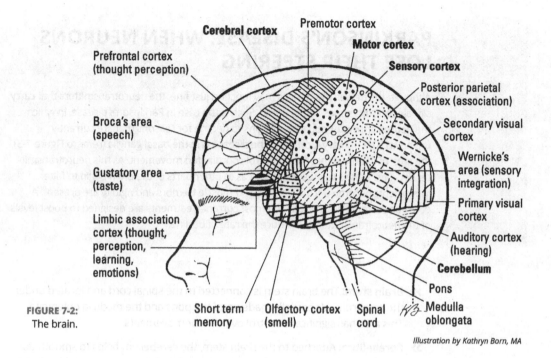

Cerebral cortex

Premotor cortex

Motor cortex

Sensory cortex

Prefrontal cortex
(thought perception)

Posterior parietal
cortex (association)

Broca's area
(speech)

Secondary visual
cortex

Wernicke's
area (sensory
integration)

Gustatory area
(taste)

Primary visual
cortex

Limbic association
cortex (thought,
perception,
learning,
emotions)

Auditory cortex
(hearing)

Cerebellum

Pons

FIGURE 7-2:
The brain.

Short term
memory

Olfactory cortex
(smell)

Spinal
cord

Medulla
oblongata

Illustration by Kathryn Born, MA

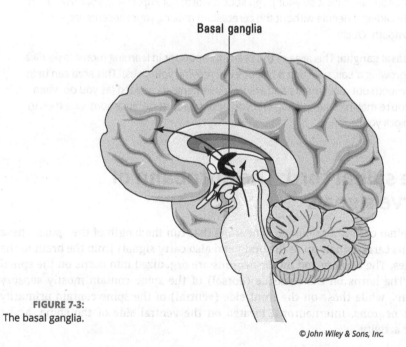

Basal ganglia

FIGURE 7-3:
The basal ganglia.

© John Wiley & Sons, Inc.

PARKINSON'S DISEASE: WHEN NEURONS LOSE THEIR STEERING

Although the nerves themselves may function just fine, the neurotransmitters that carry signals can sometimes be disrupted. Such is the case in Parkinson's disease, in which the neurotransmitter dopamine begins to decline for reasons that are currently unknown. The primary location of the disease is in the basal ganglia (refer to Figure 7-3), the area of the brain that helps control coordinated movement. As this neurotransmitter declines, signals to muscles as well as to other parts of the brain begin to falter. Movements become uncoordinated, and muscle tremors and rigidity are present. A cure has yet to be discovered, and most current treatments are designed to boost levels of the neurotransmitter and reduce the rate of decline.

>> **Brain stem:** The brain stem is connected to the spinal cord and located under the cerebrum. It's partially made up of the pons and the medulla oblongata. This area has significant control over motor movements.

>> **Cerebellum:** Attached to the brain stem, the cerebellum helps to smooth out muscle movement so your jump shot is worthy of impressing your friends. Try threading a needle without the cerebellum making your movements smooth. Ouch!

>> **Basal ganglia:** This area of the brain is important in learning motor tasks (like throwing a ball, swinging a bat, or even moving your eyes). This area can help smooth out movements and adjust movements as needed (as you do when you're making a jump shot, and you have to adjust because someone tries to block you).

The spinal cord: The autobahn of nerve signals

The spinal cord is a grouping of neurons that run the length of the spine. These neurons carry signals up to the brain and also carry signals from the brain to the muscles. The sensory and motor neurons are organized into horns on the spinal cord. The horns on the backside (dorsal) of the spine contain mostly sensory neurons, while those on the front side (ventral) of the spine contain primarily motor neurons. Interneurons, located on the ventral side of the spine, assist motor activity.

Feedback loops: Communicating between body and brain

As you move through the world walking, climbing, rolling, jumping, and doing whatever else sounds like fun, a continuous conversation takes place between what your body senses both externally and internally and the signals that the brain sends out. The brain interprets sensations and manages your motor efforts to match your desired movement. The communication between sensation and motor effort is referred to as a *feedback loop*.

TIP

A feedback loop functions something like a thermostat. If you set the thermostat to 70°F (21°C) and the room gets cool, the drop in temperature turns on the furnace, and the room heats up. When it hits 70°F, the furnace turns off. In a similar fashion, if you estimate the height of a step you're about to step on through visual clues, you prepare a motor response that lifts your leg and propels you upward to step smoothly onto the step. If you miss the step, sensory information about body position goes to the brain, and your next attempt is corrected.

Because the environment is continually changing and you're always moving, feedback loops are always in action, keeping you on track and walking upright!

The open-loop system

An open-loop system is one in which the activity is initiated, but nothing can be done to check or change the outcome. For example, you may program your sprinklers to come on every day at noon. But what if it rains? Your sprinklers still come on. An open-loop system works the same way.

The problem with an open-loop system is that no feedback exists to allow for control of the system; the system has been preprogrammed. The human body needs more control than that. For that reason, most of the feedback systems in your body are closed-loop systems.

The closed-loop system

A closed-loop system is more like a thermostat — sensory feedback helps guide the brain's response. If your body temperature goes up, the hypothalamus in your brain triggers sweating to cool you off. If your blood sugar goes up, receptors sensitive to this rise provide the brain information that provokes a stimulus to the pancreas to release insulin to help lower blood sugar.

Examples of closed-loop systems include the following reflexes, which you can read more about in the later section "Hardwiring the nervous system: Reflex control" and in Chapter 3:

>> **Muscle spindles:** Stretch the muscle too fast, and the feedback stimulus causes the muscle to contract against the stretch.

>> **The Golgi tendon:** Put the tendon under too much tension, and the feedback initiates an inhibition of muscle contraction to help ease the tension.

Your Place in Space: Sensory Information and Control of Movement

To have an effective feedback system, you need both sensory information coming into the brain and accurate motor signals being sent out to the muscles. Sensory information comes from a variety of systems, some of which provide an immediate motor response (a reflex), while others add to a list of inputs that help you coordinate some pretty sophisticated movements!

Where did I put my hand? Sensing body position

Try walking in a dark room sometime. What is your first instinct as you try to get a sense of your movement? You reach out to touch something, you search for any visible light to get a sense of up or down, and you feel the incline of the floor. Why? Because movement and performance of activity are closely linked to the sensory tools that constantly tell you where you are in space. Put together, these senses — touch, vision, and proprioception — help you perform activities with precision.

Touch

Skin may look like it's just tissue and blood vessels, but it's filled with sensors that provide vital information:

>> **Touch:** Light-touch sensors (called *Meissner's corpuscles*) provide a tactile sense that helps you apply the appropriate amount of pressure (like holding a baseball with just enough grip to throw a knuckleball). They're sensitive to very light touch and vibration.

Heavier touch can be sensed by sensors called *Pacinian corpuscles,* which are deeper within the skin. These sensors help distinguish the difference between rough and smooth.

» **Temperature:** Temperature sensors indicate hot and cold, information that can help you determine whether you want to take a sip of your coffee or blow on it a while!

» **Pressure:** Pressure sensors on the feet tell you whether you're standing and how balanced you are on your feet, for example. They also help provide feedback as you change positions (like making a cross dribble fake in basketball).

When you're swinging a bat, a golf club, or a tennis racquet, the senses of touch and pressure as you hold and hit are essential for performing well.

Vision

Vision sensation is an essential part of coordinated movement. You can always spot new dancers, for example. They're the ones staring down at their feet rather than looking at their partners. You'd almost think they need to *see* each step to be sure they're moving!

Just how useful is visual feedback? It depends on what you're looking at. Although the vision sense may be similar for individuals, how people use their visual sense may not be. Consider these examples:

» **Boxing:** An untrained boxer may watch the opponent's gloves, anticipating a punch to avoid. A trained boxer, on the other hand, may watch the opponent's trunk, hips, and shoulders in order to anticipate a punch. In the latter case, the boxer may easily avoid the punch; in the former, they may be eating a glove sandwich!

» **Baseball:** A novice baseball or softball player may watch for the ball as it approaches the plate. Expert players see the release point from the arm of the pitcher, which provides information about the angle and even the type of pitch that may be coming.

TIP

Competitors often try to disguise or deceive by providing misleading visual feedback to their opponents. They do this because they know that visual senses are essential components for guiding motor responses. An example can be the baseball pitcher who tries to hide the ball during the windup, change the angle of the arm at ball release, or change the speed of the pitch to disrupt the visual cues that the batter uses to hit the ball.

Proprioception

Have you ever been asked to close your eyes and touch your nose? Hopefully, it was just for fun! How did you know where your nose was? Or how did you know where your arm and finger were? Even without visual cues, you have internal sensors, called *proprioceptors*, that provide position sense about your limbs, head, and trunk. Like an internal Global Positioning System (GPS), proprioceptors track position, movement, and velocity.

A few key proprioceptors are the *muscle spindles*, which sense change in length and velocity of the muscle fibers, and the *Golgi tendons*, which sense the amount of tension on a tendon connecting the muscle to the bone. We explain these proprioceptors in the next section.

Hardwiring the nervous system: Reflex control

If a building catches fire, it's nice to know that the sprinklers will come on automatically. No one needs to be called for a decision! Likewise, if your tendon were being pulled on so hard that it may tear from the bone, it would be nice if your body would automatically stop the muscle from pulling harder without waiting for a decision from the brain. Such is the role of a *reflex*, a preprogrammed sensory-motor control system that is designed to protect the body. Read on to find out about a couple of key reflexes.

WHICH WAY IS UP?

The process of standing isn't as easy as it sounds. Sensory cues from pressure receptors on the feet tell you where your center of balance is. Your eyes help you orient to the upright position, and your inner ear provides more feedback regarding your position.

But what about an astronaut? In a weightless environment, every way is up! No sensory stimulus exists to provide body position or center of balance. This lack of information makes adjustment to space a difficult thing, often leading to nausea for days. Over time, however, the astronauts do adjust.

Yet when they come back to Earth, the sensory receptors have lost their "touch," so to speak, and don't initially provide enough sensory feedback to help orient the astronauts, leading to significant balance issues. Within a few days, these senses return, allowing the astronauts to once again stand up and stare at the stars.

Muscle spindles

When you think of spindles, think of speed! *Muscle spindles* are sensory fibers intertwined with muscle fibers. They look a bit like a Slinky wrapped within the muscle and moving with every change in muscle length.

Spindles sense the change in length and velocity of the muscle fibers. At slow speeds, this feedback helps you sense where your arm is in space by noting the length of the muscle. But what happens when you rapidly stretch a muscle? You trigger a stretch reflex. The spindles sense the rapid stretch of the muscle, and sensory nerves send this signal to the interneurons of the spinal cord. A stimulus to the muscle is initiated immediately, causing muscle contraction. At the same time, a signal is sent to the opposing muscle to relax so that movement can take place at the joint.

REMEMBER

You can think of the stretch reflex this way:

rapid stretch = reflex muscle contraction

When the doctor taps your knee at the patellar tendon, they're trying to induce a small, rapid stretch of the quadriceps muscle. The rapid stretch (like plucking a guitar string) results in a reflex contraction, and you notice a slight kick of the leg.

Golgi tendon organ

When you think of the Golgi tendon, think tension. The Golgi tendon monitors the amount of tension in the tendon that attaches the muscle to the bone (much like a spider feels tension in its web while waiting for the next meal to fly in).

How can tension occur at the tendon? In two ways:

>> **Lifting a heavy weight:** The force required by the muscle to lift a heavy weight pulls hard on the tendon, creating tension.

>> **Stretching a muscle:** When the muscle is placed under a prolonged stretch, the tendon experiences tension.

PLYOMETRICS: TRAINING THE MUSCLE SPINDLE FOR PEAK PERFORMANCE

One way to induce the muscle spindle to fire in the leg and gluteal muscles is by jumping down from a box. The landing motion creates a rapid stretch in the muscles, causing the muscle spindles to fire. When you then try to jump immediately after the landing, you get a "boost" from the additional muscle firing due to the spindles.

Additionally, with repeated training, you can actually speed up the time between the spindles sensing the stretch and the muscle firing. This enhancement can make a big difference in athletic performance when tenths of a second count!

A reflex response occurs in response to tension. Sensory nerves attached to the tendon sense tension and respond by inhibiting the muscles from contracting, causing the muscle to relax.

TIP

Try doing a hamstring stretch and holding the stretch position so that the muscle is placed under constant tension. Within 20 seconds, you'll notice that the muscle starts to relax. You've discovered the Golgi tendon reflex!

Now, suppose you're lifting a series of weights, each one heavier than the last. As you get to your heaviest weight, the amount of tension on the muscle and tendon is so much that the Golgi tendon is activated. As a result, your muscle can't exert any additional force (even if the muscle had the ability) because the Golgi prevents additional muscle recruitment.

TIP

If you've ever driven (or followed behind) a gas-powered golf cart, you know these vehicles go pretty slowly because a device prevents them from going faster. If you removed that device? Zoom! Well, the Golgi tendon acts in a similar way, preventing the muscle from creating too much tension. However, you can modify how the Golgi tendon responds. With training, you can increase the level of tension needed to activate the Golgi tendon, thus enabling the muscle to exert more force and making you stronger! You don't even need to grow more muscle — you're just using more of what you have.

USING MUSCLE SPINDLE AND GOLGI TENDON REFLEXES TO ENHANCE PERFORMANCE

Your built-in reflexes are meant to protect you. And if you trigger them correctly, you can use them to enhance performance. However, in some instances and with some movements, these reflexes can hurt performance. Here's what you need to know:

- **Should you hold a stretch or bounce a stretch?** Hold stretches and bouncing stretches activate different reflexes. During the hold stretch, the Golgi tendon is activated and the muscle relaxes. Yay! Nice stretch.

  During the bouncing stretch, the muscle spindles are activated (due to the rapid stretch). The reflex is a muscle contraction! Ever try to stretch a muscle that's contracting? Ouch! That can damage the muscle. Not the best stretching idea.

- **Should you do some mini-jumps to warm up or should you stretch?** Mini-jumps activate the muscle spindles, which respond by activating muscle contraction and exciting motor neurons. Yay! More muscle to jump with! Nice exercise. However, if you hold a stretch of those muscle just before the activity, the Golgi tendon responds by inhibiting muscle firing. Looks like you won't be jumping too high this time.

Threading the Needle or Shooting a Free Throw: Coordinating Movement

If you've ever played a video game that involves fast driving or flying, you know that when the path gets too complicated, you have to slow down to navigate. Things just come too quickly to make steering adjustments fast enough! Likewise, many human activities, like hitting a ball or inserting a key into a keyhole require speed, accuracy, or a combination of the two. In the next sections, we explain how speed and accuracy are coordinated.

Making the speed-accuracy trade-off

Most sport activity requires targeted movements at a particular speed (or as fast as you're able to move); pitching a ball to a batter, swinging a golf club to hit a ball, and throwing a football to a running receiver are examples. If a skill is particularly difficult because of the high level of accuracy required, like swinging a golf club to hit a ball, you sacrifice speed (slow down) in order to gain accuracy. This is known as the *speed–accuracy trade-off*.

REMEMBER

In this trade-off, any time you increase the speed of a movement, you reduce the movement's accuracy. Likewise, if you increase the accuracy needed for a movement, you sacrifice the speed at which you can perform.

So, how can a professional golfer swing a club with such a high velocity and still hit that tiny white ball? Training! Through repetitive training, you can condition your motor system to create accurate movements at very high speeds.

Following the phases in a movement

Performing an activity is a sequence of a number of events. The first phase is preparation, followed by the initial movement, followed by a terminal stage of movement. Speed and accuracy (covered in the preceding section) are dependent upon your sensory motor system making adjustments throughout all the phases, from beginning to end:

>> **The preparation phase:** In the preparation phase, you've decided upon the movement you want to initiate. If you're hitting a golf ball with a club, for example, your visual senses determine the distance to the ball and the position of the ball on the tee. Pressure sensors in your feet determine your balance on the ground, the degree of traction you have to use for force, and the direction of the intended flight path of the ball.

As you begin to draw the club back (your backswing), proprioceptors indicate where your arms are in relation to your body, the position of the club, and the velocity of the backswing, while your eyes focus on the upcoming impact point on the ball. Lower limb pressure and position sensors provide information about your windup phase. At this point, your muscles are stretching and your body is placed in a position where it can unwind in a forceful fashion.

>> **The initiation phase:** In the initiation phase, the speed of movement comes into play. Your vision maintains contact with the target object while your motor control system initiates an explosive movement to swing the club. Little adjustment in the swing is possible during this movement because it's done at such a high velocity. Just swing, baby!

>> **The terminal phase:** The terminal phase occurs just before the ball is hit at the point of contact. Using visual senses, your central nervous system can allow for subtle changes in the swing at the point of contact to adjust trajectory.

Think about all the minor swing adjustments that occur during the preparation, initiation, and terminal phases of a golf swing. Improvement in both speed and accuracy can happen only over time and with repeated swing practice. Of course, golf uses different clubs, so the swing training needs minor alterations for each club and each ground condition. No wonder golf is such a hard sport!

The field of biomechanics studies the physics of body movements (as well as the club you may be swinging) and examines the phases of movements and the aspects of the body in motion. Chapter 11 contains information on analyzing the biomechanics of movement.

Coordinating two arms: Bimanual coordination

You body likes to move its limbs (arms and legs) in a coordinated fashion (called *symmetrical coordination*), in which both arms and both legs do essentially the same thing. But what happens, for example, if the arms have to move in different ways (called *asymmetrical coordination*)? Playing the violin can be quite complicated when one hand is forming cords while the other hand (and arm) is moving a bow across the strings!

These types of movements are difficult simply because limbs prefer to work in unison. They like symmetrical movement. Consider these points:

>> The more complex a movement is for a limb, the slower the limb will move.

>> The limb doing the more complex movement influences the movement of the limb doing the less complex movement.

>> With a new complex movement that requires each limb to move separately, both limbs initially want to do the same thing.

Even though limbs want to work in unison, you can learn to move each limb separately. Here's how:

>> **Practice.** Start with slow movements and work up to the speed required. Initially, the slower movements allow for the proper sequencing of the movement. You can add speed later.

>> **Get feedback.** Find a coach who can provide instruction on proper position and initiation of movement. For the novice, attaining the proper form and position is difficult, but the practiced eye of an expert can help correct movements before they become learned in the wrong way.

>> **Try breaking the movement down into its components, and practice each component separately.** Initially, practicing the individual components of a movement can help you develop the skill. After the motor skills for each part of the movement have become ingrained, you can focus on sequencing the parts together into a more complex movement. For example, you may want to first practice tossing the volleyball in the air a bit, then practice stepping and hitting the ball, and then finally put these actions together to master your serve.

Now, you can see why walking is easy (or it *seems* easy), but dancing can be a challenge. One movement (walking) has been learned, while the other (dancing) may involve first stepping forward, then to the side, then forward again. Both movements are similar, but the movements associated with dancing haven't been ingrained. No wonder new dancers often feel like they have two left feet!

Come on, baby, do the locomotion: The rhythm of walking

Upright walking is unique to humans, and most of us get the basics down by the time we're 1 year old. Locomotion is programmed into our basic nervous system functions (we don't need to think about it). Sensory signals then help shape or modify our movements, specific to the demands. When talking about walking locomotion, the term frequently used is *gait*.

Watch how people walk. Do they simply stride with their arms at their sides in a stiff upright position? No. Instead, you'll notice a rhythm and relationship between the leg stride, arm swing, and trunk rotation. Walking is like dancing in some respects because both have a rhythm to their steps. Dancing is a bit trickier, but dance has been used as a means to improve walking and balance, due to similarities between the two.

REMEMBER
Most research indicates that the coordination of walking is a centralized nervous system control, where a pattern of signals is generated for normal walking. For this reason, a disruption in walking patterns can indicate a problem with the central nervous system.

Leg movement

Leg movement occurs in two primary phases, each completed separately by the legs (see Figure 7-4):

>> **Stance phase:** During this phase, the limb is extended and placed in contact with the ground. During ground contact, the push to move forward is generated.

>> **Swing phase:** Following the stance phase is the swing phase, during which the limb is flexed to leave the ground and then brought forward to begin the next stance phase.

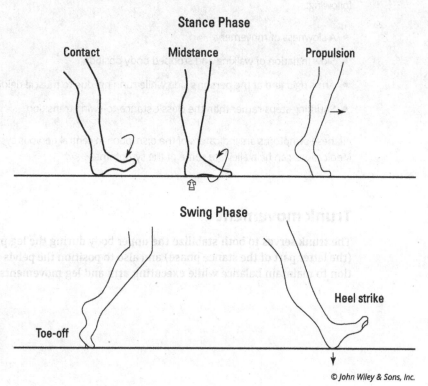

FIGURE 7-4: Leg movement is broken into stance phase (top) and swing phase (bottom).

Each leg is coordinated in the two phases separately, and faster movement is completed generally by shortening the stance phase.

Arm movement

The arms move in a synchronized fashion in relation to the legs to provide balance and propulsion. For slow walking, the arms swing twice for every leg stride, but at faster speeds, the arm-to-leg ratio is 1:1 (one arm swing to one leg swing).

OUT OF PHASE: PARKINSON'S DISEASE AND LOCOMOTION

Normal gait consists of upright posture, steady stride between the stance and swing phases, and arms rhythmically (and relaxedly) moving in opposition to the stride. Due to the neurological disruption caused by Parkinson's disease, the gait is disrupted, and normal movement is no longer evident. In people with Parkinson's disease, you see the following:

- A slowness of movement
- Slow initiation of walking and stooped body position
- Arms rigid and at the person's side while running, due to muscle rigidity
- Shuffling steps rather than the classic stance-to-swing transition

All these symptoms are indicators of the disruption in central nervous system function. Medications can help alleviate some of the symptoms.

Trunk movement

The trunk serves to both stabilize the upper body during the leg propulsion phase (the latter part of the stance phase) and also to position the pelvis in a better position to maintain balance while executing arm and leg movements.

Chapter **8**

The Nuts and Bolts of Movement

The world is continually moving. Every day you can look around and notice people doing things like walking, running, cycling, and swimming. You probably haven't given much thought to what it takes to do these activities. Few people actually examine how they or others walk, run, cycle, or swim, let alone how they can do any of these activities better — unless they've been forced to through an injury that immobilized them or they're in a field where performing at peak ability is vital.

Movement and the factors that affect motion are quite complex and require an understanding of several principles related to physics. For example, everything that you encounter is being acted on by forces. Regardless of how something may be moving (or not) — whether it's spinning, flying through the air, or sitting perfectly still — invisible forces are affecting it. This chapter provides insights into what is behind getting stronger, throwing a ball, and running faster, among other things. You'll never again think the same about how you move!

Biomechanics: The Study of Movement

You no doubt heard about Newton's laws, forces, and vectors in high school science or physics courses. When you learned about these principles, chances are, you did so in relation to nonhuman examples. Well, the field of biomechanics takes those principles and applies them to human movement.

Biomechanics is the investigation of how forces act on the human body from a mechanical perspective. The *mechanics* part of the term represents the study of physical actions, and the *bio* part refers to living organisms (in this case, humans). Examining the effects of forces, their impacts on the human body, and how the human body creates motion either internally or externally is a fascinating and very dynamic area of investigation.

By studying biomechanics, you can answer questions like, "Why do some baseball pitchers hurt their elbows?" "How can I make myself run faster (or jump higher)?" "Why don't I fall off my bike when I lean really far over as I go around a corner?" and "How come Olympic gymnasts can do such amazing acrobatic things and look so graceful?"

The role of the biomechanist

We all appreciate the grace and power that Olympians and professional athletes exhibit. But these athletes aren't as good as they are because they were born that way. Sure, genetics has something to do with their abilities, but they've also studied their skills and investigated how to improve. In a sense, they've been their own biomechanists. You can be one, too.

Shooting a basketball, walking, jumping, and skipping all sound like very simple tasks, but they're all actually quite complex skills. Executing any task involves multiple forces acting within and/or beyond the body all at once. When you break down these tasks, you may wonder how far someone should bend their elbow or knees, how big their steps should be, and which foot should go first.

REMEMBER

By understanding the types of forces and motion in relation to the structure and function of the human body, you can look for ways to stay healthy and enhance performance.

The biomechanist's problem-solving process

To assess any type of activity or task, biomechanists follow a process. Typically, this process starts with understanding the nature of the task, followed by a deliberate observation of that task in action. From this observation, data is collected and used to evaluate the performance, which ultimately leads to feedback and, if necessary, an intervention. The next sections take you through this process.

Understanding the nature and objective of the task

The first requirement in assessing a movement is to understand the task being completed. You must have this prerequisite information to fully address what's occurring as part of the movement. For example, if you want to jump, you know that you first need to bend at your knees, which causes your ankles and hips to also bend and puts you in a sort of squatting position. From this position, you then push up as hard as you can, a movement that makes your body rise and, if you have enough force behind the push, lifts you off the ground.

When you know how the joints move during the activity, you can start asking more complex questions like, "How do I jump higher?" This type of question requires not only an understanding of joint motions but also knowledge about which muscles are involved and how they're activated.

In addition to having an understanding of the task being performed, the biomechanist must understand the intent of the activity. For example, analyzing a pitcher's throwing motion can only be done with an appreciation of what the pitcher is trying to accomplish.

Observing the task and collecting data

Biomechanists must be able to collect the necessary information. Necessary data is any data that provides substantive and defendable information that is key to answering questions such as: "How can someone run faster?" "How can someone throw harder?" or "Why does their shin hurt?"

In this case, the data is anything that is observed during the motion or any measurements taken or collected during the activity. For instance, as you observe a task, you may notice that the motions necessary to improve the activity may not be in sequence. Other data like timing of the movement, amount of force exerted, or torque at a joint during the motion are also examples of data. In the end, all the data collected — both observed or captured through a measurement device — constitute "the data."

Suppose a pitcher comes into the athletic training room because of a sore elbow. The athletic trainer must collect the data necessary to answer why the pitcher's elbow hurts. Key information includes things like how often the pitcher throws, what type of pitches they throw, how they pitch and whether they were throwing long toss or off the pitching mound. The answers to these kinds of questions help the athletic trainer fully understand the situation being assessed.

Evaluating the data and making a diagnosis

After observing the task and collecting data, biomechanists use the data to make comparisons of the current situation to others like it. Everyone walks or runs differently, but certain things have consistently been proven to affect the success of the task. In this step, biomechanists compare the specific data they gathered from a subject to what they know should be occurring. Based on this information, they can recognize flaws and identify areas for improvement.

REMEMBER

The assessment is a critical aspect to answering your question. When you perform such an assessment, you must do so objectively, taking the information (data) as it is and using your findings to answer the question.

Sharing the findings with the athlete: Intervention and feedback

Concluding the process, biomechanists share their findings with their athletes. By sharing the information soon after the activity and in a way that identifies the key components, they can then develop a plan to improve performance and, in many cases, explain or avoid injury.

Kinematics: A Compass Telling You Where You Are

To assess and evaluate motion, you must understand the underlying components of human structure and the various physical and environmental components that affect everyone. *Kinematics* is the study of movement; it includes considerations of form, velocity, direction, time, acceleration, pattern, displacement, and sequencing.

TECHNICAL STUFF

Many people refer to this area of biomechanics as the descriptive or qualitative portion of motion analysis. Kinematic references are made in relation to things like direction and how fast someone may be going, or what movement is happening first and what follows. In kinematics, you don't consider the forces within the movement, which makes kinematics different from kinetics, a topic we introduce in "Studying Kinetics: May the Force Be with You!" later in this chapter.

Looking at body systems

Activities of daily living, like brushing your teeth, rising from a chair, or pouring a glass of water, are necessary to normal, everyday living. Although they're often taken for granted, especially by healthy, active people, each task is actually very complex. In fact, any movement you make, even the "ordinary" ones, requires coordination and communication between the body's muscular, skeletal, and nervous systems:

>> **The muscular system:** This system involves the soft tissue structures that are *contractile* in nature; that is, they have the ability to create tension by contracting. Muscles are connected to bones by tendons. When a muscle is contracted (see Chapter 3), it contributes to or produces an end result: Often muscle contraction results in joint movement. Other times, muscle contraction results in no motion but helps to support the body and increases stability.

>> **The skeletal system:** The skeletal system provides the framework that supports the human body. Your bones are the structural blocks that allow you to stand, sit, and walk. Your muscles attach to these bones, and when they contract, the bones are pulled by the tendons, resulting in movement of the joint.

>> **The nervous system:** The nervous system, often overlooked and largely taken for granted, involves the brain and subsequent nerve function throughout the body. Absolutely everything that you do is controlled by your nervous system. Your brain initiates movement by deciding the strategy that is needed for the particular motion, and the peripheral nervous system acts as the highway to transmit the signals among your brain, spinal cord, and the rest of your body. The brain helps determine motor patterns (for information on motor control, head to Chapter 7), and this system interprets pain, activates muscles, and controls motion.

Each of these systems has very important individual functions, but it's their coordinated work that enables you to move about every day as you do. Consider something as simple as walking. The motor patterns that dictate walking are defined in the brain from past activities and are sent to the local areas (knees, ankles, and hips), where the movement is carried out.

Here's what happens: As soon as you decide that you want to walk, your brain interprets your body position, where you are (walking up a hill, climbing stairs, and so on), and decides how best to move. Each of your muscles is activated to propel your body. While the motor pattern is being sent to the muscles that are active, other muscles are preparing for their role. At the same time, you may be pushing (propelling) yourself forward from your toes, for example, your other foot is preparing for your heel to strike the ground and your same-side hamstring group is readying to slow your leg down. All the while, your skeletal system serves as the source of support and conduit for movement.

ASSESSMENT IN ACTION: HOW DO I RUN FASTER?

Figuring out how to run faster isn't as easy as you may think. Using the process outlined in the section "The biomechanist's problem-solving process," you would approach this problem like this:

1. **Understand the nature and objective of the activity and amass the necessary prerequisite information.**

   To more deeply understand the act of running, you need to ask yourself what actually occurs during this activity. Clearly, you have to move your ankles, knees, and hips. But what other components are involved? Breaking down the running (gait) pattern can help. What about the type of running? Is the person a distance runner or a sprinter?

2. **Observe the task and collect data.**

   Typically, the gait cycle is broken down into two phases: stance and swing (refer to Chapter 7). The stance phase begins with your foot striking the ground and continues as your body weight is transferred forward. It ends when you push off at your toes to propel yourself. While one foot is in the stance phase, the other is in the air; that's the swing phase.

   The gait cycle specific to running varies from that of walking in that the heel strike doesn't exist. Instead, striking occurs at the forefoot (by the toes). Additionally, the weight transition phase is either nonexistent or occurs in a very small window of time. The interesting aspect of running is that, at times, the body is totally airborne, and no contact with the ground occurs — a situation that doesn't happen when walking.

   Understanding the motions that make up the gait cycle is important, but how those motions are achieved is equally valuable information that can help you answer the question, "How do I run faster?" Muscle actions during the gait cycle dictate the amount of push-off during propulsion at the ankle and knee. Additionally, the muscles bring a limb from the swing to the stance phase, prepare for landing, and help maintain balance throughout.

   By understanding the motion and the muscle forces that are needed to complete this task, you can begin to address the question. You now know that running speed is dependent on the length of each of your strides, the force exerted during the push-off coupled with the resistance (body weight), and how quickly you can bring your leg back after you push off.

3. Evaluate the data.

Noticing that someone may be taking strides that are entirely too long or are really bouncy gives you information that you can use to identify flaws. By comparing the current task to what you know about how the task *should* be carried out, you can identify areas for improvement. You may even notice that their shin pain seems to come from the extreme pronation that they have during the motion.

4. Provide intervention and feedback.

Given the information that you gathered and the results of the evaluation and diagnosis, you can now provide feedback and suggest an intervention program. This feedback and intervention may be as simple as telling the person to shorten their stride when running or not to bounce so high when they go from step to step, or you may determine that they need orthotic support to stop their excessive motion.

Identifying forms of motion

When analyzing motion, biomechanists often divide movement into three subcategories: linear motion (both rectilinear and curvilinear), angular motion, and general motion. Figure 8-1 shows the different types of motion.

Linear motion

In *linear motion*, all parts of an object move in the same direction at the same velocity (speed and direction). Often, this type of motion is referred to as *translation*. Linear motion can occur in two ways:

>> **Rectilinear motion** occurs when the object in its entirety is moving in a straight line. A passenger sitting still on a train that's going straight is a good example of moving in a rectilinear fashion.

>> **Curvilinear motion** results in a uniformly curved pattern of movement. Curvilinear motion exists when a stunt driver, for example, takes their car and jumps over a flaming bonfire. Because of the momentum generated while going up the ramp, the car goes up and over the fire and lands on the other side. As long as the car doesn't spin as it goes over the fire, the motion is curvilinear.

Angular motion

Moving objects don't all travel in a uniform direction. Instead, they often involve angular motion as well. Angular motion is the movement of an object around an axis of rotation or an imaginary line.

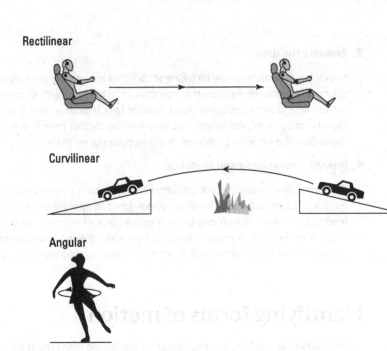

Rectilinear

Curvilinear

Angular

General

FIGURE 8-1:
Types of motion:
rectilinear,
curvilinear,
angular,
and general.

© John Wiley & Sons, Inc.

REMEMBER

Nearly every motion that occurs within the body is an example of angular motion. When muscles pull on the bones, they cause the bones or limb segments to bend or rotate at their joints. A figure skater performing a spin is an example of angular motion. The skater's entire body is spinning in relation to the axis of rotation while they balance on the ice.

General motion

General motion exists when linear and angular motions are combined. A ball thrown by a pitcher is an example of both angular and curvilinear motion: The spin of the ball is angular motion, while its trajectory as it approaches the batter is curvilinear (an arc).

REMEMBER

Human motion is almost always general motion. As you walk down the street, your joints experience angular motion (because they're swinging in an arc) while your body as a whole is moving in a straight line (*translating*) down the street in rectilinear fashion.

Defining key terms

To understand and break down the movements that exist in the world, biomechanists must have command of the vocabulary. When referring to areas of the body or movements, you do so in reference to their positioning, called *anatomical position*. Anatomical position is an upright standing position that has the feet separated shoulder-width apart, the arms hanging at the sides, and the palms facing forward (see Figure 8-2).

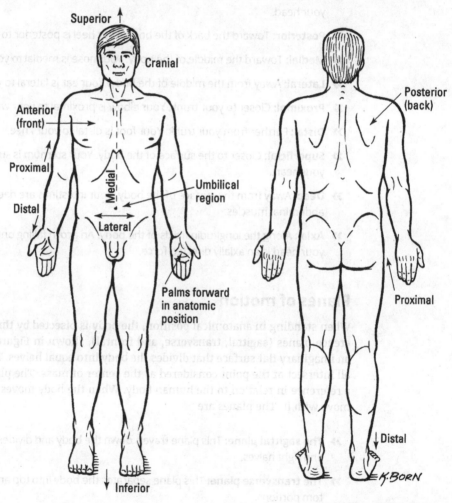

Illustration by Kathryn Born, MA

FIGURE 8-2:
Anatomical
position.

Using directional terminology

To describe how the body moves and the relationship of an object to the body, you must be able to use the following terminology:

>> **Superior:** Closer to the head, or "above." Your shoulder is superior to your hip.

>> **Inferior:** Closer to the feet, or "below." Your knee is inferior to your hip.

>> **Anterior:** Toward the front of the body. Your nose is anterior to the back of your head.

>> **Posterior:** Toward the back of the body. Your heel is posterior to your big toe.

>> **Medial:** Toward the middle of the body. Your nose is medial to your ear.

>> **Lateral:** Away from the middle of the body. Your ear is lateral to your mouth.

>> **Proximal:** Closer to your trunk. Your elbow is proximal to your wrist.

>> **Distal:** Further from your trunk. Your foot is distal to your knee.

>> **Superficial:** Closer to the surface of the body. Your sternum is superficial to your heart.

>> **Deep:** Away from the surface of the body. Your intestines are deep to your abdominal muscles.

>> **Axial:** Along the longitudinal axis of the body. An acorn falling onto the top of your head is an axially directed force.

Planes of motion

When standing in anatomical position, the body is bisected by three cardinal reference planes (sagittal, transverse, and frontal), shown in Figure 8-3. A *plane* is an imaginary flat surface that divides the body into equal halves. The three planes all intersect at the point considered as the center of mass. The planes are used as a reference in relation to the human body. When the body moves, the planes also move with it. The planes are

>> **The sagittal plane:** This plane travels down the body and divides it into left and right halves.

>> **The transverse plane:** This plane separates the body into top and bottom portions.

>> **The frontal plane:** This plane travels down and separates the body into front and back portions.

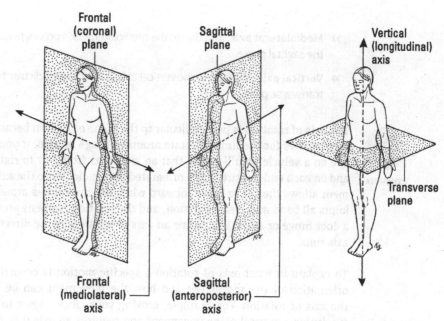

FIGURE 8-3: Cardinal planes of motion and axes of rotation.

Frontal (coronal) plane

Sagittal plane

Vertical (longitudinal) axis

Transverse plane

Frontal (mediolateral) axis

Sagittal (anteroposterior) axis

Illustration by Kathryn Born, MA

References to body motion are often based on the plane within which the motion occurs. Motion that moves in-line with a particular plane or parallel to it is typically referred to as motion occurring in that plane.

TIP

To determine in which plane the motion occurs, imagine that the motion was completed standing next to mirrors representing the planes of motion. The mirror(s) *not* broken after the movement would be considered the plane that the motion occurred in.

Jumping jacks, for example, are a frontal plane movement. During a jumping jack, your arms and legs move outward to the side from the middle of your body (*abducted* — we get to that term in a minute). If you were to do a jumping jack in front of mirrors representing the planes of motion, you would break the sagittal and transverse plane mirrors as your arms and legs moved out to the side, but your frontal plane would be untouched.

Axes of rotation

When you move your limbs (arms and legs), you do so around an imaginary axis of rotation that passes through the joint. Three axes of rotation are used in describing motion; each of the axes is orientated perpendicular to one of the three planes of motion (refer to Figure 7-3):

>> **Anteroposterior axis:** Rotation in the anteroposterior axis is perpendicular to the frontal plane.

>> **Mediolateral axis:** Rotation in the mediolateral axis occurs perpendicular to the sagittal plane.

>> **Vertical axis:** Rotation in the vertical axis occurs perpendicular to the transverse plane.

REMEMBER

The axis of rotation is perpendicular to the plane of motion because this arrangement allows for the limb to rotate around a hinge or axle. If you take a look at a tire on a vehicle, you'll notice that an axle runs from left to right under the car, and on each end is a tire that's orientated perpendicular to the axle. This arrangement allows the car to move forward when the tire rotates around the axle. Your joints all bend and create rotation, and the rotation happens around an axis (like a door hinge or axle). You define an axis of rotation by the direction in which the axis runs.

To explain in what axis of rotation a specific motion is occurring, consider the orientation of the movement and how the movement can be generated about the axis of rotation. For example, moving your elbow closer to your upper arm (*flexion*) is a sagittal plane movement and requires an axis that runs from side to side through the elbow. That axis would be the mediolateral axis.

Joint motions

Believe it or not, each movement that you make can be defined very precisely. If someone were to ask you to bend your elbow, you'd have no trouble understanding what that means, but if you think about the term *bend*, you realize it's actually pretty imprecise — too imprecise, in fact, to be used as a descriptor when you're analyzing motion. This particular motion is actually called *flexion*, a term that has a very specific meaning in motion analysis.

REMEMBER

Joint motion definitions allow you to specify what's actually happening within human movement. The term *flexion*, for example, means more than just "to bend." It also describes that the bones that make up the joint are moving closer to one another. Without the terminology to define aspects of motion to this level of specificity, biomechanists would not be able to explain types of motion in a way that guarantees understanding.

Biomechanists consider many motions, based on which cardinal plane the motion is executed in. The following sections list the most common movements.

MOVEMENTS IN THE SAGITTAL PLANE

Movements that occur in the sagittal plane are typically described as joints moving closer together in an anterior or posterior direction. Here are the most common sagittal plane motions, which you can see in Figure 8-4:

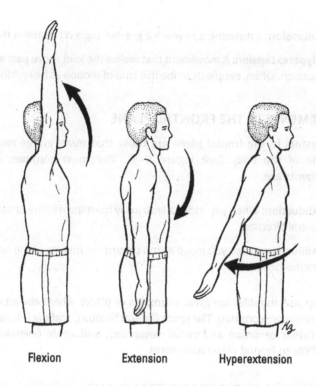

Flexion Extension Hyperextension

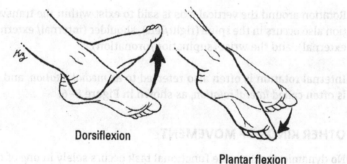

FIGURE 8-4:
Sagittal plane
movements.

Dorsiflexion

Plantar flexion

Illustration by Kathryn Born, MA

REMEMBER

>> **Flexion:** A movement within the mediolateral axes of rotation that brings the joint together or lessens the joint angle.

The term *flexion* also describes two separate motions at the ankle. *Dorsiflexion* is the act of raising your toes toward the sky, and *plantar flexion* is the act of pointing out your toes. These toe motions go directly against all the rules of describing motion, so you just need to memorize them separately.

>> **Extension:** A movement in which a greater angle is created at the joint.

>> **Hyperextension:** A movement that makes the joint move past its anatomical position. Often, people describe this kind of motion as being "double-jointed."

MOVEMENTS IN THE FRONTAL PLANE

Movements in the frontal plane are those that move either away or toward the midline of the body (see Figure 8-5). The most common of frontal plane movements are

>> **Abduction:** When you move a limb away from the midline of the body, or in a lateral direction

>> **Adduction:** When you move a limb toward the midline of the body, or in a medial direction

The hip and shoulder are great examples of places where abduction and adduction movements are common. The spine (lateral flexion), scapula (elevation/depression), wrist (ulnar deviation and radial deviation), and ankle (eversion/inversion) also contribute to frontal plane movement.

MOVEMENTS IN THE TRANSVERSE PLANE

Rotation around the vertical axis is said to exist within the transverse plane. Rotation also occurs in the spine (right/left), shoulder (internal/ external), hip (internal/ external), and the wrist (supination/pronation).

Internal rotation is often also referred to as *medial rotation,* and external rotation is often called *lateral rotation,* as shown in Figure 8-6.

OTHER KINDS OF MOVEMENT

No dynamic or otherwise functional task occurs solely in one of the three cardinal planes. Instead, a great deal of motion is diagonal. *Diagonal motion* happens when a movement occurs in more than one plane. For example, throwing a baseball is a movement that crosses the body in a diagonal fashion.

Circumduction is one of those "other" movements that don't fit within one particular plane but exists across each of them. Circumduction occurs when the limb is directed in an imaginary circle, not as in spinning around (like a top) but as in the whole segment tracing a circular pattern with the distal aspect. Imagine pinwheeling your arms. That's circumduction.

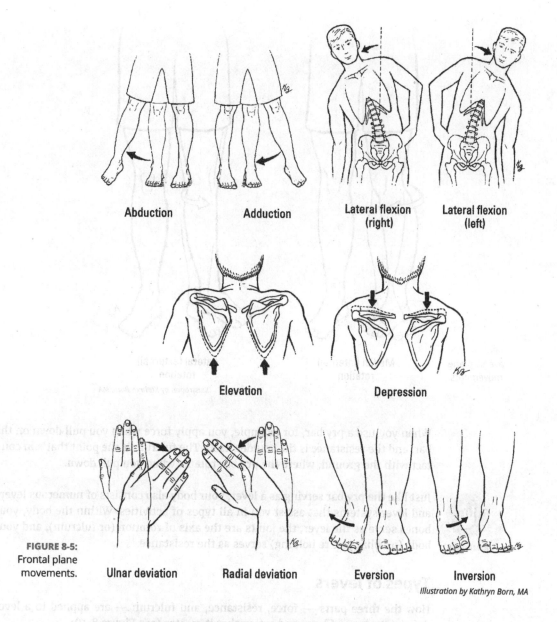

Abduction Adduction Lateral flexion (right) Lateral flexion (left)

Elevation Depression

FIGURE 8-5:
Frontal plane
movements.

Ulnar deviation Radial deviation Eversion Inversion

Illustration by Kathryn Born, MA

Working with Newton's toolkit: Lever systems

REMEMBER

Lever systems are everywhere — in the world and in your body. A lever system is a rigid segment that rotates about an axis. In this context, the axis of rotation is referred to as a *fulcrum*. A lever system relies on both a force being applied (called *effort*) and an opposing force (*resistance*) that you intend to move.

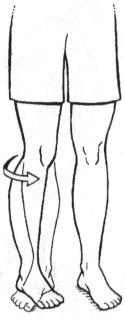
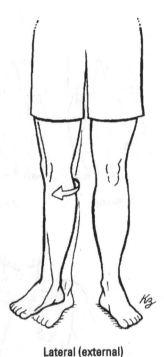

FIGURE 8-6:
Traverse plane
movements.

Medial (internal)
rotation

Lateral (external)
rotation

Illustration by Kathryn Born, MA

When you use a pry bar, for example, you apply force when you pull down on the bar, and the resistance is the boulder itself. The fulcrum is the point that's in contact with the ground, where the pry bar rotates when you pull down.

REMEMBER

Just like the pry bar serving as a lever, your body also consists of numerous levers and lever systems that assist you in all types of activities. Within the body, your bones serve as the lever, the joints are the axis of rotation (or fulcrum), and your body (or what you're holding) serves as the resistance.

Types of levers

How the three parts — force, resistance, and fulcrum — are applied to a lever defines the type of lever and action that it creates (see Figure 8-7):

>> **First-class lever:** In a first-class lever, the fulcrum is placed between the force and the resistance. A common example is the teeter-totter.

REMEMBER

An example of a first-class lever in your body is your head sitting on top of your spine. The spine serves as the fulcrum, the posterior neck muscles are the force, and the front of the head serves as the resistance.

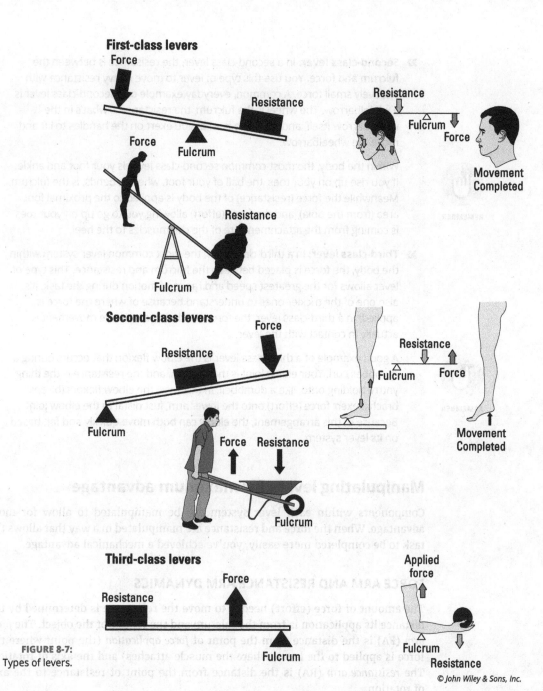

First-class levers

Force

Resistance

Force

Fulcrum

Resistance

Fulcrum

Force

Movement
Completed

Fulcrum

Resistance

Second-class levers

Force

Resistance

Fulcrum

Resistance

Fulcrum

Force

Fulcrum

Force Resistance

Movement
Completed

Fulcrum

Third-class levers

Applied
force

Force

Resistance

Fulcrum

Fulcrum

Resistance

FIGURE 8-7:
Types of levers.

© *John Wiley & Sons, Inc.*

>> **Second-class lever:** In a second-class lever, the resistance is between the fulcrum and force. You use this type of lever to move heavy resistance with relatively small force. A common, everyday example of a second-class lever is a wheelbarrow. The wheel is the fulcrum, the resistance is what's in the wheelbarrow itself, and the force is what you exert on the handles to lift and move the wheelbarrow.

Within the body, the most common second-class lever is your foot and ankle. If you rise up on your toes, the ball of your foot, where it bends, is the fulcrum. Meanwhile the force (resistance) of the body is applied to the proximal foot area (from the tibia), and the force (effort) allowing you to go up on your toes is coming from the attachment site of the calf muscles to the heel.

>> **Third-class lever:** In a third-class lever, the most common lever system within the body, the force is placed between the fulcrum and resistance. This type of lever allows for the greatest speed and range of motion during the task. It's also one of the trickier ones to understand because of where the force is applied. In a third-class lever, the force needed to create the movement is actually in contact with the lever.

A good example of a third-class lever is the elbow flexion that occurs during a dumbbell curl. Your elbow joint is the fulcrum, and the resistance is the thing you're holding onto, like a dumbbell. In this case, the elbow flexors (biceps brachii) exert force (effort) onto the lower arm, just distal to the elbow joint. Because of this arrangement, the elbow can both move quickly and far, based on its lever system.

Manipulating levers for maximum advantage

Components within each lever system can be manipulated to allow for more advantage. When the force and resistance are manipulated in a way that allows the task to be completed more easily, you've achieved a mechanical advantage.

FORCE ARM AND RESISTANCE ARM DYNAMICS

The amount of force (effort) needed to move the resistance is determined by the distance its application is from the fulcrum and the weight of the object. The *force arm* (FA) is the distance from the point of *force application* (the point where the force is applied to the lever, where the muscle attaches) and the axis of rotation. The *resistance arm* (RA) is the distance from the point of resistance to the axis of rotation.

The force needed to move an object is inversely proportional to the length of the FA. The longer the FA, the less force needed to move the object. The longer the RA, the more force is needed to move it.

Your body must be quite strong to do many of the daily tasks that you need it to, yet the human body contains many third-class levers where the RA is longer than the FA. This clearly puts you at an instant mechanical disadvantage. For example, the FA at the elbow is dictated by the biceps brachii muscles' attachment to the radius, which is only 2 inches or so away from the elbow joint (fulcrum). Because the insertion is so close to the fulcrum, the elbow's function relies on a great deal of strength. Short of surgically lengthening the FA in your joints, you can't do much about it besides strengthening yourself.

REMEMBER

Most sporting-related tasks involve several different types of levers acting at the same time to complete the task. For example, when you jump, the levers at the toe, ankle, knee, and hip joints each must work to accomplish their own unique goals while simultaneously *not* working against the other joints.

VELOCITY

Velocity refers to the speed and direction of a body or object. The longer the force arm, the more effective it is in imparting velocity. A higher velocity results in a higher force being imparted on the object at contact. For example, a baseball player can hit the ball a greater distance when they use a longer bat instead of a shorter one. But there's a trade-off: Although the longer lever imparts a higher velocity, it also increases the time needed to complete the task. (For more on velocity, head to the later section "Velocity and acceleration.")

When a thrower needs to make a faster throw to get a runner out, the thrower shortens their lever arm length (by bending their elbow) and snaps the ball out quickly. By shortening the lever, the player is able to complete the throw in a shorter time.

Although shortening the force arm helps you perform a task more quickly, it isn't the right strategy to use when you need to produce more force, like making a long throw from the outfield to home plate.

Balance, equilibrium, and stability

To affect movement, levers are dependent on the force and resistance applied to the fulcrum. Yet the goal isn't always to move an object. Sometimes, the goal is to allow an object to remain in its current state. Keeping objects in their current state requires balance, equilibrium, and stability:

>> **Equilibrium:** The state of zero acceleration, where no change occurs in the speed or direction of the body

>> **Balance:** The ability to control equilibrium, either *statically* (while still) or *dynamically* (while moving)

>> **Stability:** The resistance to a change in the body's acceleration

ARE YOU REALLY DOUBLE-JOINTED?

You've probably seen someone who can contort their body into what seem to be super-human ways; maybe you can even do this yourself. People, like the circus performer who folds themselves into a box or the classmate who bends their fingers or arms in ways that stun or disgust you, are said to be "double-jointed." In fact, no one is double-jointed.

So, how do people put themselves in these awkward positions and look so out of joint? The ability to move in such ways is usually dictated by flexibility. *Flexibility* refers to how inherently extensible the soft tissue of the body is. Your joints are held together by ligaments and other soft tissues. These tissues can vary in the amount of support they provide. The person who claims to be double-jointed is simply very flexible and probably has very lax joints.

TIP

To understand the relationship between these three factors, think about a boat being rocked back and forth by the strong ocean winds and waves. Despite being rocked back and forth, the boat must retain its balance (its original upright position). The shape of the hull and the sail allow the boat to sway side to side but maintain stability to avoid tipping over; the weight of the boat itself also provides stability by resisting the effect of the waves.

These three concepts are very important to maintaining good joint health. Your ligaments, in particular, keep the joint functioning in the direction that it is meant to. For instance, the medial collateral ligament, which runs on the inside of the knee, keeps the knee from bending inward. If stability is compromised in this ligament, the knee becomes dysfunctional and will lead to injury.

Feeling displaced and distant

In kinematics, you need to be familiar with the concepts of displacement and distance. *Distance* is the total length traveled by an object from point A to point B. *Displacement* is the length from point A to point B. Examining distance and displacement is key when you want to evaluate a task or motion for efficiency.

TIP

To understand the difference between distance and displacement, think about what happens when a punt returner catches the football: They run forward, changing direction a number of times to avoid tacklers. From beginning (catching the ball) to end (getting tackled), they may run a total of 30 yards because of all the ducking and weaving, but they may move only 10 yards forward. The 30 yards they traveled is their distance, and the 10 yards moving forward is their displacement.

Measuring kinematics

Kinematic analysis examines the *qualitative* (descriptive) and *quantitative* (numerical value) aspects of the movement. But unlike kinetics (see the next section), kinematics doesn't consider the effects of forces on the movement. Doing this type of analysis lets you evaluate limb movements, see how fast they may be moving, identify in what sequence they occur, and so on.

To gather this information, biomechanists use a high-speed video camera or digital movement capture system, which allows them to capture more frames per second than the standard video camera. The high-speed capturing systems can provide more information and allow for clearer assessments to be made.

TIP

Anyone can pull out a camera these days and record someone running, batting, or otherwise completing an activity. From the video, you're able to assess the range of motion of the joints, the sequencing of the activity, and things like limb and body orientation. True, you won't have the details that are available to professional biomechanists, but you can still get a good idea of what's going on.

Tasks like walking require specific amounts of motion to avoid injury and maximize performance. Another form of kinematic analysis happens in the rehabilitation clinic and after surgery in your doctor's office when they measure your joint range of motion. They compare this range with the normal values known for each joint.

Studying Kinetics: May the Force Be with You!

Kinetics is the study of the impact that different kinds of forces have on mechanical systems — in this context, your body. Beyond seeing the ball spinning, kinetics offers insight into how and why the ball is spinning.

The secrets of movement

Behind every great movement are the principles and components that affect it. Concepts like inertia, mass, force, center of gravity, weight, torque, impulse, velocity, and acceleration are the backbone of movement.

Inertia

Inertia is the concept that states that objects tend to want to stay in their current state of motion, whether they're still or moving, until another force acts on them.

A bowling ball sitting still on the floor, for example, will stay that way until another force (a push by a bowler) acts on it. The same holds true for a football flying through the air. It will remain in motion unless other forces, like gravity, air friction, or a wide receiver, make it stop.

Inertia is an object's resistance to change. The amount of inertia an object possesses is directly proportional to its mass. The heavier an object is, the more force required to change it from its current state.

Mass

Mass is the amount of matter contained in the object. Not all objects of the same size have the same amount of mass or the same weight. A ping-pong ball, for example, is about the same size as a golf ball, and the golf ball weighs more. So, in this context, the golf ball has more mass, making it heavier.

Force

The heavier an object is, the more force is required to move it. *Force* is the push or pull that acts on a body or object; the formula for force says that its product equals that of its mass and its acceleration:

force = mass × acceleration

Things like gravity, wind, and water are all forces that can act on you or other objects. Pushing and pulling forces are constantly applied to your body. During any movement, the joints and muscles are working to generate the right amount of force to maintain balance while walking, running, and standing. It's a complex game of push and pull — the greater the mass of an object, the more acceleration and force are required to move or overcome that force to keep your balance.

Center of gravity

The *center of gravity* is the area within an object or body that is positioned at the middle of the object's mass. The center of gravity exists regardless of an object's position and is the point by which you measure motion and the effects of any applied external forces. When biomechanists investigate motion in a gymnast, for example, they concentrate on the gymnast's center of gravity, not on their arms and legs.

Weight

How much an object weighs is determined by the amount of gravitational force being applied to it. (This is why you weigh less on the moon, which has less gravitational pull, than on Earth, which has more.) *Weight* is considered a body's relative mass or the quantity of matter contained by it.

Weight is often confused with mass. The key difference is that weight is a force, and mass is simply the amount of matter within an object. Weight is always oriented toward the center of the earth because it's directly related to gravity.

Torque

Levers are rigid systems that turn about an axis. To turn, levers rely on torque. *Torque*, the turning effect of force, is dependent on the application of an *eccentric force*, a force that is applied to an object but is not oriented with the center of rotation of the axis (see Figure 8-8). The more torque applied to the axis of rotation, the greater the turning effect of the force.

Impulse

Forces can be applied to objects in varying amounts of time. The *impulse* is the amount of force applied during a unit of time. A large force may have a relatively insignificant effect on an object if it's delivered only for a split second. Conversely, a fairly small force may have a great effect on an object if it's delivered continuously over time.

Suppose, for example, that you made the mistake of kicking a medicine ball (a large, heavy, solid ball) really hard. You probably experienced a great deal of pain in your knee because the ball didn't move. If you had used a lesser force and applied it over time, you would've discovered that moving the ball across the weight room and out of your way was relatively easy — and pain free.

Force directed downward leads to resultant rotation.

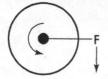

Upward directed force of the biceps on the arm results in joint rotation.

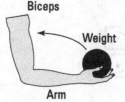

FIGURE 8-8: Torque is dependent on an eccentric force.

© *John Wiley & Sons, Inc.*

Velocity and acceleration

Forces are often *translated* (transferred) to objects. To fully understand the effects of force application, you need to explore the delivery of the force, its speed, and the direction in which the force is applied.

Velocity is the quantity that represents the speed and direction of a body or object. A concept directly related to velocity is that of *acceleration* (the rate at which an object changes velocity).

Every movement has a speed component; many are slow, and some are very, very fast. This speed in relation to movement's direction and how it may change can have significant influence on the resulting force and its effects on an object.

What a load!

Different types of forces can be delivered to the body. The effects of the forces on the body are referred to as *mechanical loads*. By understanding the types of forces and their effects on the body and its structures, you can understand regular function. Figure 8-9 shows a variety of mechanical loads.

TECHNICAL STUFF

>> **Compression:** An *axial force* (a force directed along the longitudinal axis of the object) that results in squeezing or pressing.

Did you know that in the morning you're typically taller than you are at the end of the day? You can thank compression for that. During the day, you're upright, and gravity and your body weight compress you all day long. You actually shrink over the course of a day!

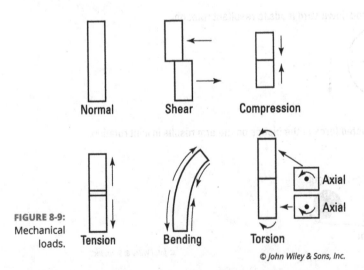

FIGURE 8-9: Mechanical loads.

© *John Wiley & Sons, Inc.*

REMEMBER

>> **Tension:** The pulling of a force on an object. The muscles often apply tension as they pull on bones to make them move. In fact, the many bumps *(tuberosities)* on your bones are a result of muscles pulling on the bone.

>> **Shear:** A force directed perpendicular to the longitudinal axis of an object. The result of a shear force allows one portion of the object to displace in relation to other portions of the object. Shear forces often result in bone fractures. If, for example, a force is delivered to the shin when your foot is fixed to the ground, one portion of the shin may be displaced in relation to the other.

>> **Bending:** The combination of tension and compression. When a non-axial force is applied to an object, bending occurs. In other words, when one side of an object experiences compression while the other side undergoes tension, it bends.

>> **Torsion:** When one end of an object is fixed and it experiences twisting at its longitudinal axis. Injuries that involve torsion are pretty common in sports, especially when the playing surface has a lot of traction.

>> **Combined loads:** When more than one type of load is delivered to an object. The human body experiences a number of different types of loads (force application) simultaneously during many activities. Combined loading is the most common in the body.

Newton's laws of motion

Throughout this chapter, we explain forces and the effects they have on objects, including the human body. In a nutshell, inanimate objects move because forces are applied to them; the body moves in the same manner. Although human bodies don't commonly roll around or fly through the air like balls do, they do move because forces — both internal and external — are applied:

>> **Internal forces are the forces generated within the body.** For example, when muscles contract, they administer a pulling force to the bones that results in movement.

>> **External forces are forces originating from outside the body.** For example, when you fall, you do so because you've lost your balance, and gravity pushes you down.

Force application and the subsequent movement or lack thereof is dependent on Newton's three laws of motion, which govern the principles of all types of motion.

Newton's first law: The law of inertia

The first law of motion states that an object at rest or in uniform motion (no acceleration) will remain at rest until acted on by an outside force. Because this law represents an object's resistance to changes in its current state (motion or still), this law is commonly referred to as the law of inertia.

TIP

Think about moving a heavy object across the garage floor. You probably notice that getting the object moving takes a lot more force than keeping it moving. The higher force needed to first move the object is an example of inertia and the object's resistance to the movement.

Newton's second law: The law of acceleration

The second law of motion states that the acceleration of an object is directly proportional to the force acting on it but inversely proportional to the mass of the body. What this means is that moving a lighter object is easier than moving a heavier one. If you've ever had to move to a new home, you can easily appreciate this law.

Newton's third law: The law of action and reaction

Newton's third law states that for every action there is an equal and opposite reaction. Translation? Whenever an object exerts a force (action) onto another object, the contacted object exerts a reaction force that is in the opposite direction and of the same magnitude.

Think about an arm wrestling contest. If both competitors are of the same strength and, therefore, exert the same amount of force, the net movement is zero. However, as the force exerted by one of the competitors lessens (because this competitor fatigues and weakens), the force exerted by the opponent increases, and they win.

TIP

Sometimes, the reaction isn't as obvious because we tend not to think of inanimate objects "exerting" anything, so thinking about what happens when you walk or jump may help you grasp the concept. During either of these tasks, you push down against the ground to propel yourself forward. When you push down, the ground "pushes" back against you with the same force, which enables you to move forward or jump up into the air.

Measuring kinetics

Just as the types and actions of forces are varied, so are the ways to measure them. Depending on the question, biomechanists determine the type of variable (the specific force) they need to measure and how to go about doing it. The methodology or process a scientist follows often determines whether the information collected will actually answer the question being asked. Part of that methodology is choosing how to measure the particular force or its effects.

Many biomechanists, for example, examine muscle activity when they want to know what exercise leads to the most amount of muscle firing. Or, they may be interested in the pattern of a person's walk (their gait), in which case, they use a force plate platform for high-speed video or motion analysis equipment.

Most of the ways to measure things within the realm of kinetics are very expensive and require very sophisticated equipment, not to mention someone who is highly trained in using the equipment.

AIN'T IT A KICK IN THE HEAD? CONCUSSIONS

You can't go anywhere today without hearing about concussions. The National Football League (NFL) has instituted many new rule changes both in the game and in how medical professionals treat patients with concussions. Additionally, many states have introduced legislation that dictates how and by whom patients can be released back into participation after sustaining a concussion.

Researchers are dedicated to investigating concussions and understanding how this injury should best be identified and treated. A recent trend in this research is investigating the actual magnitude of the blow delivered to the heads of football players. Participants in these studies are given helmets outfitted with force transducers or accelerometers that are capable of measuring the acceleration of the head and its direction. By collecting this data, researchers can examine the forces and subsequent injuries these athletes may sustain.

Some companies are now marketing this type of technology to be widely available and utilized in a number of different ways. For instance, one ad shows such a helmet being used by a young boy skiing downhill. When the boy sustains a large enough force to his helmet, a message is sent to his parents' smartphones, alerting them that the boy has been injured and advising them that he should be referred to a physician for follow-up. Using the kinetic information available through such devices can help save lives and decrease the long-lasting effects of concussion injury.

IN THIS CHAPTER

» Identifying types of joints and
   their functions

» Understanding joint stabilization

» Investigating flexibility and
   stretching techniques

Chapter 9

These Joints Are A-Jumping

Without the joints that make up your body, you wouldn't be able to move. Movement is dependent on your muscles' ability to create the forces that propel you, as well as your bones' ability to provide the necessary structural support. But imagine trying to walk up stairs while keeping your knees straight or trying to write without bending your fingers or wrist. Life as you know it depends on your body's ability to bend and twist and glide.

Movement is largely dictated by anatomical makeup, but things like flexibility or habitual movements, which differ from person to person and across occupations, can have significant impacts on how well you move and what your body is capable of.

In this chapter, we investigate the types of joints that are in the body, explain how stability is established, and delve into the influence that flexibility has on the tasks you perform every day.

Getting These Old Bones to Move: Types of Joints

Just as the body has different types of bones, the body also has different types of joints. You can become aware of these differences just by observing how your body moves or what its limitations are. Have you ever wished that you could spin your knee similarly to your neck or tried to extend your back only to realize you've gone too far? Have you ever wondered why some joints move one way and others go another way? These differences are all based on anatomical design and joint architecture. Joint architecture dictates how bones move in relation to one another and the range of motion that's created as a result.

Not all joints allow for the same amount of motion. In fact, some joints don't even move at all, whereas others move freely. Joints can be characterized by how much they move, in which directions, and to what extent. Additionally, they can be classified by structure and function and by the number of axes of rotation that they allow. The following sections have the details.

REMEMBER

A joint is a joint, but in the study of joints, you need to know and be comfortable with their technical name: *arthrosis* (singular) and *arthroses* (plural). Why? Because the terms used to classify joints by the way in which they move are based on this technical term, not the common one: *synarthroses*, *diarthroses*, and so on. Remembering these terms and what they mean will be easier if you latch onto *arthroses* now. To help you out, we use the technical and common terms throughout this section.

Structural classifications: Fibrous, cartilaginous, and synovial

Structural classifications of the arthroses, or joints, include three types:

>> **Fibrous:** In fibrous joints, fibrous tissue or cartilage connects the bones. Fibrous joints are slightly movable. An example of a fibrous joint is the lower arm (the radio-ulnar joint).

>> **Cartilaginous:** As the name implies, cartilaginous joints contain cartilage, either of the hyaline or fibrocartilage variety:

- *Hyaline cartilage,* the most common kind of cartilage, generally covers the articular surfaces of synovial joints (see the next item in this list), where it reduces friction, protects against shock, and allows the joint range of motion to be smooth.

- *Fibrocartilage* is nice and spongy, which makes it a good shock absorber. You'll find it between the vertebrae of the spine, for example.

   Cartilaginous joints move a bit more than fibrous joints. Examples include the *pubis* (a type of bone in the pelvis) and *vertebrae* (the small bones in your spine). For detailed information on cartilage, head to the later section "Enhancing Joint Stability and Longevity: Cartilage and Connective Tissues."

>> **Synovial:** Synovial joints are the most common kind of joint. They have a cartilaginous covering (hyaline cartilage) where the articulating bones meet and a *synovial cavity* (also called a *joint capsule*), which is essentially a space between the bones of the joint, where a collection of soft tissues provide stability and synovial fluid keeps everything nice and lubricated. Synovial joints possess the greatest range of motion. Examples include the elbow, wrist, hip, and shoulder joints.

Functional classifications: Synarthroses, diarthroses, and more

Classifying the joints by function allows you to separate them by how they work.

Immovable joints: Synarthroses

Synarthroses are joints that don't move. Examples of synarthroses include the following:

>> **Sutures:** This kind of joint doesn't allow for any movement. The joints between the bones of the skull are examples of sutures. The irregularly shaped bones of the skull are joined very tightly and don't move.

>> **Syndesmosis:** A *syndesmosis* is a joint that is connected by a significant amount of dense, fibrous tissue. The dense tissue surrounding this joint allows for only very limited motion. You find syndesmosis joints very tightly connecting the radius and ulna (called the *radio-ulnar joint,* in the lower arm) and the tibia and fibula (called the *tibio-fibular joint,* in the ankle).

Slightly movable joints: Amphiarthroses

Amphiarthroses are slightly movable joints connected by fibrocartilage or hyaline cartilage. Examples include the intervertebral disks, which lie between each vertebra and allow slight movement from one segment to the other. These types of joints help to absorb forces (like compression in the spine) and allow for more motion than the synarthroses.

A type of amphiarthrotic joint is the symphysis. The *symphysis* is a joint that is separated by a fibrocartilaginous disk or a very strong ligament that links two bones together. Examples of amphiarthrotic joints are the pubic symphysis of the pelvis, the spine, and the joint that connects the scapula to the clavicle in the shoulder. Each allows for only a little movement while providing support and stability for the bones they're attached to.

Freely movable joints: Diarthroses

Diarthroses, which are joined together by ligaments, are the most common type of joint in the body. They're also called *synovial joints* (refer to the earlier section "Structural classifications: Fibrous, cartilaginous, and synovial") because a cavity between the two connecting bones is lined with a synovial membrane and filled with synovial fluid, which helps to lubricate and cushion the joint. The ends of the bones are cushioned by hyaline cartilage.

Table 9-1 lists the different types of diarthrotic joints and describes the kinds of movements each type allows. You can also see these joints in Figure 9-1.

TABLE 9-1   **Types of Diarthrotic Joints**

Type of Joint	Description	Movement	Example
Ball-and-socket	The ball-shaped head of one bone fits into a depression (socket) in another bone.	Circular. The joints can move in all planes, and rotation is possible.	Shoulder, hip
Ellipsoid joint	An oval-shaped protuberance (called a *condyle*) of one bone fits into the oval-shaped cavity of another bone.	Can move in different planes but can't rotate.	Knuckles (the joints between metacarpals and phalanges)
Gliding joint	Flat or slightly curved surfaces join together.	Sliding or twisting in different planes.	Joints between carpal bones (wrist) and between tarsal bones (ankle)
Hinge joint	The convex surface of one bone joins with the concave surface of another.	Up and down motion, *flexion* (bending), and *extension* (straightening).	Elbow, knee
Pivot joint	Cylinder-shaped projection on one bone is surrounded by a ring of another bone and ligament.	Rotation is the only movement possible.	Radio-ulnar joint at the elbow (supination/pronation), atlanto-axial joint of the neck under the head (head rotation)
Saddle joint	Each bone is saddle shaped and fits into the saddle-shaped region of the opposite bone.	Many movements are possible; can move in different planes but can't rotate.	Carpo-metacarpal joint of the thumb

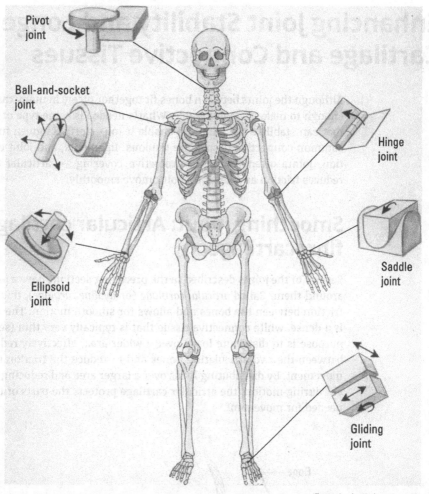

Pivot joint

Ball-and-socket joint

Hinge joint

Ellipsoid joint

Saddle joint

Gliding joint

FIGURE 9-1: Types of joints.

Illustration by Kathryn Born, MA

By degrees of freedom: Uniaxial, biaxial, and so on

Another way joints can be classified is by the number of axes of rotation that they allow, often referred to as *degrees of freedom*. Those joints that allow one, two, or three axes of rotation are referred to as *uniaxial*, *biaxial*, or *tri-axial*, respectively. A biaxial joint has two degrees of freedom; an ellipsoidal joint (knuckle), for example, can produce flexion and extension, as well as *abduction* (moving away from the body's midline) and *adduction* (moving toward the body's midline). (Refer to Chapter 8 for a complete discussion of the axes of rotation and the different types of movement.)

Enhancing Joint Stability and Longevity: Cartilage and Connective Tissues

Although the joints between bones fit together nicely in many cases, a nice fit isn't enough to make the joint stable. What's needed is some type of connective tissue that can stabilize the joint and enable it to perform its given function. The most common connective tissues are tendons, ligaments, and joint capsules. In addition, joints often possess a protective covering — articular cartilage — that reduces friction and helps the joint move smoothly.

Smoothing it out: Articular cartilage and fibrocartilage

Several of the joints described in the preceding sections have a protective covering around them. Called *articular cartilage* (or *hyaline cartilage*), this covering reduces friction between the bones and allows for smooth motion. The articular cartilage is a dense, white connective tissue that is typically very thin (see Figure 9-2). Its purpose is to distribute loads over a wider area, effectively reducing the contact between the two articulating bones and to reduce the friction that exists during movement. By distributing loads over a larger area and reducing the friction present during motion, the articular cartilage protects the parts of the bones that are needed for movement.

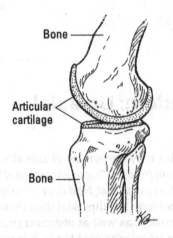

Bone

Articular cartilage

Bone

FIGURE 9-2:
Articular cartilage.

Illustration by Kathryn Born, MA

Another kind of cartilage that preserves and facilitates movement in the various joints is articular fibrocartilage. *Articular fibrocartilage* typically takes the form of a cartilaginous disk (referred to as *menisci*, or *intervertebral disks*) between the bones. These fibrocartilaginous structures help with the following:

>> Distributing loads over a joint's surface

>> Improving the fit of articulating surfaces

>> Limiting bone slip within a joint

>> Protecting the edges where articulating bones touch

>> Lubricating the articulating surfaces of bone

>> Acting as shock absorbers

TIP

Think of articular cartilage as more of a sheet covering the surface of a bone. Articular fibrocartilage, on the other hand, is typically a piece of cartilage located *within* a joint; it provides a bit more cushion during function.

REMEMBER

The articular cartilaginous structures are vital to maintaining the health of the joint throughout a person's lifespan. Yet the cartilage can be damaged when large amounts of force are delivered or when repetitive stresses are applied to the area over time.

Holding it all together: Articular connective tissue

Although the joints fit together nicely in many cases, the bony connection alone wouldn't provide enough stability to enable you to perform the many activities that you commonly engage in. Fortunately, you don't have to rely solely on how well your joints fit together because connective tissues — tendons, ligaments, and joint capsules — provide the extra support required for movement:

>> **Tendon:** A *tendon* is a soft -tissue structure that connects a muscle to bone. Often the tendon attaches the muscle to a movable aspect of the joint. The amount of movement created by the tendon depends on the size and length of the tendon, along with the type of joint it attaches to. A tendon can be overstressed, a condition referred to as *tendonitis* (inflammation of the tendon).

» **Ligament:** *Ligaments* connect bones to other bones to keep them organized and in their proper place. The wrist, for example, has a number of gliding bones. The ligaments in the wrist keep these bones from becoming disconnected and unorganized, which can result in injury and lack of use. An injured ligament is referred to as a *sprain.* People commonly sprain the ligaments in their ankles and knees.

» **Joint capsules:** In addition to the tendons and ligaments within or around a joint, a joint capsule may also exist. Joint capsules are made up of dense, soft tissues that provide stability and facilitate the function of other structures. For example, a joint capsule provides a connection among ligaments, tendons, and articular fibrocartilage, while also assisting in creating a capsule in which synovial fluid can freely assist in decreasing friction during movement.

REMEMBER

These soft-tissue structures are considered *non-contractile,* meaning they're static, providing support and assistance with movement but not exerting force themselves, which is the muscles' job. When a muscle contracts, its force is delivered to the affected bone through the muscle tendon. Like tendons, ligaments also absorb and/or deliver forces to various portions of the joint.

Tendons and ligaments are *extensible*; that is, they're able to stretch when force is applied. When the force is relatively low, they can return to their normal length; however, when the force is large enough to stretch these structures beyond their elastic limit, they become damaged and can't return to their normal length without surgery. When tendons and ligaments are stretched too often and/or too far, they become loose and their function is compromised.

Getting Physical: Understanding the Functional Basis to Moving

For your body to move the way it's supposed to, not only do the individual structures — muscles, tendons, cartilage, and bones — have to function as they're supposed to, but they also must work in an interrelated way to provide stability and normal function. This section investigates the mechanisms responsible for providing stability and explains how such a complex feat as coordinated movement is accomplished.

Perusing the factors that affect stability

Have you ever sprained your ankle, limped around on bad knees, or felt your shoulder pop out? All these events can happen if your joints lack stability. When joints are stable, they allow the bones to *articulate* (move) without a lot of displacement. In other words, the bones move the way they're supposed to — they don't "pop" out of place.

Each joint has a unique requirement for stability. As we explain in the earlier section "Functional classifications: Synarthroses, diarthroses, and more," your body contains immovable, slightly movable, and freely movable joints. Factors that play a role in stability involve the bony and soft-tissue structures that support the joint: how the bone is shaped, the arrangement of the ligaments, and more.

The shape (and contact points) of things to come

One of the factors that most influences stability is the shape of the articulating bones. Typically, bones that make up a joint are shaped as opposites to their counterparts. Where one bone ends in a socket, for example, its counterpart will end in a "ball" (refer to the earlier section "Freely movable joints: Diarthroses" for a discussion of the different kinds of articulating joints). This arrangement is often referred to as the *convex and concave orientation*, and it allows for increased stability.

Joints also tend to be more stable at certain points in their range of motion:

>> **Closed-packed position:** When the articulating surfaces of a joint are in a position where the most amount of each bone is in contact with the other, they're said to be in the *closed-packed position.* In this position, stability is increased.

>> **Loose-packed position:** When the articulating bone surfaces are in less than maximum contact, the joint is in a *loose-packed position* (also referred to as an *open-packed position*).

REMEMBER

The more surface area of contact, the more stable a joint will be. The amount of surface area contact between joints varies from person to person. Bony differences between people and past injury to the bone or soft tissue are potential causes of decreased stability.

It's articulation time: Do you know where your ligaments are?

Muscles, ligaments, and tendons all connect to the joint and provide for the delivery of or resistance to forces. The arrangement and *integrity* (condition or strength) of these structures play major roles in maintaining stability.

Ligaments, for example, attach to the bones and resist tension, thus helping to keep the bones together. When the bones are kept together within the joint, stability is enhanced. When muscles contract and exert forces on the bones via the tendon, the bones typically move closer to one another, maximizing stability.

How tight or loose are you?

Each of your joints relies heavily on the muscles around the joint to provide movement through contraction. When the muscles have adequate strength and length, the function is good. Yet a muscle imbalance around a joint — when one muscle exerts more force than the other — can actually lead to a destabilizing situation. If, for example, your knee extensors (quads) are a lot stronger than your knee flexors (hamstrings), when you contract your quads, they'll overpower your hamstrings and either injure the hamstrings or cause your joint to move beyond its normal range of motion.

REMEMBER

The muscles around a joint should be strengthened together and in a functional way. Doing so ensures that they're all strengthened for that particular function and maintains the structural balance required for stability. So, rather than just doing knee extension or flexion, for example, be sure to develop the muscles that are used for all the other motions that are involved with your activity.

Long or short? It matters

Another factor within the musculature that may impact stability is the length of the muscle. Revisiting the hamstring and quadriceps example introduced in the preceding section, if either of these muscles (or muscle groups) has limited flexibility, you won't be able to achieve the appropriate position that may be required for the activity you're attempting. If you have tight hamstrings, you may not be able to extend your knee far enough to achieve a normal heel strike while you walk, for example, a situation that has implications with the rest of the activity and, ultimately, the stability of the joint.

REMEMBER

Most ligaments and tendons attach to the joint in a way that maximizes stability, and both ligaments and tendons adapt to the forces that are applied. Over time, they may *atrophy* (shrink) or *hypertrophy* (get bigger), depending on what's required of them. Having injured a joint previously increases the chances of injury or reinjury. If you've previously sprained your ankle, for example, chances are, that loose ligament will make you prone to another injury. Maybe you'll injure another structure, or maybe you'll sprain your ankle again.

The role of other connective tissues

In addition to the ligament, tendons, and muscles, other connective tissues exist in and around your joints that impact stabilization. For instance, the joint capsule (explained in the section "Holding it all together: Articular connective tissue") and *fascia* (the connective tissue that surrounds and connects the muscles and other soft tissues) may play a role. These soft tissues themselves may help to stabilize the bones either by providing points of attachment for the tendon and/or ligaments or by helping to facilitate sensory input from the joint and muscle activity.

Understanding restraint mechanisms

Joint stability isn't the job of any single structure doing its thing in isolation. Instead, it's the result of the muscles, tendons, ligaments, bones, and other soft tissues all working in a coordinated, interrelated way. All these tissues have mechanoreceptors (see "How stimulating! The passive restraint mechanism" later in this chapter) responsible for sensing and assessing movement; they all provide a unique attribute to stability, which is enhanced when each completes its specific task and communication is facilitated between the different components.

In this section, we explore two major restraint mechanisms — the active restraint mechanism and the passive restraint mechanism — that together maintain stability, enhance activity, and help you avoid injury.

REMEMBER

To function properly and maintain stability, the active and passive restraint mechanisms need to work together. If problems exist in either mechanism (the muscles don't fire properly) or if sensory information isn't collected and processed as it should be, stability is compromised. When *both* active and passive restraint mechanisms are glitchy, the effects on stability are even more complex — and detrimental.

Muscling in: The active restraint mechanism

The *active restraint mechanism* can broadly be defined as the contractile component of joint stability — in other words, the muscles. Muscles are considered the *active* mechanism because they act on and around a particular set of structures.

Not only do the muscles that act on a joint need to provide the forces required to move or propel objects, but they also must resist forces that would otherwise cause injury. Think of a task that requires hand-eye coordination. When you reach out for and turn a doorknob, for example, all the muscles affecting your shoulder, elbow, wrist, and fingers must contract in a coordinated effort; if they don't, you won't be able to grasp the knob, twist it, and pull the door open.

To maintain stability while performing such a task, the muscles need to exert force in a coordinated fashion, do so in a timely manner, and be strong enough to generate the effect required:

>> **Working in a coordinated way:** Your muscles provide coordinated function. Through motor patterns established over time (you've opened many doors in the past, for example), tasks (movement) that you perform are already strategized. Patterns have been developed to coordinate the task at hand while minimizing distracting or opposing forces. When the efforts of all the muscles involved in a given task are coordinated, stability is maintained, and you can complete the task more successfully.

>> **Receiving and interpreting sensory information in a timely manner:** Sensory information is continually being collected from the joints involved in an activity, and the forces needed to complete the task are determined based on this information (how fast you want to go, whether you're traveling uphill or downhill, whether the ground is even or uneven, and so on).

Depending on your ability to retrieve this information, your muscles adapt accordingly. If a muscle or group of muscles isn't able to interpret the information in a timely manner, or if the muscle or muscle group is weak, then the movement pattern is thrown off and stability may be compromised. (The next section explains how these messages get to the muscles.)

>> **Reacting with adequate force:** Muscles that are too short or too long (essentially not in the ideal position) have difficulty getting the timing right or being able to develop the force necessary to either counter or facilitate the activity.

Simply contracting isn't enough. A muscle has to contract with enough force to complete its task. Many people who have had previous injuries or who have neurological problems that affect strength have a hard time stabilizing their joints. When the communication network lets the joint's support structures communicate efficiently, function is facilitated because collaboration and timeliness are enhanced. The end result? Fewer injuries and less dysfunction.

How stimulating! The passive restraint mechanism

The structures that make up the passive restraint mechanism are those that are noncontractile and involve everything *except* your muscles:

>> **The cartilage, bones, ligaments, and other connective tissues:** Refer to the earlier section "Enhancing Joint Stability and Longevity: Cartilage and Connective Tissues" for details on these structures.

>> **Mechanoreceptors:** *Mechanoreceptors* are specialized sensory receptors whose job is to detect neurological information.

Mechanoreceptors respond to mechanical stimuli such as *tension* (stretching), *pressure* (compression), and *displacement* (movement). They collect and help decipher the needed information regarding movement. For example, when pressure is applied to a bone, the mechanoreceptors transport that information to the brain to be evaluated and acted upon. Or if you've just stepped in a hole, mechanoreceptors ask certain muscles (ankle evertors) to contract to minimize how much you twist your ankle. By trying to stop the ankle from twisting, injury may be avoided.

You can find mechanoreceptors in muscles, tendons, bones, ligaments, and other soft tissues like your skin. When these structures are stimulated or affected by an activity, the information is shared and one of two things happens: Either the information elicits a reflex response (you yank your hand away from the hot burner, for example) or it triggers the brain to create a new *motor plan* (a sequence of activities like dodging a defender who is trying to block your shot).

REMEMBER

Because mechanoreceptors need to be mechanically stimulated, their responses are susceptible to injured tissue. For example, a ligament that's been sprained in the past will be a bit longer and loose. The next time you sprain your ankle, it will twist even further before the mechanoreceptors are activated and they recognize the situation.

ACL INJURY

Ligament injury is quite common in physically active people. One very common ligament injury involves the anterior cruciate ligament (ACL), in the knee. The ACL is responsible for keeping the tibia from sliding too far forward on the femur. Often the ACL gets injured when an athlete is decelerating or accelerating while simultaneously rotating, as you do when you stop and change direction quickly. ACL injury is so common in the sports world that many athletes either have or know someone who has had this injury. (Fortunately, an ACL injury isn't a career-ending one; it can be successfully rehabilitated with time and hard work.)

Several factors may predispose athletes to ACL injury. One of the most common is a muscle imbalance that exists between the quadriceps and hamstring muscle groups. Typically, the hamstrings should be one-third weaker than the quadriceps. When hamstrings are more than one-third weaker, the predisposition for ACL injury exists. Another predisposing factor is the angle at which the knee is composed, called the *Q-angle*. A large Q-angle (commonly called *knock knees*) increases your chances of suffering from an ACL injury, as does a smaller space between the *femoral condyles* (the bony protrusions on either side of the bottom of the femur), known as the *intercondylar notch*. Two others thought to play a role are the hormonal changes that occur during menstruation and having flat feet, but as yet, the evidence connecting these factors and ACL injuries isn't as strong.

(continued)

(continued)

Unfortunately, females tend to possess more of these predisposing factors than males, and, not surprisingly, females are affected more by this injury. Several preventive programs that integrate females into physical sport activity earlier have been shown to possibly curb the incidence of injury. These programs are aimed at strengthening the lower extremities. Some people speculate that beginning physical activity earlier allows the neurological system to develop earlier and helps athletes avoid injury that otherwise may occur. In the end, your best bet is to emphasize good biomechanical form, strengthening and having a physically active lifestyle.

Being flexible: You can do it!

Movement is the cornerstone of living a healthy and productive lifestyle. Whether you're getting up from a chair, walking down the stairs, throwing a baseball, or taking a jog, each task requires a certain amount of joint movement (flexibility). You need to be familiar with two types of flexibility: static and dynamic.

Static flexibility

When most folks think about how flexible they are, they usually think about static flexibility. *Static flexibility* is the amount of joint motion exhibited when you move to the end of the range of motion and hold still — such as when you bend over to touch your toes, feel the intense stretch along the back of your legs, and then hold the position. This type of flexibility is usually very controlled and emphasizes only one joint or muscle group; in the case of touching your toes, it emphasizes the hamstring group.

A static assessment of how flexible you are is helpful in understanding the amount of total joint motion that a limb is capable of. When you examine a joint from the beginning to the end of its range of motion, you get an impression of the total amount of movement allowed, called the *envelope of motion*, within a particular joint. Typically, these assessments are performed when the person is relaxed. Makes sense, doesn't it? If you're trying to stretch, you relax so that you can reach the end of the movement.

REMEMBER

Although some people seem to be more flexible than others, the amount of motion each limb and joint is capable of differs throughout the body. It's the integration of range of motion across all the joints that allows for the functional activities that you perform on a daily basis.

Dynamic flexibility

Because many joints must work in concert with others to accomplish movement, you can't simply look at static flexibility to get a holistic view of movement. Instead, you need to consider dynamic flexibility, which involves the interrelationships among joints.

Dynamic flexibility is the amount of motion experienced during movement, and it typically involves multiple joints simultaneously. Most activities that you participate in are *dynamic tasks*, meaning the movements associated with them have multiple phases and parts. To throw a ball, for example, you need movement to occur at the elbow, shoulder, wrist, spine, and legs.

Unlike static flexibility, which typically involves a controlled stretch-and-hold type of movement, dynamic flexibility relies on the interrelated joint ranges of motion required to complete the task. If a limitation is noted in one of the involved limbs, a change will likely occur elsewhere. If your elbow doesn't rotate correctly when you throw a ball, for example, the ball won't go very far.

REMEMBER

Assessing dynamic flexibility and recognizing the interrelationships that make everyday activities possible is of the utmost importance, especially for coaches and healthcare providers.

An assessment of dynamic flexibility takes into consideration the action of all the joints involved with a particular movement. For example, if you were assessing a person's dynamic flexibility by watching them walk, you would do the following:

>> Note the discrete movements that make up the overall motion.

>> Understand how each movement affects the other movements.

In this case, you may notice that the subject isn't able to fully strike on their heel when their foot contacts the ground. As a result, they're forced to make contact at the middle of the foot, the primary cause of which is that their knee doesn't extend enough to get the heel down in time.

REMEMBER

Although static flexibility is important and affects your ability to move with enough dynamic flexibility, the key component is how all the joints work together when a movement occurs. In the example related to walking, a static assessment may reveal that the subject had full range of motion when they tried to straighten their leg; the dynamic assessment reveals that, when the ankle, knee, and hip needed to move in an integrated fashion, a deficit existed that decreased the subject's range of motion.

Wrangling with range of motion

Within the musculoskeletal system, the *range of motion* (ROM) of a joint describes its flexibility (but we don't use the term *flexibility* in this context because that term is often used to describe how tight your muscles are, and it just confuses things).

Factors influencing joint flexibility

A number of different situations, events, and conditions can influence joint flexibility. The ROM of the joint is largely dictated by

>> **The type of joint:** See the earlier section "Getting These Old Bones to Move: Types of Joints" for details on the different kinds of joints.

>> **The shape of the bones forming the joint:** The hip joint, for example, is a ball-and-socket joint where the head of the femur inserts into the round cavity that is the acetabulum. Because the femur is firmly within the acetabulum, when the joint reaches extremes of flexion and extension, the bone just isn't able to move any further because, in doing so, it will contact the other articulating bone. Often clinicians refer to this stopping point as an *end feel*, and in this case, it would represent a *bony end feel*, which is abrupt, hard, and unforgiving. Another example would be elbow extension, when you simply reach the point at which your elbow can extend no further. (For more on end feel, head to the later section "Paying attention to how the end feels.")

>> **The soft tissue structures that surround the joint and stretch:** If you can't reach over and touch your toes, chances are, your hamstring muscles are too tight and don't allow you to bend far enough. This is often referred to as the *tissue stretch,* and the end feel is pretty firm. Because of the inherent elasticity of the different soft-tissue structures, some stretch, or give, more than others.

TIP

Try this example: Try bending your fingers back toward your forearm. You probably notice that this motion is relatively easy to accomplish early on, but when you approach the end range, notice the resistance, which eventually stops the motion.

>> **The soft-tissue structures that block movement:** Soft tissues can impede the ROM simply because they get in the way. Called the *soft-tissue approximation end feel,* just the squeezing of the tissue stops the motion. For example, you may not be able to bend your leg such that your heel is able to touch your bottom. In this case, the hamstring muscles are squeezed and don't allow for this motion to go so far. If you have large amounts of fat in this area, you'll have deficits in your ROM.

>> **The articular cartilage, ligaments, joint capsule, and fascia throughout the body:** These structures are constantly changing as they respond to use and disuse. Typically, if you assume a position for long periods of time or if you habitually perform a particular movement, the tissues adapt. Such

adaptations to movement can have negative effects on the health of the joint and surrounding soft tissues.

>> **The relative elasticity, extensibility, and laxity that exist within the soft tissues around the joint:** A joint that is composed of tight muscles, ligaments, or tendons tends to be tighter and has less ROM than a joint whose structures are looser. Conversely, if these structures have been injured and are more lax, the joint may experience too much motion.

WARNING

Although you may think that you can't be too loose, you absolutely can. When your joints are lax and allow more-than-normal ROM, added stress is distributed to the cartilage and bony structures. Sometimes, if the stresses are applied repetitively and at large enough levels, damage can occur.

Measuring range of motion

The ROM within a joint is based on how far you can stretch and reach. Although this method is a fine way of assessing your motion, it lacks an objective measure to compare your results to. Sometimes, you need to know the actual amount of movement that exists within the joint(s) related to both dynamic and static flexibility. For example, after an injury, you can use joint measurement to assess how well you're healing. Often after surgery, the motion in your limb is limited, and it's important that you regain what you lost. Being able to gauge your progress and know how much movement is lacking is a key part of rehabilitation.

Joint ROM is measured in units of degrees. The reference point for most measurements is the body in anatomical position. When a joint is in anatomical position (refer to Chapter 8), the joint is said to be at *zero degrees*, or *neutral*. From this point, you can measure the amount of motion that exists. The ROM for flexion of the elbow, as shown in Figure 9-3, for example, is considered to be the angle created when your limb moves from the fully extended (anatomical) position to the maximal point of flexion. To figure the amount of extension within the joint, you simply return the limb from the maximal flexion to its anatomical position.

You can measure ROM with these tools:

>> **A goniometer:** Any joint motion is able to be quantified using goniometry. *Goniometry* is the act of measuring angles — in this case, joint angles. Goniometry is usually measured using a *goniometer,* a device that, if used correctly, can easily quantify joint motion. Goniometers come in different sizes and allow for either 360 degrees or 180 degrees of motion.

>> **An inclinometer:** Inclinometers can be purchased from your local hardware store and strapped onto the limb; they simply tell you how much movement the limb has gone through. The principles for using this device are similar to those used with a goniometer.

Measuring ROM

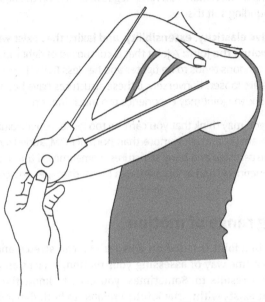

FIGURE 9-3:
Measuring range
of motion.

© John Wiley & Sons, Inc.

Paying attention to how the end feels

Each joint has an anticipated normal ROM. What constitutes "normal" is based on studies of thousands of people. When people fall beyond these norms — that is, they have either greater or lesser ROM — they experience effects within the affected joint and beyond it, a situation directly related to the idea of dynamic flexibility (explained in the earlier section "Dynamic flexibility").

Additionally, due to the anatomic makeup of each joint, a normal end feel is established. *End feel* describes how a joint comes to the terminal portion of its movement. The end feels are as follows:

>> **Bone-to-bone:** A *bone-to-bone end feel* exists when the joint's ROM is limited due to bones contacting one another. This end feel is abrupt, hard, and unforgiving. A very common example of this is an elbow extension. When the elbow extends, the hook-shaped protuberance from the ulna (called the *olecranon process*) contacts a depression on the humerus (called the *olecranon fossa*), and the motion is stopped.

>> **Soft-tissue–approximation:** A *soft-tissue–approximation end feel* involves a compression of the soft tissues around a joint that leads to the end of the motion. An example of this is elbow flexion, when the lower arm is flexed toward the shoulder. This motion is usually terminated because the biceps muscles are compressed in a way that makes further motion impossible.

>> **Tissue stretch:** *Tissue stretch* refers to a hard or firm end feel with a slight give to it. The inherent elasticity of the different soft tissue structures cause some to stretch, or give, more than others, dictating the level of end feel produced as tissue stretch. Typically, this type of end feel involves progressive tension that continues until motion is stopped, as happens, for example, when you bend your fingers back toward your forearm. Initially, the motion is relatively easy to accomplish, but as you approach the end range, resistance eventually stops the movement entirely.

TIP

You need to understand the joint's underlying anatomical makeup to know what to expect as the normal end feel for that joint and movement. If you experience an end feel other than what you expect, an injury has probably occurred. Evaluating end feel is how clinicians can tell whether you've torn a ligament, for instance. If your bone moves beyond what is normally expected, the clinician may conclude that you've damaged your ligament, which is meant to keep the joint stable.

TECHNICAL
STUFF

BEING LAX ISN'T NECESSARILY A GOOD THING!

Don't confuse being flexible with being lax. Although sometimes related, the two terms refer to slightly different concepts. *Flexibility* often refers to the range of motion of a joint, whereas *laxity* refers more directly to the movement within a particular joint. For example, being able to glide, or *translate*, your shoulder to a point where it's close to popping out is an example of laxity; the ability to reach behind you and scratch your back is more a measure of flexibility.

Laxity within a joint can be a good thing, but it can also be detrimental, negatively impacting the stability within the joint and potentially contributing to injury. Most of your joints allow for some amount of translation between the bones; many times, this translation allows the joints to move in the direction(s) you need them to. Yet, when the laxity within the joint allows for too much translation, it can result in abnormal movement and an unstable environment. For example, if a lax shoulder rotates too far back into external rotation, it will also translate, requiring the rotation to occur at the edge of the joint. When this happens, the joint is asked to perform in a position that it wasn't made to accommodate. In situations like these, the function causes undue stress, and the joint and/or articular cartilage may be damaged. In extreme cases of too much laxity, the result may be a dislocation.

To counter the effects of laxity on a joint, you need to strengthen the musculature surrounding the joint. When you strengthen the joint, you improve the stability of the joint during activity.

You Want Me to Put My What Where? Stretching Redefined!

Stretching has long been thought of as a necessity to physical activity. Before nearly every soccer or baseball practice, your coach made you stretch. (If your practices were anything like ours, you spent more time catching up on the gossip of the day than actually stretching.) Today, however, the effectiveness of stretching routines is being questioned, and there's a lot of debate about the effectiveness and type of stretching that you should do, if any.

This section explores the physiological components of stretching and answers the questions related to the types of stretching you should or shouldn't do.

Looking at what happens when you stretch

Increasing or maintaining motion in a joint requires that you use and stretch the joint on a regular basis. Why? Because the soft tissues adapt to the stresses that are applied to them, whether those stresses are caused by a sedentary lifestyle, habitual positioning, and/or repetitive activities.

In sedentary people, the soft tissues are likely to tighten and result in less joint ROM. For those who sit in a certain position for extended periods of time or who are active but complete the same task the same way over and over again, the body may have a smoother ROM in certain parts of the movement while tightening up and exhibiting restriction in others. Additionally, a decrease in ROM in a major joint may actually cause decreases in other related movements. For example, not using your thumb often leads to decreases in the motion in the wrist.

These effects occur because of the mechanisms that come into play when you move or, as the case may be, don't move. In this section, we explain these mechanisms in detail.

Making the stretch possible: Autogenic inhibition

All your muscles contain organs that are able to detect various types of sensory information. These structures are called *mechanoreceptors*. When stimulated, they communicate with the central nervous system (CNS) and tell it what's happening within that structure. The stretch reflex carries the most responsibility when stretching and relies on two primary mechanoreceptors to guide its function: the muscle spindle and Golgi tendon organs (GTOs), which are responsible for detecting changes in muscle length and tension (turn to Chapter 3 for more on these structures).

When the muscle is stretched, both mechanoreceptors begin to send signals to the spinal cord and brain. Here's what happens:

1. At first, the muscle spindles react by contracting the muscles to prevent too much stretching.

   Obviously, if you're trying to stretch, and the body responds by minimizing the stretch, it won't be very productive.

2. If the stretch is held for a few seconds — typically, ten seconds or so, — the GTO impulse overcomes the muscle spindle response.

   The job of the GTOs is to share the information about amounts of tension and length of the tissue to the spinal cord.

REMEMBER

Unlike the contraction that's initiated when the muscle spindles are activated (Step 1), the GTOs encourage relaxation of the muscle, which helps to prevent injury. By decreasing the tension within the muscle, the reflex keeps the muscle from extending beyond its limits. When the stretching muscle relaxes as a result of the GTOs within it, *autogenic inhibition* is achieved. This mechanism makes stretching possible.

Opposing muscle groups working together: Reciprocal inhibition

Activity is often dependent on opposing muscles around a joint working in concert. For example, as your quadriceps contracts, your hamstring needs to relax a bit to allow the knee to move. If both muscle groups continue to contract, they end up fighting each other, making movement inefficient at best.

REMEMBER

When a muscle group is stimulated, it may actually have a relaxation effect on the opposing muscle, a phenomenon referred to as *reciprocal inhibition*. In reciprocal inhibition, one muscle group (the *agonist-main mover*) is contracted, and the opposing muscle group (the *antagonist-opposing muscle*) is relaxed. The GTOs of the opposing muscle are stimulated and decrease the tension in that muscle, allowing for more efficient motion because the agonist doesn't have to work as hard to achieve movement. You can use both of these techniques to your advantage when implementing stretching routines. Figure 9-4 shows an example of reciprocal inhibition.

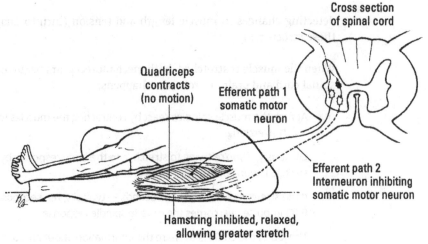

Cross section
of spinal cord

Quadriceps
contracts
(no motion)

Efferent path 1
somatic motor
neuron

Efferent path 2
Interneuron inhibiting
somatic motor neuron

Hamstring inhibited, relaxed,
allowing greater stretch

FIGURE 9-4:
Reciprocal
inhibition.

Illustration by Kathryn Born, MA

It's more than just the nerves: Collagen, elastin, actin, and myosin

Another mechanism that assists with increasing flexibility involves the muscle structure itself, which has both contractile and non-contractile components:

» **Noncontractile components:** The muscles and tendons are both composed of collagen and elastin fibers, which are noncontractile (not to be confused with static restraints, which we discuss earlier). Collagen allows the tissue to resist forces that lead to tissue manipulation, and elastin, which is composed of elastic tissues, helps the tissues return to their original shapes.

» **Contractile components:** These include actin and myosin, which are the myofilaments responsible for muscle contraction. (For more on the muscles, check out Chapter 3.)

Altogether, these portions of the tendons and muscles work together to determine the structure's ability to be stretched and return to normal after being stressed.

The collagen and elastin along with the actin and myosin seem to resist the stretch that is applied to the structure; however, the force behind the stretch and the velocity with which that force is delivered determine how far the muscle stretches. During stretching, temporary changes in the length of the structure occur. Typically, these changes are short-lived, and the muscle returns to normal.

Permanently lengthening a muscle or tendon is difficult to do safely, but it can occur when elongation exists in response to long periods of stretching or habitual movements. Although the changes that occur in the muscle's physical and mechanical structures are usually temporary, continued activity is considered beneficial if you want more permanent changes.

The push-pull of stretching: The balancing effects of agonists and antagonists

When reading and studying about stretching, you'll come across the terms *agonist* and *antagonist,* which describe what and how the muscles work to create a stretch. (We introduce these terms in the earlier section "Opposing muscle groups working together: Reciprocal inhibition.")

REMEMBER

To review, the *agonist* is the muscle that is contracted to create movement and cause a stretch. The *antagonist* is the muscle that responds to the action of the agonist by being stretched. When you flex your elbow, for example, the muscle creating flexion is the biceps, which is the agonist, and the muscle that stretches is the triceps, which is the antagonist. Balance between the agonist and antagonist is very important; otherwise, injury can occur due to muscular imbalances.

Stretching techniques

Maintaining full, unrestricted ROM is essential to your normal daily activities. The loss of flexibility in a joint can result in uncoordinated and awkward movement patterns. Although, without question, flexibility is essential to normal everyday activities and physical performance appears to be best when participants are loose, researchers disagree significantly on the effect stretching may have on performance and injury. Still, everyone agrees that joints need a certain amount of physiological ROM within them; without it, the body is affected.

The goal of stretching routines should be to increase the ROM within the joint or otherwise creating a smoother motion. In the following sections, we describe a variety of techniques that can enhance the flexibility of a particular joint. Some of these techniques are more specialized than others, and some require the help of someone else.

REMEMBER

All the stretching techniques we list can help you maintain and, if done routinely, increase ROM. However, not all types of stretching are meant for everyone. Make sure you understand the risks associated with each technique and progress appropriately through your program. When in question, consult an appropriate professional to prescribe and guide your program.

Active and passive stretching

All stretching happens either actively or passively, and some stretching techniques use both:

» **Active stretching:** In *active stretching,* you contract the agonist muscle, which creates a movement in the joint that results in the antagonist muscle stretching.

» **Passive stretching:** In *passive stretching,* you rely on gravity or the force of another person to move the joint through its ROM to the point where you feel a stretch.

Both techniques stretch the involved tissues, and because of the different functions of and structures in the body, both techniques are needed. Early in the rehabilitation program following knee surgery, for example, the best strategy may be for you to extend and flex your knee on your own (active stretching). As you progress and the pain becomes less, the clinician typically begins to push on the limb as a way to increase the range of motion in a slow and controlled, but forceful, manner (passive stretching — which is not like a torture chamber, although that may be what you're thinking!).

Static stretching

The most common stretching technique is the static stretch. In *static stretching,* you rely on gravity, your body weight, or another person to create the push that results in the stretch. The chosen antagonist muscle is pushed to a point of maximal stretch and then held in that position for a period of time. Some people say that a short (five-second) stretch is enough; others hold the stretched position for as long as a minute.

Ballistic stretching

In *ballistic stretching,* repetitive bouncing movements create an increase in ROM. This technique has been used for many years but has not been without its critics, who are concerned that the ROM created during the bouncing actually causes injury to the involved tissues, which are forced to move beyond what they may be able to handle safely.

REMEMBER

Despite the controversy, ballistic stretching is widely used and has been shown to increase ROM. When engaging in ballistic stretching, make sure that the intensity of the bouncing doesn't create undue stress on your joints, which can result in muscle or joint injury.

Dynamic stretching

Dynamic stretching is an active and controlled technique that mimics functional activity. In other words, it includes movement patterns that you actually use in the activity you're getting ready to engage in.

Dynamic stretching has grown in popularity over the past several years, especially in the sporting world. Most sporting activities require repetitive motion of a particular task — throwing a baseball in practice, for example. After throwing the ball 50 or so times during a game, for example, players often experience soreness or tightness in the muscles of their throwing arms. The active warm-up not only helps players loosen up and gain flexibility, but by getting them warmer, it also has long been considered an important aspect of getting ready to participate.

Proprioceptive neuromuscular facilitation: An advanced stretching technique

Proprioceptive neuromuscular facilitation (PNF) is a series of stretching techniques that involve particular combinations of contraction and relaxation of the agonist and antagonist muscles. We explain the more common types of PNF in this section. All are typically done with multiple (three or so) repetitions, and each phase is held for approximately ten seconds. The timing is important because it maximizes the GTO response, which is one of the primary factors in increasing flexibility in this technique (refer to the earlier section "Making the stretch possible: Autogenic inhibition").

WARNING

When using the PNF technique, heed this advice to avoid injury:

>> **Make sure your partner doesn't push too hard.** The technique *starts* at a point of maximal stretch, and further movement beyond that is the goal.

>> **Don't engage too quickly when you go from pushing to relaxing and vice versa.** As the name indicates, the transitions and contractions should occur slowly.

REMEMBER

This technique involves successive bouts of stretching and results in significant increases in the quality of motion. This can be an increase in the range of motion or simply that you can bend down and that nagging knee pain has gone — you feel better despite not gaining additional range of motion.

HOLD-RELAX PNF TECHNIQUE

The hold-relax PNF technique involves an *isometric* (no movement) contraction of the hamstrings (antagonist) at the point of stretch. After pushing against resistance for approximately ten seconds, the leg is then pushed to create further stretch. After the ten seconds of pushing, you can actually be pushed further — evidence of the antagonist muscles relaxing and allowing more movement. Although other PNF techniques may require the use of a partner, you can actually complete the hold-relax technique by yourself.

CONTRACT-RELAX PNF TECHNIQUE

The *contract-relax PNF* technique involves an *isotonic* (movement) contraction of the hamstring (antagonist) muscles. Here, the stretch begins at the point where a stretch is felt (your partner lifts your leg up in the position of a hamstring stretch); after you're at the point where you feel a stretch, you actively push your leg against your partner and then return your leg to the ground. After your leg is back on the ground, your partner again lifts the leg while you push your leg into a stretch, most likely moving past where the last stretch occurred.

SLOW-REVERSAL-HOLD-RELAX PNF TECHNIQUE

The *slow-reversal-hold-relax* technique, shown in Figure 9-5, involves a little more coordination and communication between the person being stretched and their partner, as these steps show (we use the hamstring stretch here, but the process is generally the same when using this technique to stretch other muscles):

1. **Your partner moves your knee and hip back to a point where you experience a stretch.**

    Usually felt behind the knee and at the back of the leg, this is where the antagonist is.

2. **Upon feeling the point of stretch, you actively try to straighten your leg back out and push down toward the ground, but your partner doesn't allow your leg to move.**

    This goes on for about ten seconds.

3. **You contract your agonist (quadriceps) and pull your leg actively back toward your head to intensify the stretch. While you actively pull your leg back, your partner applies a slight overpressure and helps you continue to move back.**

    Working together, you and your partner are able to achieve a maximal stretch of the antagonist muscle in that direction.

4. **When a new point of hip flexion and an increased stretch have been achieved, you relax while your partner holds the stretch for about ten seconds, or so.**

5. **After the rest period, you repeat the preceding steps from the new position.**

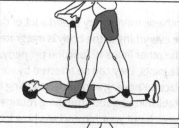

1. Passive stretch

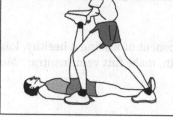

2. Contract against resistance

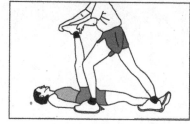

3. Relax passive stretch

FIGURE 9-5:
The PNF
stretching
technique.

© John Wiley & Sons, Inc.

Other things to keep in mind about stretches and stretching

The benefits of stretching go beyond just what happens in the muscle; they also extend to the involved tendons and joint capsules. Here are some other things to know about stretching and stretching regimens:

» **Although an increase in ROM is likely the goal of a stretching program, it isn't always needed to get the results you want.** In many cases, just simply encouraging and facilitating the muscles to relax or loosen up helps the joints that they attach to. Many runners, for example, experience *runner's knee,* in which, over time, they experience pain on the outside of the knee. The culprit is typically a tight iliotibial (IT) band. In treating this injury, increasing the knee's ROM itself doesn't eliminate the pain. Instead, you can loosen up the particular muscle so that it can go through the full ROM required by the activity without absorbing too much stress or having to overwork.

» **You can often achieve desired results by focusing on areas other than the problematic joint.** For example, you may have discomfort in your knee, but a physical therapist or athletic trainer may spend a lot of time stretching out your hip. That's because everything in the body is integrated; the knee (in this example) is reliant on the other limbs to function properly. Because your muscles often cross multiple joints, they can be affected by various components at several different places. Knowing and understanding how your anatomy works is key to establishing a good stretching routine. The next time you have knee pain, try to stretch out your hip and see how it makes your knee feel!

TIP

Good joint health is a key component of leading a healthy, long life. So, for your joints and for your overall health, make this your mantra: "Move in all ways and always move!"

Chapter **10**

Assessing Movement: Motion Analysis

A nalyzing human movement is something we bet you do all the time, although you probably don't think of it that way. If you've ever people-watched and said to yourself, "Wow, they're really limping," or "Huh, that jogger is certainly bouncing down the street," you've been analyzing movement.

As it turns out, an entire discipline is devoted to just this task. In this chapter, we explore a movement analysis process that makes evaluating movement easier. We also share some of the important principles and concepts to remember when you do so.

Investigating Movement: The Basics

Some of the most common reasons why people use motion analysis is to improve performance (for example, they want to get quicker, faster, or more efficient) and to prevent or treat injury. To adequately analyze movement to achieve these goals, you need an approach that follows a defined process. This process, combined with information about the actual task, enables you to discover some very helpful and valuable information.

One of the biggest pitfalls related to motion analysis lies with the practitioner who, after eyeballing a task in real time, makes judgments without having knowledge of the specific task or its purpose, and without really understanding the person being studied. Each person is a unique individual, with their own past histories of injury, levels of strength, previous training, and unique goals and activities.

Choosing an approach

Motion analysis typically takes one of two forms — either quantitative or qualitative. Occasionally, a mixture of the two is used.

Each type of analysis requires the examiner to have a sufficient level of understanding of the task at hand and the intended outcomes of the performance. And each is essential to motion analysis efforts and has its own set of benefits and drawbacks, which we explain in the following sections.

Qualitative analysis

Qualitative analysis offers general motion analysis assessment and feedback pertaining to the movement. A pitching coach, for example, may notice that one of their athletes is really leaning to the side during the pitch. The coach may ask the athlete to straighten up and direct their body toward home plate when throwing and to avoid leaning so much. This type of feedback is considered qualitative.

Qualitative assessment is the most common type of assessment for these reasons:

>> **It doesn't require high-tech instruments.** A qualitative analysis can be made simply by watching the movement, either in real time or on some type of video device for replay.

>> **It doesn't require a particularly high level of skill.** As long as the examiner knows how the body can move, knows how it should move optimally to perform the task, and can pick up the key positions, they can complete the analysis.

In most cases — when a quick look is needed — a qualitative assessment is appropriate. Typically, this is going to be the only way a Little League coach or physical education teacher may be able to examine their athletes or students. Whether watching the movement in real time or watching a replay, people can carry out qualitative assessments easily and quickly.

Quantitative analysis

Quantitative analysis involves using actual measurement to gauge performance. If, instead of providing general assessment and guidance, the pitching coach records the motion with a high-speed video camera, uses analysis software in their evaluation of the movement, and then says to the pitcher something like, "You're leaning 18 degrees when you release the ball. You need to straighten up so that you don't lean more than 5 degrees," the coach is using quantitative analysis. In this case, the specific measurements that were made of the motion inform the coach's recommendations.

REMEMBER

When the clinician needs more information about the amount of force, the velocity, or the angles of a movement — information that a qualitative analysis just can't provide — then a quantitative analysis is the better option.

Knowing types of tasks and feedback mechanisms

Motion analysis can be overwhelming if you don't really know how to go about it and don't know what to look at. If you're a novice, you may find yourself staring awkwardly at your subject, not really knowing where to begin. Unless you have an established process that includes knowledge of the person completing the task, the components of the movement being evaluated, and an understanding of feedback mechanisms, your analysis isn't likely to provide much useful information.

In the following sections, we explain what you need to know about the person you're evaluating and how understanding the different types of tasks (simple and complex) and feedback mechanisms (open and closed) is vital to making a sound evaluation and providing useful feedback. Head to the later section "Breaking Down an Analysis Model" for a process you can follow when the time comes to put your knowledge to work.

Comparing simple and complex tasks

Not all movements have the same difficulty or require similar amounts of preparation to execute. Simple movements require very little or no thought, and they aren't dependent on another body part completing its movement first. A good example of a simple task is picking up a ball.

Complex tasks, on the other hand, require thought and regular practice. They're made up of several individual components that must be completed in a particular way to produce a successful end result. An example of a complex task is pitching;

it involves a coordinated effort between the legs, torso, and upper extremities. Each activity required for a successful pitch depends on another part of the body doing its job. Consider this sequence of movements:

1. The pitcher pushes off their back foot to move their body forward.

2. Their hips begin to twist to facilitate the sling-like motion at the root of throwing.

3. While their body twists from the hips up through the torso (core), they move the ball forward and hurl it at the target.

If any flaws occur within the chain of activity, the pitcher's performance — and potentially their health — may be in jeopardy.

Paying attention to open- versus closed-feedback mechanisms

Some tasks are difficult to alter while they're being performed; others are easily changed. The type of information that the body must process and the way in which it processes that information — its *feedback mechanism* — determines whether an activity can be changed midcourse. There are two types of feedback mechanisms:

>> **Open-feedback mechanism:** A task that has an open-feedback mechanism (or *open task*) can be changed in real time. During this type of movement, the body collects information and then alters the movement to maximize its success in that particular situation. For example, if you're going up for a jump shot and someone makes contact with you, you're able to change how you shoot the ball in midair.

>> **Closed-feedback mechanism:** A task that has a closed-feedback mechanism (or *closed task*) can't be altered after it's started. Closed tasks are those that, once turned on, can't be turned off. A free throw is a good example. The only way to be more successful with free-throw shooting is to practice it over and over and over again.

Breaking Down an Analysis Model

To make analyzing movement easier and more efficient, you use a defined analysis model. A typical model for analysis involves knowing the nature and objective of the movement, observing and evaluating the movement, and providing recommendations based on the performance outcomes. We outline the different parts of the analysis model in this section.

REMEMBER

The outcomes vary extensively and can include information to help achieve different goals, like improving performance or avoiding injury. They can also focus on the whole task (how to better jump for maximum distance, for example) or specific components of a given task (informing a pitcher, for example, that they may be experiencing elbow pain during a pitch because they drop their arm slot when throwing).

Gaining background knowledge

As a basis for the beginning of the movement analysis, the examiner (coach, clinician, or personal trainer) must have some background knowledge about the task to be completed. Understanding what the performer is trying to accomplish and having an understanding of the components needed to be successful are essential to the analysis. Background knowledge, explained in the following sections, helps you to identify the key elements of the movement that need focus.

How to perform the task

You need to know the mechanics of the movement, its purpose, and the most efficient and safest ways to go about it. This knowledge makes you a more effective assessor.

REMEMBER

Although having performed the task yourself can sometimes be helpful, it's not essential. Some of the best coaches weren't the greatest or most successful athletes; instead, their study of the game and its elements enables them to be successful. If you haven't personally performed the task you're evaluating, make sure you perform sufficient research into the mechanics and purpose of the task.

WARNING

Many folks that analyze motion or provide coaching do so without considering how and what information they're basing their advice on. A clue that you're dealing with one of these people is someone who says, "I know good mechanics when I see them" and then, when asked to define good mechanics, isn't able to do so.

The objective of the movement and each of its components

The objective of a movement may be singular and relatively simple — performing a dumbbell curl, for example, which simply requires bending the elbow and repeating. Or the movement can *seem* simple, like getting the batter out, but is actually quite complex. Consider the individual components of a pitch:

>> **How the pitcher stands on the rubber as they prepare to throw:** The stance provides the foundation for what's to come. Good balance and a controlled windup allow for a successful throwing motion.

>> **How the pitcher moves their torso, hips, legs, and arms as they lead up to releasing the ball:** These motions generate the force leading up to the pitcher letting go of the ball.

>> **How the pitcher moves their torso, hips, legs, and arms during the pitch itself:** These movements help dictate where the ball is going and what kind of movement (curve, slider, and so on) it may have.

>> **How the pitcher slows everything down after the pitch:** At this point, the muscles have to stop the arm. If the pitcher has their body in the right position, some of the pressure is taken off of the shoulder muscles.

REMEMBER

To accurately assess a task and ultimately provide feedback for improvement, you must understand the end goal and the individual components that make up that task.

The specific attributes of the performer

You must consider the level of skill, strength, range of motion, age, gender, and fitness level of the person you're evaluating. Each of these characteristics not only has a significant impact on how a particular task is executed, but also determines whether the athlete is actually even able to perform the desired activity. For example, someone who lacks good balance isn't ready to complete many functional activities like kicking a soccer ball, diving from a platform, or high-jumping. Instead, the athlete needs to be coached on specific techniques aimed at improving balance, like having them practice balancing in various positions. Such tasks enhance body awareness and allow the athlete to be more efficient and to avoid crazy movements that distract from the intended purpose.

WARNING

Unfortunately, folks are too often put in situations that only lead to failure or injury. When we see patients for elbow or shoulder pain, we invariably find that they don't have the core strength or balance needed to safely complete the task — like throwing a shot put — repetitively. By taking a systematic approach to preparing a person for a particular activity — helping the athlete develop the necessary strength, dexterity, or agility, for example — you can often avoid a bad situation.

REMEMBER

Be sure to ask what the athlete's individual goals are. To improve performance? Avoid injury? Reduce existing pain or rehabilitate after an injury? The evaluation you perform for an athlete with performance-related goals is very different from the evaluation you perform for one who wants to reduce their pain. For the athlete recovering from an injury, you examine not only the actual movement but also the training regimen and number of rest days, whereas for the athlete just wanting to get more movement on their curveball, you focus on the mechanics of the movement to determine whether an adjustment needs to be made.

Observing the subject in action

Obviously, you can't make an assessment of a movement, let alone provide feedback, without seeing the person perform the task. In this section, we tell you how to make this observation and what to look for during each phase of the movement. Depending on what you're looking for, you may use a power-and-return model, a three-phase model, or a model that breaks the movements down even more. The following sections go into more detail on the power-and-return and three-phase models, ones that you'll use most often.

Three-phase model

To make sense of what you see, you need to break the movement down into various segments, or phases. All complex movements require *preparation*, *execution*, and *follow-through* components, and each of these phases has a series of movements that must occur in order for the next phase to follow and be successful. When you break a movement into these components, you're using the *three-phase model*:

> » **Preparation phase:** Before each movement or task, preparatory work needs to be done. (For the purposes of this discussion, the preparation that we're talking about is the actual activity, not previous training and that sort of thing.) Getting into a position that facilitates the impending movement is the key to this phase. Proper preparation provides a firm foundation on which the athlete can perform the task competently and safely. To prepare for a standing long jump, for example, you squat down by bending at the knees, hips, and ankles — a position that maximizes the muscular force output (refer to Chapter 3 for information about the length-tension relationship). This stance helps you push off in a way that lets you jump as far as you can.

REMEMBER

Other important considerations include timing and positioning on the court, field, or track. For example, the angle at which you release the javelin is also critical to successfully executing the task. Although it may not be directly related to the task (the jump) itself, it's closely related to the success or failure of the event.

>> **Execution phase:** During this phase, the athlete's body executes the movement. They propel the object or jump up and complete that triple axel on the ice. The appropriate timing, strength, and flexibility are required to maximize their performance and avoid injury.

>> **Follow-through phase:** During this phase, the athlete slows down and returns to a normal (starting) position. The follow-through often requires deceleration of the limbs and continuation of the momentum as the body transitions to another task. For example, when you kick a soccer ball, your leg doesn't just stop after you strike the ball. Instead, it continues to move forward as your body follows and transitions to a step, typically followed by running.

Power-and-return model

Some professionals use a *power-and-return model* (also called the *two-phase model*). This model is broken down into — you guessed it — the power and return phases. The *power phase* includes the execution of the task, and the *return phase* encompasses the preparatory phase. (*Note:* Despite the name implying that the power phase happens before the return phase, it does not.)

REMEMBER

This model typically doesn't offer insight into the follow-through of the task as the three-phase model does. If your purpose is to evaluate the outcomes of the task rather than the intricacies that make it up, the power-and-return model may be sufficient; however, if your goal is to look deeply into the task, a three-phase approach is more appropriate.

A step-by-step guide to observing movement

Follow this process when observing the movement (remember, what you look for depends on why you're doing the evaluation or the objective of the performance):

1. **Break the activity up into phases with clear beginnings and endings, if possible.**

   REMEMBER

   TIP

   Most activities are complex in nature; they consist of many movements that need to be sequenced in a particular way. Identify the different phases and break the activity into two, three, or, if needed, more phases.

   Looking deeper into the movement, most examiners also break up each individual phase and define what should happen within each. For instance, the gait cycle of walking consists broadly of the swing and stance phases. However, many biomechanists may break those phases up even further to include pre-swing, heel strike, weight acceptance, push off, and so on. In this case, more detailed assessment occurs, but this strategy isn't typical for most folks or tasks.

2. **Examine the participant as they perform the movement and note whether they move through all the phases and whether they do so in the correct manner.**

For example, if you're evaluating someone throwing, look to make sure the elbow and shoulder are doing what they're supposed to do when they're supposed to do it. Comparing what you see with the established norms (which you know either by personal experience or through research), you identify flaws, which can help you determine whether more complex issues exist. A complex issue commonly seen in throwers, for example, is that they don't move their hips early enough, which usually causes the arm to drag behind as the body moves forward. The end result is a lot of stress on the elbow and less velocity on the ball when released.

TIP

Exploring every aspect of each and every task can be daunting and so time-consuming and complex that it's pretty much impossible. To avoid this trap, try these strategies:

>> **Answer the particular question at hand.** Taking a targeted approach ("Why does my ball hook every time I hit the golf ball," for example) can provide the necessary focus.

>> **Break the motion up into the appropriate phases, based on your purpose.** By incorporating the key elements within each phase, you can appropriately and efficiently analyze their sequencing.

>> **Identify common flaws.** Experts typically have their own abbreviated lists of movement flaws (stance, shoulder positioning, wrist rotation, and club alignment, for example) that they look for. Usually, these common flaws or critical elements have been proven to cause other issues, like poor performance or injury.

REMEMBER

A pitfall that many novice examiners fall into is that they observe the task from only one vantage point, even though most tasks occur in multiple planes of motion (refer to Chapter 8). For example, if you sit behind the backstop, you can see the front of the pitcher and they may look just fine, but when you examine the same pitcher from first base, you may notice they seem to have an extraordinarily long stride. Without witnessing the motion in all planes, you can't make a full assessment. To avoid this trap, look at the task from each of these vantage points. Identifying flaws in any of the three planes of movement is the only way to fully evaluate the movement.

Making your evaluation and diagnosis

Ultimately, the purpose of motion analysis is to correct or improve the performance or avoid injury. To do so, you evaluate the subject's performance, identifying specific flaws and making diagnoses. You may notice, for example, that while shooting a free throw, the athlete doesn't appear to be bending their knees as they should. By evaluating critical elements of the free throw, you're able to diagnosis the movement flaw as a lack of knee movement.

The evaluation process typically involves comparing the athlete's actual performance against predefined critical factors. If the person repeatedly falls outside the normal range for that factor, you note that finding, and intervention can then follow. Read on for things to keep in mind as you perform your evaluation and make your diagnosis.

Being mindful of personal differences

One of the difficulties that exists with motion analysis in living things is that each person is unique. The organic influences of the actual performance — height, strength, previous history of injury, and so on — differ from person to person. Because of these variations, no one looks exactly like anyone else when completing the same task. Even the critical elements of a particular task can vary a bit, which is why a range exists in normal subjects.

WARNING

Just because someone is successful or pain free doesn't mean that person's technique is the right one to emulate. For example, you may think that you should model pitching mechanics after Major Leaguers. After all, they're successful and have lots of media attention. Yet, despite being incredibly effective pitchers, many Major League pitchers are fighting mechanical flaws that ultimately have led to career-ending injuries. If you emulate them, you may find yourself promoting a technique that leads to repetitive injury that can ultimately be the end of a pitching career!

REMEMBER

Mechanics are highly specialized in each individual and don't always translate well to others.

Tying recommendations to the purpose of the analysis

Preventing injury, enhancing performance, and overcoming discomfort are some of the reasons people have their movements analyzed. Each of these reasons requires a unique look into the task, and the diagnosis and intervention recommendations should be related to the analysis's purpose. "How do I jump higher?" is a very different question from "Why does my knee hurt when I jump?," and it requires the examination of a different set of key elements (even though, at times, they may be related).

Taking into account repetition and situation variability

Take a look at multiple repetitions in both practice and game situations. Examining someone during a practice yields different information than you get if you examine that person during a game. Also, if you take a look at only one repetition of the task, you can't be sure that what you see is actually what the athlete typically does. What you see between the scenarios is sure to surprise you — and make your analysis more accurate and helpful.

WARNING

One thing you're sure to experience is that of *analyst bias*. We all have our own ways of looking at things and our own perspectives that impact what we think constitute critical factors and optimal performance. Analysts who don't take into account the whole person during an evaluation and who try to fit everyone into the same model are missing the boat. Cookie-cutter analysts just don't get the big picture of the individual.

A seasoned expert identifies the unique factors of each participant and paints a full picture of both that person's performance and their flaws. In the end, the well-researched practitioner who stays up-to-date on the most current literature and trends in performance analysis is best able to provide the most robust assessment.

Providing intervention and feedback

What good is coming up with a diagnosis of the flaws in someone's mechanics if you don't provide feedback and intervention strategies? Saying what's wrong with someone's motion is generally easy; figuring out how to correct it is a bit more challenging. Key to providing feedback and intervention is having deep knowledge of the task at hand; relevant information about the participant's strength, injury status, and performance; and an understanding of the participant's goals.

Giving feedback

Based on what you know about the client, you can prioritize the feedback you give. Basically, you want to make deliberate decisions about what information to share and when. Here are some tips to keep in mind:

>> **Prioritize the information.** Your client may not be able to absorb all the information or correct all their flaws at one time; therefore, you need to

decide what information to share and when. For example, when you do mechanical analyses on patients with multiple critical flaws, you may provide feedback only on the most critical flaws and/or the ones that, if remediated, can help improve other aspects.

>> **Organize the feedback in specific phases or in an order that facilitates growth or improvement.** Some tasks require significant practice and a step-by-step approach to be accomplished. As you decide what information to provide your clients, consider things like the best way to improve a skill, the level of difficulty of the different components, which tasks support others, the sequence in which the tasks are performed, which actions are key to preventing injury, and so on.

For instance, say that you want to attempt a new dive off of the high jump; you don't just climb up the ladder and jump off. Instead, you spend lots of time on the ground, working on the phases and the motion sequences to build up the strength or range of motion necessary to complete the dive. After the ground-level work, you progress to a trampoline, and then you go into the pool. Considering a progression of skills is important when you establish plans for integration back to the activity.

>> **Provide examples, where necessary.** For improvement to be successful, the participant must have proficiency in the movement, know what's expected, and know how the movement is broken down. Providing solid examples like videos or still images is invaluable.

TIP

With tablet applications and digital image sharing, providing these examples is incredibly easy. Make sure, however, that your clients truly understand what you're sharing. If you use visual models, consider walking them through what you're looking at on-screen to make sure they're clear about what you're pointing out.

>> **Speak the lingo.** Every sport has its nuances and technical jargon, and part of your effectiveness as an examiner depends on your ability to speak the lingo. Doing so helps you build trust and give the participant confidence in your recommendations.

TIP

Engage patients or players and help them see the importance of improving their performance. Being told that they just aren't as good as they may have thought or that they're at risk of significant injury can be overwhelming or crushing emotionally. Some people will just quit and move on; others will be so overwhelmed that they won't know where to start. That's where your encouragement and feedback are vital.

Studying Motion Analysis Examples

In this section, we include a few common tasks to demonstrate how movement analysis works. By going through both simple and complex tasks, you can see how to apply motion analysis to activities you experience regularly. The model we use here breaks down the activities into phases, as well as identifies the joint actions within each. For a review of the different analysis models and the phases in them, refer to the earlier section "Observing the subject in action."

Note: Some models go as far as listing the muscles that cause each joint action and explaining how those muscles work. Although this information can be very valuable to the examiner, especially when giving feedback, for our purposes, we just stick to the phase breakdown and the individual movements that cause each.

TIP

By using the processes presented earlier in this chapter and following the examples we include here, you should be able to complete your very own motion analysis. Of course, you'll need to decide what the goal is (for example, performance enhancement or injury prevention). But after you decide on those factors, you'll be on your way to being a full-fledged biomechanist. Here are some activities you can try:

» Making a free throw

» Standing from a seated position

» Shoveling dirt

» Swinging a golf club

» Making a tennis serve

Analyzing a squat

The squat is considered a key exercise in the sporting world because it strengthens a lot of the lower-extremity muscles. A number of sporting activities are jumping and running related, so this exercise is a good one. However, if done incorrectly, injury can result.

In Figure 10-1, you can see how a relatively simple task can easily be broken down, using the power-and-return model. In this case, the analysis begins when the athlete is in the upright position and gets the bar off the rack. (The act of lowering to a full squat position can also be referred to as a *preparatory activity*.) In the power phase of the squat, the athlete rises up from a squat position, and in the return phase, they lower back down to a squat. Here are the details:

>> **In the power phase:** The individual joint motions in this phase include knee extension, hip extension, back extension, and ankle plantar flexion. Because the back doesn't really move during this phase, its action is *isometric* (muscle contraction without movement); the other actions are all moving.

>> **In the return phase:** This phase is generally the opposite to the power phase. The knee flexion, hip flexion, back extension (again), and ankle dorsiflexion occur. The muscles in the back that cause the extension do so isometrically, which is why they don't cause motion.

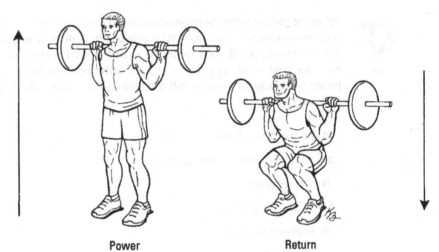

FIGURE 10-1:
Power and-return phases of the squat exercise.

Power   Return

Illustration by Kathryn Born, MA

Some of the common flaws when doing a squat include the following:

>> A poor base of support, in which the feet are placed either too close together or too far apart. Typically, they should be shoulder-width apart.

>> People come down too far during the return phase, putting undue stress on their hips and knees.

>> During the power phase, people begin to lean forward and rely on their backs to pull them upright again — a real killer on those muscles! By looking straight ahead instead of at the ground, they can help avoid the problem of leaning forward.

Checking out your gait (walking)

Unlike a squat, walking is a considerably complex task. Walking challenges every aspect of your balance because it involves continually shifting your weight and executing complex sequences of motions for each joint involved. It's no wonder that, as people age, they tend to fall more and more frequently.

In this example, we break the gait cycle into eight phases (although it can be broken into more or less, based on the preferences of the person doing the analysis). In the gait cycle, the phases include both legs, typically one in contact with the ground and the other in a swinging phase. As you can tell from Figure 10-2, as one leg completes a particular phase, that same phase begins on the other leg, a pattern that occurs over and over and over again as you walk.

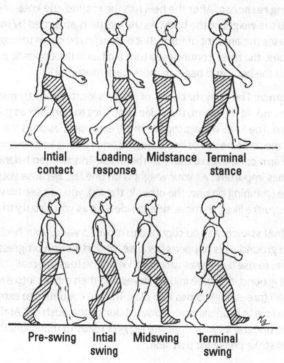

Intial contact   **Loading response**   **Midstance**   **Terminal stance**

Pre-swing   **Intial swing**   **Midswing**   **Terminal swing**

FIGURE 10-2: The phases of walking.

Illustration by Kathryn Born, MA

Here's what's happening during the different phases:

>> **Initial contact:** The heel of one leg makes contact with the ground. To achieve initial contact, the leg needs to get to the point where the heel can land. For this to occur, the hip flexes and pulls the leg forward (an action we discuss further in the swing) as the knee extends and the ankle is dorsiflexed in an attempt to get the heel ready to hit. Further up the chain, take a look at the torso and arms. You can see that the arm opposite the striking heel is swinging forward while the torso rotates toward that front foot. *Note:* Some people call this motion the *heel strike;* we use the term *initial contact* because more than just the heel is affected here.

In *dorsiflexion,* or as you *dorsiflex,* your toes get closer to your shin, even though you aren't lifting your toes up.

>> **Loading response:** After the heel hits the ground, the knee and hip flex to absorb the weight of the body. As the weight is absorbed by this process, it decreases the amount of force that is transferred down through the heel. At this point, the torso continues to turn a bit, and the opposite arms are still in front of the body and begin to move back (posterior).

>> **Midstance:** The body, or center of mass, is located directly over the foot on the ground. At this point, the ankle continues to dorsiflex as the body moves forward. The knee moves toward more extension, as does the hip. At this point, the torso becomes more neutral and returns to its beginning position as the arm continues to move farther back. This is when balance really becomes important. All your weight is on one leg. Because your legs are side by side (standing on one, the other in the air), you can see how, during this phase, you're likely to move side to side a bit as you also try to move forward.

>> **Terminal stance:** As you continue to move forward, your heel begins to lift off the ground. This happens because, as dorsiflexion progresses, it causes the heel to rise (known as *windlass*). When the toes are really the only things on the ground, the knee initially flexes and then moves into extension as the push-off (pre-swing) comes into play. The hip continues to extend back and plays a role in propelling you forward during the push-off. At this point, you remain upright, as your opposite leg gets ready to move into the initial contact or heel strike phase for that side.

>> **Pre-swing:** The pre-swing phase is pretty much the same as the terminal stance, but the emphasis is different. The goal of the terminal stance phase is to achieve a position in which the toes are the only thing on the ground. In the pre-swing phase, the focus is on the act of propelling you forward. To achieve transition to the next phase, push-off must occur, and it's achieved with *plantar flexion* at the ankle (which points the ankle and toes to the ground), extension at the knee and hip, and, once again, an upright posture at the torso and head. Some people also refer to this phase as *push-off* or *propulsion.*

>> **Initial swing:** The pre-swing's effect on propelling the person forward demands that the foot be picked up higher so that it doesn't drag or catch on the ground. In the initial swing phase, the ankle is dorsiflexed (lifting the ankle and foot up) to clear the ground and not trip. Meanwhile, the knee is flexed, as is the hip; a lag in either of these motions causes you to catch your toe and trip. At this point, the same-side shoulder is flexed but moving back, and the opposite side arm is back and, like the leg, is moving forward.

>> **Midswing:** The continuing forward motion of the leg makes up the midswing. In this phase, the hip continues to flex while the knee begins to extend and prep for the terminal phases and heel strike. The same-side arm continues to move back while the opposite arm moves forward; the torso rotates toward the leg that is up. The ankle is still dorsiflexed to make sure the foot is clearing the ground.

>> **Terminal swing:** At the terminal swing phase, the leg slows down its forward momentum a little to achieve an optimal stride length. If the terminal swing phase doesn't control momentum of the leg moving forward as it should, you overstep. The hip continues to flex, the knee extends to maximize the stride without overstretching, and the ankle begins to plantar flex. Stepping with too short of a stride causes the impending initial contact to occur too early, and you won't land on your heel as you should.

The surface you're walking on has effects on each of these phases and the extent to which some of the motions occur. For example, if you're walking on a sandy beach, you have to push a lot harder in the terminal stance and pre-swing phases, but the loading response creates less knee and hip flexion because soft ground has fewer forces.

REMEMBER

The key difference between walking and running is that, when running, at some point, the whole body is off the ground, usually referred to as *flight*. Additionally, you usually don't see the heel hitting the ground when you run; instead, the contact almost exclusively occurs at the front of the foot and toes.

As complex as walking is, you don't really think about it much. Pretty cool, huh? Chalk that up to your amazing body!

Observing a kick in action

Another complex developmental task most kids use growing up is the kick. A kick involves integrating movements between both upper and lower extremities, as well as between left and right limbs, and it requires precision upon execution. Heck, who doesn't want to score a goal? Timing and sequencing of each phase are integral.

To keep things relatively simple, we use a penalty kick approach as the example (see Figure 10-3). With a penalty kick, the athlete doesn't have to negotiate around a defender, moving targets, and so on. The logical way to break this task up is into the preparation (approach), execution (kick), and follow-through phases.

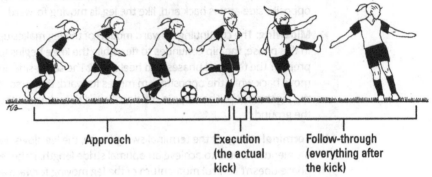

FIGURE 10-3:
The phases of a soccer kick.

Approach

Execution
(the actual kick)

Follow-through
(everything after the kick)

The approach

The approach, illustrated by the first four motions shown in Figure 10-3, includes movements from stepping up to the ball to planting next to the ball in preparation for the strike (when you put one foot next to the ball and begin to kick it with the other one).

Refer to the preceding section, "Checking out your gait (walking)," to understand the movements of the knee, hip, and ankle during this phase. Where the approach begins to differ is in the way you begin to lean forward and rotate your body as you move toward planting next to the ball.

When you plant, you have to maintain your balance on one side. In this case, the actions are largely isometric in the planted leg. The striking (kicking) leg begins to draw back to wind up by flexing at the knee and extending at the hip as the torso rotates to the side of the planted foot. The torso's leaning forward facilitates the explosiveness of the strike and is an important aspect of this phase.

The execution

In the execution phase (which happens between the fourth and fifth image in Figure 10-3), the kicking-side knee extends and the hip flexes as the ankle plantar flexes until it makes contact with the ball. While the leg is being brought forward, the torso begins to rotate quickly toward the striking leg, a movement that helps produce a more powerful kick. The arms follow the torso and rotate, and the non-kicking-side shoulder flexes and *adducts* (comes toward the middle of the body) horizontally while the kicking leg shoulder *abducts* (moves away from the body) horizontally and extends, both with extended elbows.

TECHNICAL STUFF

An interesting side note is that, just before contact, the foot appears fully plantar flexed, but upon making contact with the ball, it's pushed even further into this position because of the force of the contact.

The follow-through

After striking the ball, the torso recoils back to its original position, in essence rotating back away from the kicking-leg side, and the arms return to their original starting position, as the final image in Figure 10-3 shows. The kicking leg then returns to the ground as the hip and knee on the kicking side extend and the kicking ankle dorsiflexes to return to its original position. The non-kicking side pretty much remains the same and continues to stabilize and balance the body.

Analyzing phases in throwing

Considered a survival skill, throwing has various developmental patterns. Although the throwing action can happen in several different ways (shot put, javelin, and so on), here we explore the baseball pitch because it's a good example of a complex task that is highly dependent on sequencing and timing. Pitching a baseball involves and relies heavily on the coordination between the lower and upper extremities, as well as coordination between both sides of the body. While the throwing side does one thing, the glove hand does another.

Even though baseball pitchers often pitch in two different types of motions (the windup and the stretch), we limit the discussion here to the throwing motion related to the windup mechanism. In this example, we break the pitch up into six separate phases (see Figure 10-4): windup, early cocking, late cocking, acceleration, deceleration, and follow-through.

The windup

Despite being the namesake of the entire process, the windup can also be one of the individual phases within this analysis technique. This particular portion of the pitch sequence includes all movement that occurs up until the ball is removed from the glove.

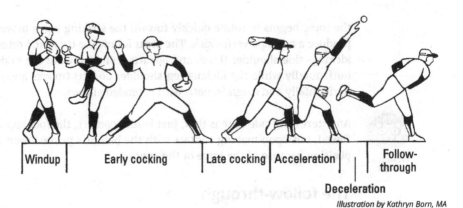

Illustration by Kathryn Born, MA

FIGURE 10-4:
The phases of a
baseball pitch.

| Windup | Early cocking | Late cocking | Acceleration | Follow-through |

Deceleration

The pitcher gets to the top of the pitching mound and stands on the rubber. At this point, everything starts. Here's what happens during this phase:

1. **Standing on the rubber, the pitcher begins to step backward and then rotates and brings their leg up in preparation to step toward the plate and throw.**

2. **To achieve the upright position, the player flexes their hip and knee while their ankle is on the stepping, or** *lead,* **leg (the one in front) typically plantar flexes. At the same time, the abdominal muscles, the gluteal muscles (buttocks), and the back all work to maintain a balanced position.**

   In this stage, the glove hand and ball hand are in the mitt with the elbows flexed and upper arms at the sides.

3. **The pitcher begins to push off the rubber, with the planting foot (the foot on the same side as the throwing arm) toward the plate and batter.**

   To push off, the planting ankle dorsiflexes initially and then quickly changes over to plantar flexion while the knee and hip both extend on that side. As with the gait cycle, the leg that was initially raised is being driven toward home plate and extended at the knee and hip while the torso begins to rotate. Additionally, the hip is abducted in an attempt to make the necessary lateral move toward the plate.

Early cocking

When the ball is removed from the glove, the early cocking phase begins. The movements between the upper and lower extremities must be integrated during this phase:

>> **Lower extremity:** The front leg continues to move toward the plate while the back (push-off) leg propels the body forward. In the front leg, the ankle is plantar flexing, the knee is extending, and the hip is both abducting (moving away from the body to the side) and externally rotating. In the push-off leg, the knee and hip are both extending as the ankle plantar flexes. One of the keys to this phase is that the abdominals must contract, effectively rotating the torso to the side of the body opposite from the ball.

>> **Upper extremity:** In the throwing arm, the shoulder joint is being both horizontally abducted and externally rotated. The elbow moves from a flexed position to an extended position. On the glove side, the shoulder flexes and rotates externally, and the elbow extends as the pitcher prepares to move the glove toward the target.

Late cocking

Just as with the early-cocking phase, both upper and lower extremities are involved in the late-cocking phase. Remember that, throughout this phase, the ball is still in the hand:

>> **Lower extremity:** The center of mass (torso) has moved forward significantly, and the front leg begins to assume a lot of the body's weight. The foot is in full contact with the ground, and the ankle is more dorsiflexed than previously. The knee flexes to absorb the body weight, and the hip flexes and rotates internally. Continuing its movement from the early-cocking phase, the torso continues to rotate, effectively transferring energy from the lower extremity to the upper extremity.

>> **Upper extremity:** The arm moves backward, even as the lower extremity moves forward a good bit. To generate velocity, the torso twists. The throwing-side shoulder joint (the glenohumeral joint) continues to rotate externally and abduct horizontally while the elbow begins to flex as the body moves forward. The glove arm now is being drawn back as the shoulder extends and the elbow flexes.

REMEMBER

This phase is important for three reasons:

>> This is the primary phase where energy is transitioned between the lower and upper extremities.

>> In this phase, the shoulder is asked to go abruptly from external rotation to internal rotation in preparation for the acceleration phase.

>> How the athlete performs during this phase of the pitch is integral to avoiding shoulder injury and instability.

Acceleration

Acceleration is characterized by the ball finally moving forward until it leaves the hand. Again, both lower and upper extremities play key roles in this phase of the pitch:

>> **Lower extremity:** Through knee flexion, ankle dorsiflexion, hip flexion, and internal rotation, the front leg continues to absorb the weight of the body as the center of mass moves forward. Meanwhile, the back leg finally pushes off the rubber by extending the hip and knee and plantar flexing the ankle. After the initial push-off, the knee flexes and the hip continues to extend until the deceleration begins to happen.

>> **Upper extremity:** During this phase, the ball moves forward from behind the body. The throwing arm adducts horizontally and rotates internally to propel the ball forward. In addition, the elbow of the throwing arm extends while the torso continues to rotate to the opposite side. The glove arm essentially isn't doing much besides tucking itself toward the side of the torso and holding still.

TECHNICAL
STUFF

Believe it or not, this phase isn't the one that has the most muscle activity. That accolade goes to the deceleration phase (explained next). What does happen of note here is that the shoulder rotates the fastest during this phase.

Deceleration and follow-through

Although typically referred to as two separate phases, the motions of deceleration and follow-through are pretty much the same, with a key difference: The deceleration phase includes a very distinct difference in muscle activity.

The arm needs to slow down at this point in the pitch; therefore, the muscles fire a lot to brake (slow) the internal rotation and horizontal adduction that's occurring. This braking occurs in the deceleration phase, whereas the follow-through is a continuation of the motion, but the muscle activity quiets down tremendously. In fact, the deceleration phase is where most muscle activity occurs.

Here's what happens in both the lower and upper extremities:

>> **Lower extremity:** As the body continues to move forward, the lead leg still accepts the weight through knee flexion, ankle dorsiflexion, and hip internal rotation and flexion. In addition, in this phase specifically, the torso begins to flex forward in an attempt to absorb and help slow down the body after ball release. The back leg now begins to rise up behind the body by extending the hip and flexing the knee as the body leans forward.

>> **Upper extremity:** Long after the ball has been released, these two phases result in the throwing shoulder continuing to adduct horizontally and rotate internally, while the elbow finishes in flexion. The glove hand sustains its position next to the torso, and the phase ends with the player assuming a position where they're ready to field the ball.

Common pitching flaws

Some major flaws that can be identified during this activity include:

>> **The lack of balance during the windup:** If you aren't able to maintain balance during windup, you begin to lean, throwing everything else off.

>> **Pitchers not initiating their hips early enough:** This problem commonly occurs in the early-and late-cocking phases and leads to a decrease in external rotation. Often, throwers don't move their hips as they rotate. Instead, they try to accomplish all that rotation in their spine, which isn't designed for that.

>> **Players dropping their elbows and nearly pushing the ball:** This issue occurs during the acceleration phase.

WARNING

Because this flaw can potentially be catastrophic, causing ligament damage, it needs to be addressed early.

>> **Lack of follow-through:** Mitigating the forces created during the entire motion is important; otherwise, you end up relying on the little rotator cuff muscles to slow everything down. Proper body positioning and going through the necessary follow-through phase lets the arm slow down without putting undue stress on the limb.

4

Improving Fitness and Performance: Putting It All Together

Chapter **11**

Improving Physical Fitness: Training Wisely

There is no one-size-fits-all method for designing exercise programs. Everyone's goals may be different. Want to lose weight? Set a personal best in the 10K? Need to gain strength, or just be strong enough to handle your work tasks? We may all be exercising for different reasons, but the tools we use to design our programs are the same. The trick is to match the exercise training to the individual's goals, progress safely and wisely, and let time help them achieve their goals. This chapter introduces the components of exercise planning, along with the basic exercise prescription guidelines to help you get started on developing your training plan.

Thinking of Exercise like a Dose of Medicine

When you're prescribed medication, the drug is usually given by the size of the dose (intensity), the number of times per day to take it (frequency), and how long the drug will last (duration). If you look at exercise as a treatment, we also use similar "dosing" strategies. Depending on the individual, the intensity of the exercise will vary, as well as the frequency and the duration. Should you take your medicine all at once, like a high-intensity exercise done for a short period? Or should the dose be spread out at a lower intensity over time? You have to design a program that is tolerable and makes sense for the person doing it!

REMEMBER

Don't just copy someone else's training program. Everyone has a unique body, different levels of fitness, and different goals. Design for the individual who's doing the training.

WARNING

Before getting started, you should know as much about the individual as you can. Have they been to a doctor for their annual physical? Is the physician aware that they're starting an exercise program? What old injuries do they have that may present a challenge? Any heart, lung, or other health issues such as diabetes? These conditions mean that more care and planning are needed in the program. Training wisely means training safely. Be sure to communicate with other health professionals working with the individual.

How much aerobic exercise is enough? The minimum dose for health

Any amount of aerobic exercise is better than nothing, so don't fixate on amounts like it's all or nothing. Just get them moving! Also, remember that the accumulation of work is what matters, so 5 minutes walking the hallways at work, another 10 minutes walking to that lunch spot, maybe a nice 30-minute walk after lunch, a 15-minute dog walk after work. . . . That's one hour of exercise! Do that three days a week, and they have 180 minutes. People need to see that this is doable!

TIP

Ease them in. You probably don't just jump into a cold swimming pool. Most people ease in, get used to it, and then go in deeper. If exercise is new for someone, ease them in! They don't have to be at their full exercise intensity initially — get them used to moving and allow some time for a little soreness to go away. Let the body adjust! They have time — after all, this exercise program should be with them for a long time to come.

Parts of the aerobic exercise plan: Frequency, intensity, time, type

Any exercise program involves a stimulus (workout) with recovery time. Consistent exercise-recovery periods lead to conditioning. The frequency of the exercise helps to spread out the exercise and allow recovery time, while modifying the duration (time) of exercise adds to the overall volume of the workout. Probably the hardest to get just right is the intensity of exercise: Too light, and you don't get a training effect. Too heavy, and they may be too fatigued to do the next workout! Finally, the mode or type of exercise can be adjusted for comfort, to accommodate any physical limitation, or simply to choose something fun! The following sections look at these components and some basic guidelines.

Frequency

The total volume of exercise is the most important aspect of gaining health benefits from exercise. Frequency is something that can be modified both within a single day of exercise, as well as across a week.

What's better: a 30-minute workout, or three 10-minute workouts across a single day? Both are fine! It's the total minutes accumulated that matters. You can modify the frequency even within a single day.

REMEMBER

The goal is to get at least 150 minutes of moderate intensity exercise, so three to five days of exercise is recommended. That may be a lot to start with. If so, start with two or three days, and as you gain conditioning, try to add a day. They can also do 75 minutes of vigorous activity to attain the same dose. Perhaps a combination of each may suit them best.

Intensity

How hard should you exercise? This is often the big question — and often misunderstood. Many people feel that exercise must be "hard" to be good, and that's simply not true. In fact, for the very unfit, even light exercise intensity can provide health benefits. Exercise intensity choices may vary depending on your goals:

>> **Light intensity:** Good for people with very low levels of fitness and who are just getting started. You may also exercise at a light intensity if the exercise is new to you and you need to gain some skill, or perhaps you're nursing a strain.

>> **Moderate intensity:** Good for people trying to accumulate their 150 minutes per week. Maybe you're trying to lose body fat, and moderate-intensity exercise maximizes fat use. Moderate intensity is beneficial for both general conditioning and body composition control.

>> **Vigorous:** Good for people who are going for 75 minutes of vigorous activity per week. Maybe you're training for a 5k, a 10k, or some type of event where performance is measured. Maybe you're trying to accelerate gains in fitness.

Choose the intensity that best suits your goals and is something you can manage. Don't jump into high-intensity exercise right away.

Often, exercise intensity is based on some peaks measurement, like heart rate or VO_2 max. But there are other ways as well. Some are good for general exercisers and others are better for athletes. The following sections cover some common ones.

HEART RATE METHODS

Typically, heart rate zones first need some maximal heart rate value to start from. If you can't get this measured, then estimated (based on age) maximal heart rate can be used. The most common basic formula is 220 – age. So, for example, a 35-year-old would have an estimated maximal heart rate of 220 – 35 = 185 beats per minute (bpm).

After you have a maximal heart rate, there are two common heart rate prescription methods:

» **Percent HR max:** Multiply your maximal heart rate by a percentage (as a decimal) to determine intensity:

- **Light intensity:** 57 percent to 63 percent of max heart rate

- **Moderate intensity:** 64 percent to 76 percent of max heart rate

- **Vigorous intensity:** 77 percent to 95 percent of max heart rate

Using the example of a 35-year-old, at a moderate intensity of 67 percent of max heart rate would be 185 × 0.67 = 124 bpm. A single heart rate value is hard to get to, so give them a +/–5-beat range on each side of the value (so 119 to 129 bpm).

» **Heart rate reserve method:** This method factors in resting heart rate, so you need to measure that. Let's say that 35-year-old has a resting heart rate of 65 bpm. The formula is a little more tricky:

Heart rate= [(max heart rate – resting heart rate) × intensity as decimal] + resting HR

If we use that 35-year-old and an intensity of 67 percent (moderate) here is what we get

Heart rate = [185 – 65) × 0.67] + 65

[120 × 0.67] + 65

80 + 65

145 bpm

Factoring in a +/–5-beat range to gives you a heart rate training zone of 140 to 150 bpm.

Notice how the same intensity gives different heart rate ranges with different methods? The methods differ because one is including resting heart rate. More data is better, so if you can get a resting heart rate, then using the heart rate reserve method is preferable.

PERCEPTUAL METHOD

Have you ever gone for a run and just picked your own intensity, maybe based on your internal feelings of physical stress, effort, and fatigue? If so, you were using a perceptual method of intensity regulation. Nice work! It takes practice to cue into those sensations, but there is a perceptual scale you can use to help.

The verbal cues associated with the numbers (see Table 11-1) help you select either the intensity you're experiencing or the intensity you're trying to attain. You can always use that scale to find your comfortable intensity and then measure your heart rate to get additional information.

TABLE 11-1 **Effort Perception Scale**

Scale	Label	Description
10	Maximum effort	It feels almost impossible to keep going. You're completely out of breath and unable to talk. You can't maintain this level of activity more than a very short length of time.
9	Very hard	It's very difficult to maintain this exercise intensity. You can barely breathe, and you can speak only a few words.
7–8	Vigorous	This level of activity is borderline uncomfortable. You're short of breath, and you can speak only a sentence.
4–6	Moderate	You're breathing heavily, but you can carry on a short conversation. You're still somewhat comfortable, but the activity is becoming noticeably more challenging.
2–3	Light	You feel like you can maintain this activity for hours. It's easy to breathe and carry on a conversation.
1	Very light	This level of activity requires hardly any exertion, but it does involve more than sleeping, watching TV, or reading a book.

VO₂ MAX METHOD

For aerobic athletes, you may want to select intensity using more sophisticated methods. Chapter 4 talks about VO_2 max as the measure of maximal aerobic fitness. Having that maximal value (usually measured in a lab) can help identify your peak fitness. Intensity is then based on a percentage of max.

TALKING THE TALK: EXERCISE INTENSITY TERMINOLOGY

On a treadmill, it's easy to find the exercise intensity measurements (such as heart rate and perception of effort) or work rate measurements (such as speed and grade). But when you're prescribing exercise on a leg ergometer, for example, or basing the prescription on oxygen consumption, you need to understand a couple of terms:

- **Metabolic equivalents (METs):** Resting oxygen consumption is 3.5 mL of oxygen for each kilogram of body weight. So, instead of calculating a specific value for training, you can use a system that equates work in terms of resting metabolism. One MET is equal to the oxygen used while at rest; three METs is an intensity three times that of rest. In this way, you can give a cost to an activity. Walking at a moderate pace may be 3.5 METs. When prescribing exercise, you can set a MET intensity target for training, and then find activities or work intensities that match the goal.

- **Watts:** If you ever exercise on stationary cycles, ellipticals, and other aerobic training devices, you may see exercise intensity identified in watts. This is the standard measurement for power, or work that is done per unit time. Add more load, and watts increase. Pedal faster, and watts increase. Do both, and watts *really* increase. For prescribing exercise, watts are used to set specific levels of work on an exercise device for an individual.

Exercise training intensities based on percent of VO_2 max would be the following:

- » **Light intensity:** 37 percent to 45 percent
- » **Moderate intensity:** 46 percent to 63 percent
- » **Vigorous intensity:** 64 percent to 90 percent

ANAEROBIC THRESHOLD METHOD

VO_2 max is the primary measure of fitness, but the anaerobic threshold (AT; see Chapter 4) is an excellent tool for establishing the highest aerobic work intensity without the accumulation of lactic acid. Often, race pace for distance events 10K or longer is strongly linked to this intensity; it can also be used as a center point for interval training.

The AT can be identified using repeated blood lactic acid measures during a VO_2 max stress test. The sudden rise in lactic acid levels help identify the AT work rate. In athletes under normal dietary conditions, we can also use sudden changes in CO_2 accumulation or ventilation (respiratory rate × tidal volume), because some lactic acid is converted to CO_2, which makes you breathe more heavily. This is the basis for the "talk test," which suggests that if you can't hold a conversation while running, you may be beyond your AT. Figure 11-1 gives an example of identifying the running speed at the AT. The solid lines are regression lines of fit through the data. The intersection of these lines represents the onset of the AT.

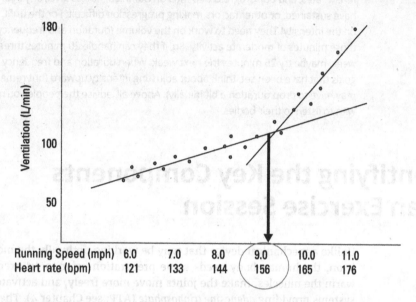

| Running Speed (mph) | 6.0 | 7.0 | 8.0 | 9.0 | 10.0 | 11.0 |
| Heart rate (bpm) | 121 | 133 | 144 | 156 | 165 | 176 |

FIGURE 11-1: Identifying the running speed and heart rate at the anaerobic threshold.

Time

The duration and intensity of exercise are inversely related to each other. If you're working at a heavy intensity, the duration must be shorter. Lighter work can be done much longer. So, factor intensity of the exercise as you consider the duration. Also, factor in your goals. If you're aiming for fat loss, low to moderate intensity exercise is warranted, because fat burning is maximized and duration of exercise can be longer.

Type

You can get a training effect using a range of aerobic activities. One common element among these is that large muscle groups are used. The more active the muscle, the greater the calorie burning and conditioning of the heart. Activities can range from walking, cycling, and water aerobics to more sport or conditioning modes, such as jogging or running, rowing, cycling, elliptical training, stair-stepping, swimming, hiking, or cross-country skiing. You can also try recreation activities for conditioning like dancing, racquet sports, basketball, soccer, and so on.

Progression has a big "It depends" attached to it. This is because we all progress at different rates, and our progress depends on our initial fitness level, any injuries we may have sustained, or other factors making progression difficult. For the unfit, take it easy on the intensity! They need to work on the volume (duration and frequency) to try to get those minutes of moderate activity. So, if they can handle 20 minutes three times a week, maybe try 25 minutes the next week. When duration and frequency meet the goals that have been set, think about adjusting intensity upward (but remember you may have to drop duration a bit initially). Above all, advise the people you're working with to listen to their bodies.

Identifying the Key Components of an Exercise Session

Unlike a mechanical device that may be working optimally the moment you turn it on, the human body needs some preparation prior to an exercise session to warm the muscles, make the joints move more freely, and activate the metabolic systems providing *adenosine triphosphate* (ATP; see Chapter 4). The warm-up session is an important part of any exercise session. Following the exercise session, there are waste products of exercise and elevated systems that need to be brought back to a resting state, and standing still is not the answer! The cooldown session is important to safely transition from exercise to rest.

This section offers some key information about the warm-up, exercise, and cooldown sessions.

The warmup

The warmup consists of light movement, often the intended activity but at a lower intensity. Warming the body helps energy systems produce ATP faster, helps the muscles become more flexible, draws blood to the muscles being used for activity and allows the sympathetic nervous system to kick in, preparing the body for movement. Warmups can last 5 to 15 minutes, or longer if you need them. Always ease yourself into activity.

The exercise session

The exercise session may last 10 minutes to 60 minutes or even longer! Individuals should be aware of how they feel during the session. They should monitor training intensity (running pace, watts of work, METs), as well as physical measurements like heart rate and feelings of exertion. How do their legs, joints, and body temperature feel? Should they go slower today? Feeling a bit energetic? Modify as needed.

REMEMBER

Tailor each session to the individual instead of assuming each person can complete a specific workout.

The cooldown

In Chapter 4, we explain that slow-twitch muscle fibers can help clear lactic acid. Use these fibers during a low-intensity cooldown. You may walk, go for a light jog, or reduce the intensity of whatever you were doing during your exercise session. Allow your heart rate and blood pressure to slowly return to near resting levels. Like the warmup, the cooldown can last 5 to 15 minutes or more depending on the activity.

WARNING

Don't just stand still. Blood will pool in your extremities, and your blood pressure may drop. You don't want to get dizzy. But you do want to clear the waste products of exercise.

Building Strength

Weakness and frailty are indicators of poor health outcomes, especially for older individuals. The lack of strength to perform daily activities and to have the strength reserve to handle a major health event (for example, injury, flu, or cancer) points to a low quality of life. Strength matters for people of all ages.

This section addresses the basic principles of strength training, the benefits of strength, the basic guidelines for strength training, as well as some differences in training programming depending on goals.

Understanding the importance of strength training

Fitness isn't just about cardiovascular health — muscular fitness, which is the strength, power, and endurance, also matters. It can be developed only by giving the muscles a load that is heavy enough to induce stress on the muscles, and by activating all the muscle fibers to a point near fatigue. With time, adaptations take place that can add to your overall fitness:

>> Increased bone mass

>> Reducing the risk of falling by preserving powerful fast-twitch fibers

>> Reducing the effort needed for everyday tasks

>> Recovering function lost after an injury or surgery

>> Maintaining function and ability well past 60 years of age

Strength from resistance training gives us a reserve of strength that can help you through illness and age, maintaining your health span and quality of life. Everyone should be doing it!

Strength programming plans for health, performance, and balance

Strength training has common principles for everyone who does it, but there will be differences in the intensity, volume, and even type of exercise according to the individual's fitness and their training goals. Here are some guidelines for strength training across different fitness goals.

Strength training for health and daily function

For beginning lifters, aim for at least two nonconsecutive days per week for each major muscle group. This schedule allows for a stimulus of stress and some rest time for growth. Keep in mind that not every muscle group needs to be exercised on the same day. You can break up days (split the routine), but still aim for two days per week for a muscle group.

Like cardiovascular training, intensity is often a hard one to get just right without some testing. Typically, the intensity is based upon how much you can lift one time, known as your *one-repetition maximum* (1RM).

Beginning lifters should aim for a load that is 60 percent to 70 percent of 1RM. This would be a load that you can lift 12 to 15 times before fatiguing. If a one-rep max isn't possible, try reversing the concept: Find a load you can only lift 12 to 15 times before fatiguing. The key is to have a load heavy enough and to lift to *near fatigue* (fatigue without a change in your lift form).

How many sets of lifts should you do? Well, even one set can help increase strength, especially deconditioned individuals. Two to three sets are recommended and should be sufficient to cause the stress and strain on the muscle to stimulate growth.

There are a variety of ways to create load stress on a muscle group. For general strength, lifts that use multiple joints will involve many muscle groups. However, some exercises may require only a single muscle to be worked, so plan your lift according to your needs. Some types of resistance loads include:

» Body weight

» Elastic bands or tubes

» Resistance poles

» Free weights

» Machine weights

HOW TO PROGRESS IN STRENGTH TRAINING

Progress is easier to chart than you think. When you first start lifting that 20-pound bicep curl, maybe you can do 12 repetitions, and now you can do 15. You're measurably stronger! That means increase the load. How much should you increase it? Well, that depends on the size of the muscle and just how you want to add more overload. Some options include:

- **Increasing the number of sets:** Keep the load the same but just overload by more sets. That may be a safe way to add training stress.

- **Increasing the load by 5 percent:** Maybe that brings the 15 repetitions you did down to only 11 repetitions. Well, now you have a new load stress. Work up to more repetitions!

- **Adding an additional day of training for the muscle group:** Depending on how fast you're recovering, you may be able to add another training day with the same load. Monitor how you feel and how you recover.

Monitor your progress, how your muscles feel, and how you recover. Be ready to adapt or add more challenge.

Strength training for athletic performance

For trained individuals seeking larger improvements in *hypertrophy* (growth in muscle fiber size) and strength, larger training intensities are warranted. Loads as high as 80 percent to 90 percent 1RM with one to six repetitions to fatigue are often used. This is a lot of stress! Be sure to provide those muscles adequate rest to grow between training sessions. Risk of injury goes up with heavier loads.

Training for power requires lighter loads, because heavy loads can't be moved very fast. Loads from 30 percent to 60 percent 1RM are used, and the lifts are done at maximum velocity. With a lighter load, you can move at greater speeds and activate the fast-twitch muscle fibers, which are important to maintain balance and for power performance. For example, maybe an individual has a maximal squat of 200 pounds (that's their 1RM). For strength and hypertrophy training, you may work them at 60 percent of 1RM (200 × 0.60= 120 pounds). But if power development is the goal, you'll emphasize fast movement with a lighter load, say 30 percent of 1RM (200 × 0.30= 60 pounds).

Strength training for balance

Balance is not just about being strong enough to hold your body upright. It's also about coordinating muscles to restore balance when some type of event occurs that knocks you off balance, such as tripping, walking on uneven terrain, or experiencing a sudden shift in your center of mass, like bumping into someone. Training core muscle, such as the abdominal muscle and back muscles can help hold the core steady and help the limbs reestablish balance. Using the principle of specificity of training, something that destabilizes you may be a good training tool. Some methods include:

>> Lifting light loads while sitting on a Swiss exercise ball

>> Standing on a Bosu ball (flat on the bottom, half-ball on the top) and trying to maintain balance

>> Lifting water-filled "slosh tubes" that create turbulence and force you to maintain stability during a lift

In the case of balance training, neural adaptations can play a large role in improving your function. Strength is important, but balance-related exercises are generally not done with a heavy load and not done to complete fatigue. Balance training is often an additional training tool alongside traditional strength training.

VARIATION IN EXERCISES CAN HELP IMPROVE STRENGTH AND FUNCTION

The neuromuscular system adapts within a few weeks to a new lift. You may be wobbly at first, but soon you'll lift smoothly like a pro. That's great! But creating conditions where the muscle and the neuromuscular system must adapt is a helpful training tool. Mix it up a bit. How many ways can you train the bicep? Try some variations. Change the angle of your arm — try a pulling-down motion that uses the shoulder as well as the bicep. These different challenges may help to force different adaptations while also giving some functional adaptations. They may just keep you from becoming bored, too, so that's a plus!

Working on Flexibility Training

Flexibility is the ability to move a joint through its full range of motion. When joints are free to move, you're better able to control your body movement, mobility, and balance. Limitations in flexibility can lead to a reduced ability to move, balance problems, falls, and injuries. Maintaining flexible joints is part of any comprehensive fitness plan.

Flexibility training for functional movement

As part of the principle of specificity of training goes, if you want a joint to keep moving, you must keep moving the joint. Joint flexibility can decline due to inactivity, aging, injury, or a chronic condition such as osteoarthritis. So, the first thing to do if you want to maintain joint range of motion is to *keep moving!*

TIP

To improve joint flexibility, work the following into your fitness plan:

>> **Static stretching:** This is a classic approach to improve joint range of motion by placing the muscles around the joint in a stretched position and holding for 10 to 30 seconds. This activates the Golgi tendon reflex to help relax the muscles (see Chapter 9). You can do this alone in held positions or in yoga-type poses. You can also do it passively, for example, by using a bar to support your leg or by having a partner apply the force to cause the stretch.

>> **Dynamic movement stretching:** Tai chi is a good example of this type of stretching. The exerciser moves slowly from one position to the next, gradually increasing the movement at the joint. This can assist in developing balance while also developing joint flexibility.

>> **Proprioceptive neuromuscular facilitation (PNF) stretching:** This is a contract-relax, partner-assisted type of stretching. The exerciser contracts the muscle they want to stretch against a resistance for 2 to 5 seconds. Then their partner moves the joint through a range of motion until the muscle is placed in a static stretch; this stretch is held for 10 to 30 seconds.

Flexibility training to avoid injury

Many times, injury can happen during exercise or sport when the joint is suddenly placed in a position outside the usual range of motion. If the muscles around the joint aren't adequately prepared, you may be in for a muscle pull, a muscle strain, or worse! The best way to use flexibility training to avoid this is by incorporating it into your workout plan:

>> **The warmup:** The exercise warmup before the activity or event isn't just for turning on energy systems and diverting blood flow. It also warms the muscles, making them more pliable and adding range of motion around the joint. Simply warming up can add a great deal to your range of movement.

>> **Post-warmup stretch:** After the warmup is complete, take a few minutes to utilize one of the stretching methods mentioned in the previous section. Do some static stretches and some gentle movements that take your body through the range of motions you'll be using in the activity. Maybe have a partner help with some specific stretches for muscles particularly at risk of strain.

>> **Post-exercise cooldown:** After you've finished the workout or activity, your muscles may be strained and tight, but still warm. This is a great time to stretch! Take some time to statically stretch muscles that have been put through the workout. Ease the tension in the muscles and help prevent later stiffness. This will help you relax better and let go of any post-exercise tension and strain you may still have.

Chapter **12**

Managing Your Body, Not the Other Way Around

Most people try to get some level of physical activity most days, whether they're taking the stairs on the way up to the office, working in the yard, or training to compete in that upcoming marathon. And odds are, they've all experienced some kind of pain in the process. Sometimes, that pain is bad enough that they can't do the things they want to; other times, it's just a nagging problem that they wish they didn't need to worry about.

In this chapter, we break down some of the common structures that contribute to that discomfort or injury and answer some questions like, "How do I know if I'm injured or hurt?" and "What can I do to make this calf pain go away after my runs?"

Note: This chapter is targeted specifically to individuals getting back into shape or wanting to maximize their fitness. If you're an exercise science student or professional, you can use this chapter to help the people you work with.

Staying Healthy While Staying Active

When you get going and create a routine that you can fit into your everyday life, you don't want it to be derailed or stopped altogether by injury. The key is planning a program that you're ready for and that doesn't require you to do too much too fast. All too often, people jump into a routine full-force, but that can be problematic if your body isn't ready for what you're asking it to do. A well-planned program will put you on the right path.

Getting started

Whether you're thinking about starting to exercise or you're getting back into the gym or onto the court again, consider your goals. Do you want to be the next world-champion pickleball player, or do you just want to get more active and feel a little better? Both are great goals to have, but they require very different paths to achieving them. Do your homework and maybe talk to a personal trainer or other professional who can help you create a pathway to accomplish your goals. In the end, you want to achieve those goals without having unnecessary setbacks and hiccups that ultimately may frustrate you and result in having to stop altogether.

Taking small steps

The easiest way to injure yourself is to do too much too fast. Take your time and let your body adapt to what you're doing. It's normal to feel pretty sore when you start doing exercises or activities you aren't used to. That soreness you feel a couple of days after you do a new activity is called delayed onset muscled soreness (DOMS), and it's common. Soreness is okay — it can even be a good guide that can tell you when you've done too much. Don't be scared that you'll hurt yourself, but be mindful of doing far too much too early. Your body will usually tell you when something isn't going right.

A simple rule is to start somewhat slow and light, meaning if you're running, you should start with a short distance; if you're doing a new lift, start light and work your way to a heavier load after you've mastered the technique and seen how your body has responded. At that point, you can increase your resistance or intensity.

Conditioning best practices

Just because your football, soccer, or basketball coach used to have you run until you got sick doesn't mean that's the best way to work out and get back in shape.

If you were to do that as an adult, you'd probably just get hurt. Instead, plan your program by determining your goals and what you want to accomplish. This is the topic of our conversations with people when we're helping them recover from an injury and get back to their activity goals. Getting into shape is really no different, except you haven't been injured yet.

After you've identified your goals, you'll be able to figure out how to achieve them. For instance, if you want to run for a longer period of time, you need to challenge your endurance, your cardiovascular fitness, and the strength in your legs to allow you to run longer. Your program would include gradual increases in running distances and intensities coupled with strengthening. By planning a program so you vary the workouts every day, you limit the chances of injury while maximizing the chances that you'll reach your goals. As you build on that volume and intensity and you get stronger, you'll notice your body recovering and responding well to the stress you're putting on it.

TIP

You know that you're recovering well and ready for the next increased intensity when, after the workout, your body feels good and isn't too sore and you continue to feel stronger and stronger. It's when you feel like your body is breaking down, not recovering as you'd hoped or when you continue to move forward with your plan when you're feeling some discomfort when injury occurs.

Warming up and cooling down

Most recreational athletes either don't know the importance of the warm-up and cooldown or, if they do, they conveniently forget it. Most people are pressed for time — they just want to walk into the gym and get started working out. And when they're done with the workout, they want to hit the locker room and head on to the next thing on their to-do list. Unfortunately, that's a recipe for disaster.

Your body needs to be prepared to work out. You may be starting your workout minutes after you rolled out of bed, or you may be coming straight from the office where you've been sitting all day. If your muscles haven't really come alive in hours, they can't just turn on like a light switch — they need to be warmed up.

A warm-up doesn't need to take an hour — you just need to get some blood flowing to the muscle groups that you'll be working. A few minutes of dedicated time to prime the muscle groups that you'll be using is plenty. You can even do a general warm-up like walking on a treadmill for a few minutes and then doing some stretching (see Chapter 9).

After a workout, a lot of blood and other fluids have been vigorously circulating through the body. If you just stop and do nothing to help those fluids return to their normal state, you may experience pooling of blood in the extremities, which may cause you to feel lightheaded or dizzy. Additionally, exercise causes micro-damage of the muscles (which you want!), and it's important to facilitate good blood flow return so that new blood, rich in various nutrients, can return to the muscles and help them recover, ultimately facilitating functional gains and decreased soreness.

TIP

A cooldown should include a short low-intensity exercise like walking, swimming, or biking followed by stretching the muscles that were just involved in the workout. It takes about 10 to 15 minutes for most exercises, but with higher intensities consider a more specific and longer cooldown.

Managing discomfort and injury

Discomfort and injury are two different things, and knowing the difference between the two is important. An injury involves damaged tissue that needs rest and some type of treatment or intervention to help it heal and get better. Discomfort, on the other hand, is when you begin to get a little tighter and maybe have some DOMS from the expected micro-tearing in the muscles used in your workouts. Feeling discomfort is something to pay attention to, but you may be fine by modifying your workout or adjusting your volume or intensities to allow the sore tissues to recover. If you continue to push through discomfort, it certainly can become an injury.

If you're truly injured, you shouldn't try to work through the injury to see if it gets better — because it won't. On the other hand, if you're not injured, and you're experiencing some discomfort, that's a normal and expected part of working out, especially if you've recently made a change in your routine. Still, you should pay attention to your body's discomfort and figure out what's contributing to it. Maybe you haven't given yourself enough recovery time after the past few workouts, and now you're starting to feel some discomfort.

REMEMBER

Discomfort can get worse until it reaches the point of an injury — the key is to try to prevent that from happening.

Whenever you're experiencing pain, you may want to seek professional advice from a doctor, athletic trainer, or physical therapist. If you can adjust your workout or technique a bit, you may be just fine.

Understanding Your Body: What Is It Made of and What Force Can It Take?

Movement is all about using the forces that are generated from our muscles and those that are experienced from our environments, and they need to be accommodated for in order to complete the movements or tasks that we do. Every aspect of the musculoskeletal system is built to endure forces, either by generating or mitigating them. Technique is a key factor in ensuring that you remain healthy, whether that's how you walk, throw a ball, or lift a weight. When muscles and the tissues that support movement work together in a unified way, we reach efficiency and minimize the risk of injury or discomfort. In this section, we cover common forces and how they affect the body's function.

Mechanisms of injury

When you're injured, figuring out what happened often requires a bit of detective work. Part of that process is identifying the mechanism of injury, which involves identifying key characteristics that may have led to the injury. Painting that picture requires you to answer questions like:

>> What type of pain do you have?

>> When did you first notice it? What kind of activity were you doing over the few days leading up to the injury?

>> How did the injury happen? For example, do you twist your ankle? Or did you wake up with knee pain?

>> Which direction did your joint turn? How did you land?

>> Did you hear or feel anything at the time of the injury?

>> What has made the injury feel better or worse?

>> Have you ever injured yourself before? How does this injury compare?

By answering questions like these, you can start to collect the data you need to determine how, what, when, and why you're feeling the pain. You can then address the situation and either avoid the contributing factor or otherwise determine the best treatment or rehabilitation plan to get better.

WARNING

If your pain persists or limits what you can do, stop and consult a medical professional for help.

Common structures involved in injury

The bones provide structure and support, while the muscles, tendons, and ligaments (along with other soft tissues like fascia) work together to hold it all together; collectively, they achieve movement and the functions you demand as a functional person. But when one or more of those structures begins to fail or otherwise becomes compromised, the whole systems begins to fold. In the following sections, we explain more about these structures.

Bones

Most people think of bones as hard, unforgiving structures. What they often overlook is just how dynamic and accommodating bones really are. Much of a bone's structure is defined and dictated by its function. As you look closely at a picture of a skeleton, you can see that some bones are intended to assist with load bearing (like walking and running), and others aren't.

You can generally recognize whether a bone is load bearing or not by its size and shape. Load-bearing bones are typically bigger and thicker, whereas non-load-bearing bones are usually smaller. But the outside appearance of the bone isn't the only indication of its function; the inside also provides clues.

The foundations of most bones are:

>> **Calcium carbonate and calcium phosphate:** These are the minerals primarily responsible for bone strength, and they account for approximately 60 percent to 70 percent of a bone's weight. They help dictate its *stiffness* (the extent to which it resists deformation from a force) and *compressive strength* (its ability to resist being squeezed or otherwise shortened), both of which are important determinants of a bone's function. Although these materials play a primary role in a bone's makeup, other materials such as sodium, magnesium, and fluoride also help.

>> **Collagen:** A protein, collagen is responsible for the bone's flexibility and ability to resist *tension* (a pulling force).

>> **Water:** Water enhances the strength of the materials that make up the bone and contributes significantly to nutrient delivery and waste removal. Water accounts for about 25 percent to 30 percent of a healthy bone's weight. When the water content decreases, as it does with aging, bones become more brittle.

The percentage of each of these substances varies by the function, age, and relative health of the person and the bone itself.

To appreciate the various roles bones can play in supporting and contributing to movement and supporting the body, look at their structural components (see Figure 12-1).

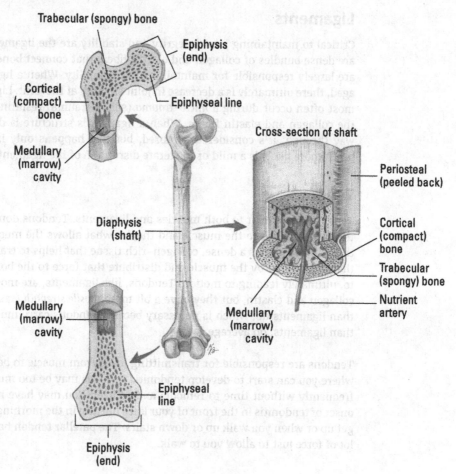

Trabecular (spongy) bone

Epiphysis (end)

Cortical (compact) bone

Epiphyseal line

Medullary (marrow) cavity

Cross-section of shaft

Periosteal (peeled back)

Diaphysis (shaft)

Cortical (compact) bone

Trabecular (spongy) bone

Nutrient artery

Medullary (marrow) cavity

Medullary (marrow) cavity

Epiphyseal line

Epiphysis (end)

FIGURE 12-1: Long bone structure.

Illustration by Kathryn Born, MA

Muscles

Muscles attach to bones via tendons. They create motion or otherwise help stabilize a joint when they contract. In Chapter 3, we cover the structural makeup of muscle and how muscles contract and otherwise contribute to joint motion. Muscles are the primary contributor to providing movement and controlling that movement. While covering joints in Chapter 9, we also explain how muscles contribute to providing stability and work with the ligaments and other soft tissues to make sure the joints remain stable. The size of the *site of insertion* (where the muscle meets the joint), *pennation type* (muscle fiber angular orientation), and location will dictate if the muscle is primarily responsible for providing motion or stability at that joint. Rarely do muscles work independently.

Ligaments

Critical to maintaining joint integrity and stability are the ligaments. Ligaments are dense bundles of collagen and elastin fibers that connect bones to bones and are largely responsible for maintaining joint stability. When a ligament is damaged, there ultimately is a decrease in joint stability at the joint. Ligament injuries most often occur during a *micro-trauma* (subtle trauma) resulting in damage to the collagen and elastin fibers. When a ligament's structure is damaged all the way through, it's considered ruptured, but this happens only in severe cases; much more likely is a mild or moderate disruption of the ligament.

Tendons

Tendons are similar to both muscles and ligaments. Tendons don't contract, but they are attached to the muscle and they're what allows the muscle to attach to the bone. Tendon is a dense, collagen-rich tissue that helps to translate the force that is produced by the muscle and distribute that force to the bone it's attached to, ultimately leading to motion. Tendons, like ligaments, are mostly made up of collagen and elastin, but they have a bit more *tensile strength* (resistance to pull) than ligaments do, which is necessary because tendons carry much higher loads than ligaments, on average.

Tendons are responsible for transmitting loads from muscle to bones, but this is where you can start to develop tendonitis — loads may be too much or occur too frequently without time to remodel and recover. You may have noticed an early onset of tendonitis in the front of your knee hurting in the morning when you first get up or when you walk up or down stairs. The patellar tendon has to deal with a lot of force just to allow you to walk.

Types of stresses and common overloads leading to injury

Each of the structures we mention earlier has a threshold, which determines how much and what kind of force can be applied to it before it fails or positively responds. The threshold is realized by the bones, muscles, ligaments, and tendons being able to accommodate a certain type and amount of force; when forces equal the threshold in both direction and amount, no change in structure occurs, but when the tissue experiences a greater amount, growth can be stimulated. When that force becomes even greater, tissue may break down and become damaged. In essence, muscle, ligament, bone, and tendon have been uniquely designed to handle that activity.

Changing the type or intensity of an activity results in forces exceeding the threshold and stimulating either bone development or collagen synthesis through *fibroblasts* (cells contributing to tissue growth) that exist in the tissues. When forces delivered to the bones decrease and produce less demand, bone mineralization lessens and collagen strength decreases, leading to weakened structures. You need just the right amount of activity and force to keep the structures healthy — too much and they break down, too little and they get weaker. But if they're just right, tissues respond well to the demands placed on them.

Normal weight-bearing and everyday activities, like walking and standing, exert a variety of forces on the bones and soft tissues, including compression, tension, torsion, and shearing:

>> **Compression:** The squeezing force that occurs through normal weight bearing, as your body weight and gravity push down on your frame.

>> **Tension:** The stretch that happens during normal weight-bearing and other physical activities. Tension occurs when a muscle or tendon pulls on a bone at its attachment site to create movement or increase stability. Extending your knee, for example, creates tension on the tibial tuberosity.

>> **Torsion:** A twisting effect. When you're standing and you twist to change directions, torsion is exerted on the *tibia* (leg bone). This twisting is usually combated by the strength in the bone, but sometimes the bone may break.

>> **Shearing:** The tearing across the longitudinal axis. When you stop abruptly and your foot extends in front of you to stop your forward momentum, your leg bone experiences a shear force. Part of the bone wants to continue going in the same direction as your body's momentum, but the foot stopping your forward movement pushes it back.

Identifying Common Injuries

Throughout the course of your life, you'll inevitably experience some sort of injury to your joints. Some will be mildly debilitating; others may require significant rehabilitation and possibly surgery. In the following sections, we cover some of the more common issues that you may find yourself dealing with.

Sprains

A *sprain* involves the disruption of a ligament within a joint. A ligament connects bony structures to other bony structures. Most sprains are not extraordinarily debilitating and only require a few days to recover. However, in some cases, the injury can be severe enough to warrant surgery, either to repair the ligament itself or to repair other structures that were damaged because of the sprain.

TIP

If you sprain a joint, rest it. A compression wrap can help deal with the impending swelling, as can ice. Wrap the joint above and below the injury, keep it elevated, and ice it for 20 minutes or so (but not much longer). Try to move it if you can do so free of pain — that way, you'll help the swelling exit the area so good nutrient-rich blood can get to the joint to help it heal.

Dislocations

A *dislocation* occurs when a joint becoming separated — the two articulating bones come apart, leading to deformity and lack of function. Fingers are commonly dislocated at the joint when baseball players slide headfirst into the base. Another joint commonly dislocated is the shoulder joint (the glenohumeral joint) where it "pops out" and hurts really badly.

WARNING

A dislocation is different from a fracture, even though they often look similar. For that reason, never attempt to *reduce* (pop back in) a dislocation. Without X-rays, you just never know whether you're dealing with a pure dislocation or a fracture that, if moved, may cause significant damage.

Bursitis

Bursas provide lubrication and padding to many joints. Think of them as little oil cans that secrete synovial fluid (see Chapter 9) into the joint when squeezed. The synovial fluid lubricates the joint and its structures. Many folks, especially older people, experience *bursitis* (inflammation of the *bursa*, a small sac between the bone and tendon). Bursitis commonly occurs in the elbows and knees. You may feel discomfort when you move and notice what looks like a rounded squishy growth protruding from the joint. In most cases, bursitis is caused from overuse or not appropriately increasing the intensity of exercise.

Arthritis

Inflammation and pain experienced within a joint is often diagnosed as arthritis. The most common type of arthritis is *osteoarthritis*, a degenerative joint disease caused by the damage to articular (joint) cartilage (see Chapter 9). When healthy, the bones that make up your joints appear white and shiny. As a protective measure, the articular cartilage absorbs forces, lubricates, and provides for better contact within the joint.

Over time or because of injury, this cartilage may become damaged and/or degenerate. When this happens, the *hyaline cartilage* (the cover coating the bones has to absorb these forces and provide the function of the articular cartilage. Unfortunately, it's not made to do this, so it quickly begins to degenerate, resulting in pain, inflammation, and additionally bony changes. These changes continue to be aggravated with physical activity and often lead to the need for a joint replacement.

Tendonitis

Tendonitis (inflammation of the tendons) can cause significant discomfort. Typically, tendonitis is an overuse type of an injury, where the tendons have experienced a lot of stressful activity without a suitable amount of time to recover. It can happen when you do too much too fast, have poor technique, are too tight, or just don't have enough strength for the activities you want to do. Typically, there is a bit of a progression where you start to feel something minor in the tendon after exercise and stay sitting still for a bit after working out. But when you start moving again, it seems to get better or it hurts at the start of your workout but seems to get better quickly. The condition progresses to lasting for longer and affecting more aspects of your day.

TIP

If you notice this progression, first try to alter your activity and perhaps take a rest for a couple of days, which usually helps it. Make sure to get a good warm-up before working out, possibly including the use of a warm pack. After the activity, cool down and possibly ice the area. A good stretching routine may help with tendonitis, too.

Strains

A *strain* is an injury of the muscle or its tendon. When the muscles are overloaded, they can tear and result in a strained muscle. These injuries can be pretty debilitating and range from a minor tear, where only a few fibers are torn, to a major strain, where a majority of the fibers are torn or fully displaced from the bone (known as *ruptures*). When the tendons are involved in a strain, they experience a tearing of the fibers that compose the tendon. Strains usually occur when a muscle is overloaded acutely, is continuously stressed and overloaded over time, or is overstretched.

TIP

If you experience a strain, stop what you're doing and protect the injury by resting it or using a wrap or brace to keep the muscle or tendon from being tensed again.

Fractures

Fractures, officially defined as "a disruption in the continuity of the bone," are the most common type of bone injury. Often referred to as *breaks,* fractures can be debilitating and very painful. Some fractures are minor, requiring only minimal treatment; others are very complex and require surgical treatment.

The kind and severity of the fracture you end up with is dependent on several factors: the type, direction, amount, and timing of the force(s) delivered to the bone, as well as the maturity, nutrition, and hydration of the bone. Figure 12-2 shows what some of those different types of fractures look like.

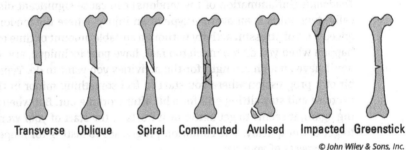

FIGURE 12-2:
Types of bone fractures.

Transverse   Oblique   Spiral   Comminuted   Avulsed   Impacted   Greenstick

© John Wiley & Sons, Inc.

TECHNICAL STUFF

With *stress fractures,* bony deformation doesn't occur, but the bone is damaged because of the repetitive microtrauma. A common reaction to the repetitive microtrauma involves cells known as *osteoclasts* being delivered to the area to absorb the damaged tissue, while cells known as *osteoblasts* follow to deliver new bone to the site. When the bone isn't able to go through a full stress reaction that involves bone absorption and delivery, the cumulative effect is a stress fracture.

Treating Injuries

There are simple but meaningful things that you can do to get better on your own when you're injured. Stretching, strengthening, rest, and recovery are key, but you need to use them at the right time and in the right way or you may not see good results. We cover a few of the common methods for treating injuries in the following sections.

Ice

Swelling is nearly always present when there is an injury, and ice can help reduce swelling. Ice also often helps to decrease pain. But it also makes you feel tight and shouldn't be used just before you go for a workout. The common method of ice application is a bag of ice, but you can use ice cups, ice baths, ice packs, or cold sprays, too.

TIP

Ice when you have inflammation and need to control the negative effects of swelling, like *cell hypoxia*, which occurs when cells don't get enough oxygen, or lack of nutrient delivery to the injured tissue.

TECHNICAL STUFF

Ice helps by decreasing the metabolic needs of the damaged tissues. By decreasing the temperature of the tissue, the tissue needs less oxygen and nutrients.

Heat

Heat is great for preparing the body for activity, especially in the case of tendonitis or for tight muscles. However, heat also increases swelling, which can lead to too much swelling in a damaged area. If you have too much swelling in an area, it can make it difficult or impossible for new oxygen- and nutrient-rich blood to get to the area. Avoid heat — including hot tubs — when you have a recent injury that's still swollen.

TIP

Use heat to stimulate blood flow to a muscle group when you're tight, sore, and stiff from DOMS or otherwise need to loosen up.

Stretching, foam rolling, and massage

The stretching techniques discussed in Chapter 9 are the more common ways you can increase range of motion (ROM) and flexibility in your muscles and joints. However, plenty of other common activities can result in the same increases in flexibility. Many people, for example, regularly engage in pilates and yoga; these exercises and overall health and wellness programs incorporate similar strategies that are aimed at increasing both strength and flexibility.

Another technique that is gaining a lot of popularity, especially with runners, is *soft-tissue mobilization.* Although not necessarily a stretching technique, soft-tissue mobilization can increase the ROM of a joint and create added flexibility in a muscle. It involves self-massage (usually via large foam rollers or balls, but anything that can provide pressure in an area will do the job, like a softball, your elbow or thumb, a massage gun, and so on) and muscle relaxation. By enhancing blood flow and the Golgi tendon organ (GTO) response for muscle relaxation, this technique helps the affected muscle loosen up so it can move better and with less discomfort. Most people use this technique at the *gluteal* (buttocks), *hamstring* (back of upper leg), and iliotibial (*IT*) *band* (outside of upper leg) areas, but any muscle group can benefit.

Another really popular way to accomplish the same goals is to just go and get a massage. In that case, it's a little easier because you can just lay still while the massage therapist does all of the work.

Chapter **13**

Molding the Clay: Body Composition and Weight Management

W e live in a fast-fix society, where there seems to be a "hack" for everything. That may work for a faster way to fold a shirt, but the human body doesn't respond very well to dramatic, short-term weight management programs. The body is a complex system of different tissue types that function together and influence each other. What you try to change in one tissue may influence another. So, any approach to weight loss and weight gain needs to take into consideration how the body adapts to conditions of reduced calorie consumption and exercise. There are limits! Likewise, weight gain is usually focused on muscle and bone mass gain, but some approaches can instead mean putting on a lot of fat!

In this chapter, we take this one step at a time and look at the tissue of the human body, methods of assessing body tissue status, and guidelines for managing weight.

Knowing What Makes Up the Human Body: Body Composition

Humans come in all shapes and sizes, but we consist of the same components. Surprisingly, most of our mass is water! On average, water makes up about 60 percent of our body (more if you're young, less if you're old). Our shape would have no structure without bone, which is another 7 percent to 15 percent of our mass. The remaining mass is split between muscle and fat and tends to change the most. Managing weight really means managing the components of body composition. Some parts we don't want to lose, while others are free to go!

Fat: Subcutaneous, visceral, and more

Human evolution has been a history of food scarcity. When we found food, we had to eat up while we could and then store the rest as fat in the body for later! Fat is essential for formation of nerves, cell membranes, and hormones, and it's a dense-storage form of a lot of energy. Fat-soluble vitamins can't be stored without fat, and fat protects organs and insulates the body from heat and cold. Fat is the least dense of the tissues and contains almost no water.

Location matters! Where we store our fat can contribute to heart disease risk:

>> **Subcutaneous fat:** As the name suggests, this is the fat under the skin. It's the stuff you can pinch. The arms, hips, legs, and belly hold subcutaneous fat.

>> **Visceral fat:** Visceral fat is deep within the body, often covering organs. It's the bad kind of fat. When the distribution is in the upper body, the risk of heart disease is higher than those who hold the fat more in the lower body.

>> **Other locations:** Fat covers many nerves for faster signal transfer. Fat is also in bone marrow. And did you know that 60 percent of your brain is made of fat!

TECHNICAL STUFF

Distribution of fat in the body differs based on hormone profile (estrogen versus testosterone), sex, and age. Women tend to store more fat in the lower body (referred to as being *pear-shaped*), while men often store more fat in the upper body (referred to as *apple-shaped*). As you get older, more fat is stored as visceral fat, so fat becomes even riskier in excess as you age.

Muscle

Dense and waterlogged, muscle is heavy! But muscle is the key to movement. Without adequate muscle mass, we can't do normal daily activities, play, run, jump, avoid falls, or go dancing. Muscle mass is active tissue, and it eats up calories to do its work. The more muscle we have, the more work we can do and the more calories we can use up.

Muscle is composed of various types of proteins. Some are connective-tissue proteins such as collagen, while others are used in the contraction cycle that shortens muscles and produces force. Making muscle takes energy in the form of carbohydrates as well as protein. It also takes work. The signals to produce muscle only come when the body is challenged with work. Weight training is an excellent stimulus tool to help start the muscle-making process.

Bone

The Eiffel Tower is only as strong as its iron beams, and our skeletons are only as strong as our bones. Bones are dense, filled with minerals to make them strong, and yet they also have some flexibility so they can bend before breaking. The hardness comes from the mineral calcium, in the form of hydroxyapatite crystals within the bone. Flexibility comes from collagen fibers made from protein. Bones have their own blood supply and are in a constant state of change.

Wouldn't it be nice to have a pothole-filled street repaved every year? What a nice road that would be! Bone is "repaved" constantly. *Osteoclasts* are the cells that can dissolve and break down damaged bone, making way for new bone formation. *Osteoblasts* are the cells that drive new bone to be formed. Normally, there is a balance between osteoclast and osteoblast activity such that the bone mass stays about the same. However, there are factors that can mess up the balance between the two, and it may result in either bone mass gain or loss.

Bone mass gain is often the result of:

>> **Compressive, pulsatile forces that load the bone:** Things like walking, jogging, or stair climbing load the bone in this way.

>> **Exercise that uses the muscles, which pull on the bone and cause the stress and strain that helps add bone:** Strength training is an excellent exercise to both stress the muscles and load the bone.

Bone mass loss is often linked to:

>> **Low estrogen levels:** This can happen in young women who are overtrained and in menopausal women. Estrogen helps keep osteoclast formation down to promote bone growth and closure of the growth plates (epiphyseal plates) at the ends of growing bones in adolescence. So, reduced estrogen increases

osteoclast formation and accelerates bone breakdown. This can lead to a loss in bone mass.

>> **Lack of physical activity:** Bones need loading stimuli to help keep bone growth moving. Sitting unloads the bone, and the signals for bone growth go away. You may think your bones are getting weaker due to age, when really it's just years of doing no activity!

>> **Lack of key dietary nutrients:** Important bone-building nutrients, such as calcium, vitamin D, potassium, and protein are all essential to ensure that bones get the building blocks they need. Stressing the bone is not effective if you don't have the dietary "mortar" to make the bone!

Water

Water is essential for all chemical reactions within the body. Without water, we can't maintain our organ function, move our blood, or digest and absorb nutrients. The list of water's value is endless. The problem is, we lose water continuously via breathing, sweating, urinating, and breaking chemical bonds to make energy. Dehydration is the enemy of normal physical function.

You can get water from the following sources:

>> **Food:** Fruits and vegetables are 75 percent to 99 percent water, so a diet that is high in fruits and vegetables provides a lot of water. High-fat foods may have only 15 percent to 30 percent water, so eating a high-fat diet may mean you aren't getting enough water.

>> **Fluids:** Drinking water is, of course, a great way to consume water. But drinking water isn't the only way to hydrate. For example, milk is about 85 percent water! Soda, coffee, and fruit juices all are sources of water. Just use good judgment when choosing the drink — other things in the drink, such as sugar, caffeine, and even fat, may not be as good for you.

Measuring Body Composition

Most people who want to know about their body composition want to know how much fat and muscle (lean tissue) they have. Being able to track these components in conjunction with their diet and exercise offers insights into their body's makeup and tells them if their new behaviors are paying off.

In this section, we look into a few of the more common methods for measuring body composition and give you some insights on the various techniques.

Body mass index: Uses and misuses

Body mass index (BMI) was first described in 1832 by Adolphe Quetelet, a statistician, astronomer, and mathematician whose work was based on the idea that weight is relative to height and that an "ideal" weight can be calculated based on height. In the 1950s, the index began to be used by the Metropolitan Life Insurance Company to establish tables of "normal" weights for clients after the company began to note that more and more claims were coming from obese policyholders. Categorizing clients into three categories based on their frame — small, medium, and large — was done to determine insurability and premiums. Today insurance companies continue to use this method for determining premiums and eligibility for coverage.

Here are some limitations and misuses of BMI:

WARNING

>> BMI was developed using bodies of non-Hispanic white men, which doesn't allow for association across different cultures.

>> BMI doesn't account for body composition, such as the ratio of fat, muscle, and bone. Often, athletes have high BMIs despite having low body fat because they have much more muscle than a non-exercising person.

>> Based on current BMI practices, someone may be classified as being overweight without any accurate body fat measure. On the other hand, an individual who is frail and has little muscle but more fat may have a normal BMI but be at risk for osteoporosis and falling.

So, BMI is not a measure of the composition of the body. Instead, it's a measure of the body's size (height and weight). For uses with a given individual, BMI can't replace a true measurement of the components of the body's mass (fat, muscle, and bone). For individuals with more muscle mass than a typical non-weight-training individual, the BMI gives misleading information. But when you look at the United States as a whole, most of the population is inactive and non-weight-training, and if you track large populations (like the entire country), large BMI values most likely indicate people with excess body fat as the reason for the increased BMI. In other words, there is a place for BMI in the toolkit for examining obesity — just use it wisely.

Skinfold body fat

Subcutaneous fat can be measured using skinfold techniques. A *skinfold caliper* is a tool used to measure the thickness of a fold of skin and the underlying fat. By pinching and folding the skin at specific spots on the body, measurements can be used to estimate total body fat. Several sites have been established around the body for skinfold assessment, but most often the triceps and *subscapular* (below the shoulder blades) locations are used. The examiner pinches the skin and tries to include the subcutaneous fat that exists below the skin and then applies the caliper, measuring the thickness of the skin and fat. (Most calipers are limited to measuring about 50mm, so this technique isn't possible on those with more fat present.) The examiner can compare the amount of fat measured at the chosen site to established normative values. The normative values are based on national reference data and utilize a statistical computation to provide information about body fat percentage.

REMEMBER

You may find this technique useful for establishing a body fat percentage value, but remember that everyone's body is unique. This technique is not a direct measure of body fat but rather a collection of individual site data that's computed into a final percentage.

Dual-energy X-ray absorptiometry

Dual energy X-ray absorptiometry (DEXA) is a very common and well-accepted solution for looking at fat, lean mass, and bony tissues. It uses two low-energy levels to examine the differentiation between tissues, which allows it to differentiate between fat and lean mass while also being able to examine bone mineral density. Although this technique is relatively fast and safe, it isn't readily available and is costly to have done. DEXA also relies on mathematical algorithms to calculate and estimate fat and lean tissue, but it's far more accurate than other available measures.

To have a scan, you lie within the DEXA scanner for about 10 to 20 minutes while your body is scanned from head to toe. Most people are able to undergo DEXA, but some people may be too large to fit within the scanner.

Hydrostatic weighing

Hydrostatic weighing, also known as underwater weighing, measures body volume and estimates body composition. This technique uses body weight, body volume, and residual lung volume to calculate body density and body fatness. Hydrostatic weighing requires the subject to get into a tub of water, submerse themselves all the way under the water, and exhale as much air as possible from their lungs while their mass is collected.

Hydrostatic weighing has been used for many years in research and clinical settings, but it has limitations. Many people are uncomfortable getting into a bathing suit. Some people can't fit into the water tank. Some people are very uncomfortable exhaling all their breath while submerged.

Air displacement plethysmography

Air displacement plethysmography uses the relationship between pressure and volume to establish the body volume of a subject who is seated within an enclosed chamber. The BodPod is one such device that has been developed to calculate body volume while using measurements of body mass to establish density and an estimation of percent fat and lean mass. The BodPod measures body volume by air displacement, not much different from how hydrostatic weighing (see the preceding section) uses water displacement to measure volume. A benefit in using the BodPod is that it's quick, and it can measure many people in a short amount of time. Plus, it doesn't require people to get into a bathing suit or hold their breath underwater. The participant simply sits inside the enclosed BodPod for a couple of minutes and then, based on its established algorithms, estimates aspects of body composition.

Bioelectric impedance

Another indirect measure of body composition is that of bioelectric impedance (BIA). Unlike some of the other methods described earlier, BIA measures resistance within the body by sending a very small electrical current through it. Based on the amount of resistance that is measured when the electrical current is passed through the body, BIA can estimate total body water, fat-free mass, and fat mass. Based on pre-established indexes and equations, body composition values are calculated. BIA is highly dependent on hydration status and, because it doesn't measure any "biologic" structure but rather electrical impedance, it relies heavily on statistical associations. A lot of research has questioned the validity and reliability of this body composition method. However, because of the availability of BIA on the market (you can even buy a scale that has BIA in addition to body weight) and how easy it is to be scanned, the technique is used widely.

Managing Your Body Composition

As we have just reviewed, the scale is not any indication of the composition of the body, and our desire for fat loss or muscle gain (maybe a bit of both?) aren't always seen on the scale. A well thought-out and reasonable approach to changing body composition is required — well, that and a bit of patience!

When you want to lose weight

Losing weight really means losing fat weight, and this is where people go a bit overboard on some of their weight-loss tactics. Muscle is quite dense, but losing muscle mass is *not* something you want. So, how do you keep the muscle and lose just the fat?

Research has shown that dieting alone doesn't work well, because it results in muscle mass loss. The best approach is a combination of exercise and diet adjustments to reduce body fat. Current weight loss guidelines suggest a plan that will cause a 1- to 2-pound weight loss per week. Losing more than that results in losses of muscle mass, slowing of metabolic rate, and the fat returning.

Exercise guidelines

Current exercise guidelines for improving health are 150 minutes of moderate exercise each week, but if you want to reduce body weight, that's probably not enough. Instead, aim for 150 to 450 minutes of physical activity each week, or up to about an hour per day of moderate activity.

Aim for about 1,200 to 2,000 calories of activity per week, or 170 to 285 calories per day. This is the equivalent of walking 1.5 to 3 miles each day depending on body weight.

The best type of exercise for burning calories is one that uses the most muscle mass. Get those muscles engaged in activity and keep them moving. Moderate activities may include:

>> **Walking:** You can walk outside or on a treadmill. To burn more calories, increase the incline a bit.

>> **Jogging:** Jogging is often too difficult for overweight and out-of-shape people, so only consider jogging if it feels like moderate exercise that you can do daily. Beginners sometimes split up their workout into walk-jog interval segments as a way to work themselves up to continuous jogging.

>> **Cycling:** You can ride a stationary bike or cycle outdoors.

>> **Hiking:** Hiking is a great way to work your muscles, be out in nature, and burn calories.

>> **Skiing:** Cross-country skiing uses the arms and legs and is a great exercise for burning calories.

>> **Swimming:** If you can swim with enough skill to maintain a steady pace, swimming is an excellent whole-body movement activity that uses a lot of muscle mass.

WHAT ABOUT RESISTANCE TRAINING AND WEIGHT LOSS?

Resistance training is essential to maintain functional ability and bone strength, but is it great for weight loss? Adding muscle mass may increase resting metabolism, which definitely helps, but the actual act of weight training doesn't burn many calories. When you engage in regular resistance training, you may add muscle and see the number on the scale go up, so be wary of using the scale as your guide — it's not the best at giving you an accurate picture of what's going on with your body.

>> **Sports:** Game play is a great way to burn calories, as long as it engages a lot of muscle groups. So, whether you're hitting the pickleball courts or playing a game of basketball with friends, it counts as activity.

>> **Dancing:** Dancing is an activity requiring coordination as well as physical movement — social interaction, movement, and balance training all in one. A few hours of social dancing can add up to a lot of calories.

You can mix and match and try different activities every day. Maybe you walk the dog every morning, play pickleball on Saturday afternoons, go dancing Friday nights, and hike Sunday mornings. The key is to accumulate minutes of activity and expend those calories. Moderate activity burns the most fat, so just keep at it!

Dietary guidelines

Human metabolism functions best when it has all the energy nutrients available. You need to maintain a diet that has some fat, plenty of healthy carbohydrates and protein, all in amounts that support fat loss and muscle growth. (Chapter 15 has specifics on nutrition.)

Most people can easily get all the nutrients they need while also reducing total caloric intake. Just a 250-calorie reduction in daily calories is equivalent to ½ pound of fat lost per week. You can probably reduce more than 250 calories per day.

Current dietary guidelines recommend a reduction in daily calories between 500 and 1,000 calories, but take into account your current calorie status before jumping to the big numbers. According to research, long-term weight loss has been most successful when the diet is low in fat (20 percent or fewer calories from fat) with the remaining calories from complete carbohydrates and lean proteins. Because fat is so calorie dense, look for the highest-fat food in your diet as a good starting place to find the calorie reductions.

Here are some other strategies for calorie reduction:

>> **Reduce your portion size.** Portion control is an easy way to cut calories without affecting food choices, and it can really make a difference.

>> **Increase the frequency of your meals.** Eating one large meal gives you far more calories than your body needs in the moment; as a result, more of it is stored as fat. So, increase the frequency of smaller meals to four to six meals per day. Smaller meals may initially make you feel hungry, but you get the meals more frequently. This can help prevent large fluctuations in blood sugar and may help keep you satisfied throughout the day. It may also keep you from binge eating.

>> **Use meal replacements as an alternative.** If you find it difficult to manage six meals per day, you may consider eating a meal replacement as one or two of the meals during the day. Meal replacements contain known amounts of calories and nutrients, so they can be an effective part of your daily plan.

>> **Make smart food substitutions.** Do you read labels? Are there other options for dressings, pizza toppings, that special drink? Diet isn't about eliminating foods entirely, but rather making wise choices and perhaps strategically substituting foods to reduce caloric intake. Some examples include:

- Baked tortillas instead of fried
- Broth-based soups instead of creamy soups
- Baked potato instead of french fries (just watch the toppings!)
- Plain Greek yogurt with fruit instead of sweetened yogurt

A combination of reducing portion size and making food substitutions can go a long way toward reducing fat intake and overall calories. It may take some planning, but isn't the fat loss worth the time?

TECHNICAL STUFF

WHAT ABOUT THE KETOGENIC DIET?

The ketogenic diet (which is a very low-carbohydrate diet) is a fad these days. The idea behind keto is that if you take away carbohydrates (glucose), your body will have no choice but to burn fat. But carbohydrates are essential for brain function and even fat burning. If you take away carbohydrates, fat can't be completely metabolized, and as a result, it's converted to ketones. The body can use ketones for energy, but *ketosis* (the buildup of acetoacetic acid, from the incomplete breakdown of fats) slows metabolic rate, and the lack of carbohydrates makes any physical activity very difficult.

The other problem with the keto diet is the potential loss of muscle mass. Most of the protein in your body is in the form of muscle, and when there is a lack of glucose in the diet, protein can be broken down into its smaller, amino acid building blocks and used to make glucose. So, as a result of excessive restriction of carbohydrates, muscle mass is lost. You may like what the scale says, but you're losing the wrong type of mass. A better strategy is to consume high-nutrient, complex carbohydrates but not overeat. If you avoid ketosis and the breakdown of muscle mass, most of the weight loss will be fat.

Putting the plan together

Here is a hypothetical example of weight loss planning to get to a goal of 1 to 2 pounds of fat loss per week:

REMEMBER

>> **Exercise:** Start with 20 minutes of walking per day (that's about a 1-mile walk).

As you get more comfortable walking 20 minutes a day, increase the length of your walks until you're getting an hourlong walk every day. Or, add other forms of aerobic exercise in addition to your 20-minute walk. In addition, two days per week, do resistance training working your major muscle groups (for example, bench press, lat pull, and leg press to train the chest, back, and legs, respectively).

>> **Diet:** Eating is one of those things people sometimes do without thinking. A good first step may be to log what you eat and how much you eat. From there, you can estimate calories consumed. Based on the information, you can adjust portion size and some food substitutions to reduce caloric intake. A good starting point can be a 300 calories per day reduction. Try smaller, more frequent meals to help adjust to smaller portions.

The estimated impact of these changes is a loss of 700 calories per week through exercise (if you're walking 20 minutes a day and doing resistance training twice a week) and a loss of 2,100 calories per week through diet, for a total of 2,800 calories per week, or about 0.8 pounds of fat.

When you want to gain weight

Some people seem to burn through calories and just can't seem to gain any weight. As they get older, frailty and very low body weight are a risk factor for weak bones and falls, so gaining muscle mass is important for many people. These folks need resistance training to create the stimulus for muscle growth and the right nutrients to drive muscle mass increases. (Chapter 11 covers resistance training guidelines, and Chapter 3 provides information about muscles and how they adapt.)

In order to grow muscle mass, you need to start with an adequate stimulus to the muscle to turn on the muscle-building process. Strength training should be done at least two or three days per week, involving all of the major muscle groups. Loads should be at least 60 percent of the one-repetition maximum, and the loads should be lifted to fatigue (or near fatigue). Loads of 70 percent to 80 percent may result in faster gains. More advanced weight lifters may have to add additional strategies involving varied cycles of loads and intensity (known as periodized training).

You have a plan to induce the muscle-building process, but you won't see any growth in muscle mass if the body doesn't have adequate energy and building materials for the muscles. Here's where dietary adjustments are needed:

>> **Total calories:** Add 500 calories to your diet per day. These calories should come mostly from protein and carbohydrate — don't reach for the fatty foods! You need carbohydrates to fuel the growth process and protein to provide the structure for the muscle tissue. Fat just adds, well, fat!

>> **Protein:** For those who consistently strength train, the protein requirement is about twice that of a sedentary individual. Recommendations are about 1.6 to 1.7 grams of protein per kilogram of body weight. For a 160-pound (72.7-kilogram) person, that's 116 to 123 grams of protein per day. Track your diet. Maybe you're already getting this much protein, or maybe you're not eating enough protein rich-foods to reach this amount and need to do some adjusting.

>> **Carbohydrates:** It takes energy to both satisfy your daily energy needs *and* provide the extra energy for muscle building. Carbohydrates are essential. Ideally, the carbs you consume will be low-fat, high-fiber complex carbohydrates providing all the nutrients you need in addition to the extra calories.

WHAT ABOUT PROTEIN DRINKS?

Getting all of the protein you need just from meals may be pretty tough, especially if you have a lot of complex carbs in the meal. (They fill you up!) There is a place for protein drinks within a diet plan. Getting the extra protein you need from a drink is quick and easy. Just don't make protein drinks your primary source of protein — you still need carbohydrates.

Be sure to read labels on supplemental protein products. Products labeled as weight gain supplements have enough protein, but they often add calories by adding simple sugars and fat to the mix. Those added calories don't provide much bang for your nutritional buck, so choose protein drinks that give you protein, with lower fat and sugar. You can get the other nutrients in your diet, or add them to the protein drink and make a smoothie.

WEIGHT MISMANAGEMENT: WEIGHT LOSS ISSUES IN SPORT

Some sports have historically been known to focus more on weight and aesthetics than others. Focusing on weight as a singular factor in healthfulness or readiness for competition can be problematic. Coaches often tell athletes that if they lost some weight, they'd be faster or if they gained weight they'd be stronger. Beyond the psychological damage this may do to an aspiring athlete, it just isn't the case and can lead to unhealthy behaviors like cutting calories or overeating to tip the scale. Many disordered eating situations are precipitated by comments like these. Athletes are in competitive environments, and they often strive for the pinnacle of success and will often do anything to achieve those outcomes.

Weight mismanagement in sport can lead to unhealthy calorie restriction, dehydration, and injury from muscle weakness. Eat a balanced diet, hydrate well, and consult a qualified professional who isn't your coach to establish a plan if weight loss or gain is necessary.

Chapter **14**

Measuring Performance: Fitness Trackers and the Wearables Craze

Most people who are physically active are curious about their bodies and find themselves trying to find new ways to get in shape or perform just a little bit better. Historically, most people have relied on fairly anecdotal information to guide them as they developed their programs and assessed their performance. Over the past several years, there has been a monumental growth in technology that allows the average person to look much deeper into what's happening during exercise or movement in general.

In this chapter, we explore how you can measure performance through wearable devices. We explain the different ways these tools work, what types of devices exist, and how to use them.

If you're using wearable technology, you may want to be careful about the data you share about yourself with the makers of that technology. When you start using a wearable device, read the fine print and make sure you understand how they store and use your data.

Seeing What Wearables Can Do

In the past, if you wanted to know information about your body when you were exercising, you had to go to a research lab and go through a pretty involved process. Today, it's easier than ever to not only explore what's happening to your body when you exercise but get real-time information while you're in the middle of the activity. Measuring performance isn't just important to Olympic athletes trying to shave a tenth of a second off their time; the average person who just wants to improve their fitness may find benefit in tracking their steps or monitoring their heart rate when working out.

Wearable sensors come in various forms, including wrist straps, watches, smart clothing, and GPS sensors, to name a few. The information spans physiologic (sweat, pulse oximetry, respiration); inertial (forces, angular rate); Global Positioning System, or GPS (direction, distance); and in some cases, video. No matter what your goals are, you can find a device that will give you the information you need.

Looking at different types of wearable devices

With literally hundreds of different options on the market to measure performance, the first step is knowing what you want to measure. Most devices these days measure all kinds of things — maybe more than you even care to know. For example, if you have an Apple Watch, you see how many hours you slept last night, how many steps you've taken, your heart rate, the noise level around you, and more. Table 14-1 lists the different types of wearable devices and what kind of information you can expect to get from them.

There are hundreds of manufacturers of wearable devices, and each device works a little differently. If you're overwhelmed by the options, just ask yourself: What do I want to know, and what do I want to wear?

TABLE 14-1 **Types of Wearable Devices**

Type of Device	What It Measures
Smart watches	Time, sleep, distance, location, heart rate, oxygen level, number of steps, calories expended, amount of activity
Fitness trackers	Physical activity, sleep, heart rate, calories expended, oxygen level, distance, movement specifics like acceleration and changes in direction, number of steps, heart rate variability (HRV)
Smart jewelry (rings, necklaces, bracelets, earrings, and so on, with embedded technology)	Activity, sleep, heart rate, HRV, oxygen level, fitness levels, calories
Smart clothing	Heart rate, body temperature, respiration rate, movement patterns, sweat, environmental conditions, falls, stress levels
Health/physiologic trackers	Electrocardiogram (ECG), electroencephalogram (EEG), body temperature, stress levels, hydration, sweat rate, breathing rate, skin temperature
Biomechanical trackers	Body movement, joint angles, accelerations, change in direction, electromyography (EMG)

Understanding how the technology works

You can think of wearables as having three layers to them: sensors, processing, and the network. Think of the sensors and processing as everything that occurs on the electronic hardware itself. The sensors are the part of the device that collects the particular information that they were designed for. The information collected by the sensor is transmitted as a signal to the processor. The processor then has to decipher the signals and ultimately convert the information into the data that you ultimately use.

Each device has unique computing needs and protocols for communicating the information and how it's ultimately incorporated as part of the wearable. Depending on the device, a series of sensors and multiple processing techniques may be used all at once.

Three main types of information are provided by wearables — physiologic, biomechanical, and GPS — and the technology is different for each kind of information being gathered.

Physiologic information

A broad area of wearable devices and embedded technology involves collecting physiologic information (information that relates to the body's functions). Physiologic information provides insights into your health, performance, or overall condition. The following sections cover sensors that are used to provide physiologic information.

FUNCTIONAL NEAR-INFRARED SPECTROSCOPY

Functional near-infrared spectroscopy (fNIRS) provides information about human brain function. You wear a device that looks like a winter hat with fiber-optic lights attached to it, and we can examine blood flow in the brain, which is a functional measure of brain activity.

OXIMETERS

You may have noticed a light shining from the back of your smart watch. The light is used by a technology called *photoplethysmography* to measure blood flow and heart rate. It does this by using *diodes* (electrical components that measure the flow of electrical current) to measure how much light is absorbed. The wavelength of that light provides information to the processor and helps you to assess oxygen levels (pulse oximetry), pulse rate, respirations, and variability associated with heart rate.

BLOOD PRESSURE SENSORS

When you go to the doctor and have your blood pressure taken, you have to sit still, be quiet, and wait for them to pump up the sleeve and listen for sounds, which identify the levels of pressure. If you want to know your blood pressure while you're active, that's impossible without a wearable device. Wearables that monitor blood pressure work similarly to what happens in a doctor's office, but usually in the form of a small inflatable cuff or wristband. The device is inflated until the arterial blood flow is stopped (the systolic value, or the upper number of your blood pressure; when the heart beats); then as the device deflates, the wearable can pick up the heartbeat, which represents cardiac contractions. When the heartbeat is no longer detectable, that equals the diastolic value (the lower number of your blood pressure; when the heart is not beating). Together, these numbers represent your blood pressure.

GALVANIC SKIN RESPONSE

Galvin skin response (GSR) is used to measure the volume of sweat that is excreted through the skin.

RESPIRATORY MONITORING SENSORS

In many sports and clinical applications, respiratory responses need to be measured. These include rate, depth, and patterns measured in real time in order to better understand a person's performance, exercise capacity, and energy expenditure.

Optical, mechanical, and electromagnetic sensors can be placed on the chest to measure variations in light or electromagnetic waves that are caused by breathing. Obviously, breathing is important and dictates much about exercise and what a person can do physically, so there are other very technical options, too. Some of those include smart masks, gas sensors, flow sensors, and heart rate sensors — all aimed at providing information related to aerobic capacity (Chapter 4), anaerobic threshold (Chapter 4), energy expenditure, respiratory efficiency, lung function, and substrate utilization (how the body uses energy from fuels) to name a few.

These devices become pretty technical, but the point is that wearables and, in some cases, an additional piece of equipment that communicates with the wearable can provide very detailed and necessary information in real time.

OTHER TECHNOLOGIES

Other important physiologic measures that can be incorporated into wearables is that of electromyography (EMG), which measures the muscles; electrocardiogram (ECG), which measures the heart; and electroencephalogram (EEG), which measures the brain. Electrical currents are detected at the intended structure or organ by placing electrodes on the body. For instance, when electrodes are placed on a muscle, the signals the muscle gives off while it's working are detected and interpreted to show the amplitude, length, and variability of the muscle activity. This technology is often used by sport scientists to measure muscle strength or responsiveness. A similar process is used for EKG and EEG. The techniques for all these methods are clinical, meaning they're usually done in a place like a doctor's office in order to capture very precise signals that then are interpreted to assess function or dysfunction, but with updates to technology, they're now more widely available.

Biomechanical information

When you're interested in how you're moving, you're likely to use something called an *inertial measurement unit* (IMU) to give you information about what's happening. These sensors measure variables of the movement of the body, such as acceleration, deceleration, forces that are absorbed, and displacements. The three main types of IMUs are:

>> **Accelerometers:** Provide information about linear forces — how fast you get going or slow down.

>> **Gyroscopes:** Measure angular velocities. Rather than only measuring how you move in a straight line, angular velocities give us information about how the body is turning.

>> **Magnetometers:** Provide information about the direction of movement oriented to the earth's north.

Collectively, we explore some of the more common uses for IMUs later in this chapter and see how they're considered "biomechanical" sensors.

Global Positioning System information

Another common type of information provided by wearables is GPS. Wearables that provide this information aren't much different from the GPS devices you may use to find your way around. These GPS devices utilize information from nearby satellites to provide information about your location. GPS devices are used by marathoners to map their runs and calculate their splits, and they've become widely used in sport performance by providing a quantification for activity profiles — coaches or sports scientists can track where and when certain players are on the field and better evaluate their various strategies or examine the players' movement profile during a game. Maybe the team has a breakdown in their defense or a specific player is dealing with a bad hamstring. GPS information can be used to assess their performance.

Pedometers

Pedometers are perhaps one of the oldest wearables on the market. These are pretty simplistic devices that measure the number of steps that we take. An accelerometer is inside of a pedometer and acts like a teeter-totter. Each time the teeter-totter touches down, an electronic circuit is completed and counts a step. We've evolved from wearing pedometers on our hips to now having pedometers integrated into most smartphones.

RELIABILITY AND VALIDITY: THE TWO ESSENTIALS

Not only do wearables consist of sensors that directly measure a variable, but many wearables use a combination of sensors or algorithms to calculate values that they then share as an *indirect measure* (or a representative of a measure). Companies that develop wearables tend to keep most of their information top-secret. They consider their information proprietary, so we don't really know how they come up with the information they do. This is mostly okay, and it doesn't inhibit the user from drawing conclusions that are meaningful to them, but some users may be interested in the nuances within the data, and for those types of users, it may be impossible to fully understand what and how the device truly is working and what information it is sharing.

As a current or future user of a wearable, keep two terms in your mind:

- **Reliability:** The ability for a measure to be repeated on multiple occasions and produce relatively similar results. This tells you if the device is able to measure a variable at a particular time and be able to reproduce the same finding when that same activity occurs again at a different time. For instance, you want your body-weight to be the same if you measure it three times in a row on the same scale. That's reliability.

- **Validity:** Whether a measure, in fact, assesses what we believe it to measure. If you're using a device to assess heart rate through an optical assessment technique, you'd expect that the technology of using optical measures for measuring heart rate does, in fact measure, heart rate and isn't a derivation of other data that then is called "heart rate."

In the end, you want devices that can be both reliable and valid. For the typical user, simply reading the user's manual and instructions for use may suffice, but for others looking for more technical information, you should definitely do your homework before drawing conclusions form the data you receive.

Measuring Activity and Performance

Now that you know what technology exists, you're ready to put it to work for you. Wearables are useful to coaches and participants and, in some cases, medical professionals. It's commonplace now for higher-level sporting organizations to use wearables to optimize training and competitions, collect biological and physiologic data, and monitor workloads on their players.

Managing workload

Every recreational or competitive athlete is different. So, if that's the case, why have teams trained each of their athletes the same? Traditionally, all the athletes on a team have lifted, run, and practiced the same because we weren't able to easily assess each athlete in real time. All we had were static measures of how strong they were, how long they can run, or how fast they can run. If you pushed someone too hard in their workout or during a game, they ran the risk of breaking down and not being as effective or, even worse, getting injured. Coaches now dedicate a lot of time to managing the workloads and recovery of their athletes.

When you're thinking about workload, it's all about acute, chronic, and a ratio between the two. First, let's define these terms:

>> **Acute workload:** The efforts exerted over a short period of time. This is typically related to a single session, but it may extend as long as a week. Acute workload takes into account the load experienced both during training and during competition. Many professionals use the acute workload value as a measure of fatigue.

>> **Chronic workload:** The loads experienced over a period of three weeks or longer. Chronic loads give an impression of the effort you've given up until the training or match session. Chronic workload is usually calculated as a rolling average from the past few weeks and is a representation of your overall fitness level and how much training stress you're accustomed to over time.

Here's the thing: You can work out hard one day but not be very fit. So, to control for this, some people use the *acute-to-chronic workload ratio,* which provides a measure of the training performed by the participant in relation to their capacity. The ratio allows you to examine if you're overworking or underworking.

When assessing your workload, some of the things that you may pay attention to are variables like distance, velocity, acceleration, and oxygen saturation. A number of studies have been done over the years that have tried to establish the best measures to assess workload. Some of those are heart rate, rate of perceived exertion (RPE), repetitions, amount of weight, speed, distance, velocity, HRV, and power output.

Many devices are capable of measuring any one or some of the factors related to workload, but most sport scientists agree that in order to accurately assess workloads and make associations about performance or risk for injury, many variables should be used to draw those associations. The devices that high-level teams use not only collect the distance, acceleration, and change in direction of an athlete, but also have algorithms that are used to create a score or series of scores that are interpreted by a sports scientist or coach to give them a measure of the workload.

WARNING

Some manufacturers claim that their devices can predict injury or performance based on workload measures and underlying metric values that are calculated, that's more of a marketing claim than anything backed by science. Assessing workload absolutely has a place when you're looking for ways to improve team and individual performance and get an edge over your competitor. Management of workload is important — if workload isn't assessed and monitored, you risk overworking your team and creating injuries or having them be too tired and fatigued to perform well.

Tracking your sleep and recovery after training

Some wearables use heart rate, accelerometers, and body temperature to collectively measure your sleep. Some simply give you a graph that represents motion while you're sleeping; others provide insights into the quality of your sleep. Most manufacturers won't tell you exactly what information they collect or how they provide a measure of your sleep quality, but they're using algorithms that they've tested and feel represent phases of the sleep cycle. With that data, they can look over time to make comparisons, giving you insights into your sleep history.

Sleep is definitely an important variable when you're looking at recovery. Recovery is a complex and interrelated measure. Coaches, personal trainers, and others should be keenly interested in maximizing their participants' performance. It's no secret that if you're pushed and pushed, and you don't ever get a chance to recover, your body will break down and likely become injured.

From a simplistic standpoint you can use nearly any measure to assess your recovery. Comparing your current values (heart rate, oxygen levels, and acceleration during activity) to your normal metrics is a way to see if you've recovered or returned to your normal state.

A really common and popular measure these days is HRV, which is used to measure stress and recovery by assessing the variability in time between your heartbeats. Most research will say that a higher HRV (one that shows variability in the timing between heartbeats) indicates better recovery and a lower one (less variability in timing between beats) indicates worse recovery, stress, and fatigue. HRV can be measured by wearing a wristband, ring, through EKG, or a smart phone application. All of these devices probably use different algorithms to come up with your HRV. Coaches and personal trainers use HRV to indicate the readiness of an athlete for the impending workout or competition. Many sport scientists will come up with individual workouts based on HRV. Because HRV is often calculated over time, with rolling averages to establish a normal range, the HRV measure gains accuracy over time.

Staying hydrated

For short-duration activity where there are lots of breaks and chances to drink, hydration isn't too much of a concern (unless you're in extreme heat). But if you're engaged in high-demand activities that span hours or days, with either heat or cold elements, maintaining your hydration is critical not only to performance but to overall health.

Currently, wearables are able to use photoplethysmography to measure fluid in the body and, indirectly, hydration. Other devices are able to assess sweat rate and the analyte (chemical substance) concentration within that sweat — basically, how much you are sweating and how salty your sweat is. That, coupled with how much fluid you've ingested, gives you an understanding of how hydrated you are.

Returning to play after injury

If you've ever suffered an injury, you may have wondered if you're ready to return to your normal activities. Sometimes, you can't know for sure, but some metrics found through wearables may help.

If you have access to pre-injury data or how you used to be before getting hurt, that can be helpful in knowing how close you are post-injury to where you once were. This is especially true for people who have been out for a long time because of an injury or surgery. Acceleration, total distances during an exercise bout, oxygenation during the activity, heart and respiration rate, and changes in direction can all be used to assess an athlete's readiness to return.

TIP

When data isn't available, you can always compare yourself to others on the team to get an idea of your status in comparison to a teammate's.

While you're working to return from an injury, be sure to manage your workload. Managing increases in activity while also tracking recovery are essential to progressing to full activity. As you're progressing through rehabilitation, you or your therapist may find benefit in using an IMU device to track distances, changes in direction, and velocities. Other measures that give more of an indication on someone's fitness to actually compete are variables related to heart rate, oxygen levels, and HRV. These metrics may be really beneficial in sharing progressions and give a measure of how much and how hard you're working. Especially when you're able to compare these values to teammates or their pre-injury data it will be helpful to assess readiness.

REMEMBER

Each sport is different and requires specialization from a qualified clinician to help manage the process and provide guidance as you navigate the key factors of the injury recovery paradigm (workload management, hydration and fatigue, cardiovascular health, sleep and recovery, musculoskeletal response/healing).

Enhancing Performance

No matter what type of activity you participate in, whether it be for recreation or competition, you probably want to be as good as you can be. Not everyone will put in hours and hours to gain a tenth of a second on their sprint times, but we all like the feeling of improving. A few years ago, when activity monitoring became possible, counting steps was all the rage. Before you knew it, there were pedometer challenges, and clinicians and scientists began to look at links between how many steps people took and their overall health.

One of the benefits of being able to track steps was that it was possible to have a real metric of how much activity you did in a day. You didn't have to guess — you had an actual count. This translated to better adherence to regular activity and ultimately positive responses in resting heart rates, oxygen consumption, and overall fitness.

Two common areas where we can experience improvements that will translate to activities are in aerobic and anaerobic fitness. Aerobic activity uses the body's large muscle groups over longer time spans that is rhythmic and repetitive. Anaerobic activity consists of activities that are short, fast, and high intensity. Assessing and working to improve your fitness in these two global areas is accomplished by taking the variables that you can collect with wearable devices and putting them to use in aerobic or anaerobic activities. The following sections explain how you can do that.

Improving your aerobic fitness

When you're looking to enhance aerobic fitness, some of the metrics that you may be interested in are heart rate, oxygen consumption, VO2 max, and energy expenditure.

Heart rate

Heart rate has been a staple in exercise monitoring and as a way to assess the kind of shape you're in. Typically, a lower heart rate at rest and during activity indicates that your cardiovascular system is working efficiently to supply blood and oxygen and other nutrients to supply the working muscles. The higher your heart rate, the harder your system is working, and ultimately the more inefficient it is. Of course there is a limit — you can't lower your heart rate too far without passing out or not supplying enough blood and nutrients to the body. It's a fine-tuned system that gets better as you exercise more and more.

Oxygen consumption

One of the factors that dictates your heart rate is in how much oxygen is delivered to the muscles and the rest of the body. If the lungs aren't oxygenating enough blood quickly enough to be transported to the rest of the body, then your heart rate stays high to try to push more blood through the body. By training, the respiratory and cardiovascular systems can work together to maximize the amount of oxygen and nutrient delivery to the necessary portions of the body. Pulse oximetry is a measure of how much oxygen is in the blood. It has been integrated into lots of wearables to make it easier to track.

VO2 max

VO2 max is an assessment of maximal oxygen uptake. It's regularly used when athletes are training for distances or sustained exercises. The more oxygen you can transport through the body, the better for maintaining intense and demanding exercise. Unfortunately, there is no way to measure VO2 max directly with wearables, so, like some of the other variables we've discussed, what you'll get is an estimated or calculated value.

REMEMBER

Because a number of factors go into estimating VO2 max through a wearable, the calculation may not be reliable as the body continues to adapt to the exercise. In other words, a change in running biomechanics alone may lead to a higher estimated VO2 max, but perhaps the body itself hasn't experienced an increase in oxygen uptake. As long as you're aware that what you're seeing is really just an estimate, you can make your own judgments on the information you're given.

Energy expenditure

When you're jogging on a treadmill, riding a stationary bike, or using an elliptical machine, you've probably noticed the calorie output. Clearly, this number involves a little bit of guesswork by the machine. You may have told the machine how much you weigh and, by knowing your heart rate and the intensity and/or resistance the machine is providing, it can estimate how much energy you've used.

Wearables are a little better than those machines because they've been designed to collect those physiologic (oxygen, blood flow) measures in addition to the biomechanic (acceleration, distance) aspects of your activity. By taking those physiologic and biomechanic values along with what the wearable knows about your height, weight, and hydration, among other things, it can provide an estimate of how much energy you're expending.

TIP

Energy expenditure to complete a task can be a measure of fitness improving, but it likely serves as a good way to monitor exercise and helps your personal trainer know how hard you're working during the session.

Boosting your anaerobic power

Anaerobic exercise is related to short, fast, and high-intensity exercise that doesn't require the body to use oxygen. It uses glucose to fuel the activity, but this can only happen for a short period of time. Some anaerobic activities include weightlifting, jumping, sprinting, and high-intensity interval training. There are plenty of other examples, but pretty much anything that's done quickly and at a high intensity would be characterized as anaerobic.

Power is a factor of how much force you can exert over a short period of time. The stronger you are and the better your body is at exerting that force in a shorter amount of time, the more anaerobic power you have. We don't all have to be weightlifters or sprinters, but increasing your anaerobic strength will help you maintain a functional lifestyle.

IMU devices provide data including direction, changes in that direction, and velocities. When they're integrated with GPS, you can see distances more accurately represented. All these measures can be used to provide estimates of anaerobic power for athletes. Other metrics can come through accelerometers or magnetometers and may go beyond just something that you're wearing on your wrist. Today in Major League Baseball, for instance, a lot of attention is placed on swing speed and power. By placing an IMU device on the batting handle, coaches can get an indicator of the power, direction, and speed of a player's swing. These metrics are then translated into launch angle, bat speed, and exit velocity off the bat. Similarly, pitchers are wearing arm sleeves with embedded IMU technology that are providing players and coaches with information about arm angle, arm velocities, and intensity of throwing exercise. This information is used not only for performance enhancement and real-time data understanding, but in management of volumes and intensities across bouts of throwing, ultimately limiting injury.

Chapter **15**

Eating for Success: Sports Nutrition

Many people don't really think about what they eat or how it affects their bodies. But nutrition is essential for peak physical performance. Poor nutrition can mean reduced sports performance and poor recovery from exercise; it can even lead to chronic conditions that affect your overall life. Understanding how to use nutrition to improve exercise performance can mean the difference between winning and losing!

In this chapter, we explore how nutrients impact the body's function. We explore nutrients that fuel performance and build strength. We also look at nutrition as medicine to help the body recover from heavy exercise and maintain health.

Macronutrients: Carbohydrates, Fat, and Protein

The body is a system of organs that can process *nutrients*, the chemicals necessary for life. Some nutrients — such as fat, cholesterol, and some amino acids — can be made by the body. But many nutrients must be obtained through proper nutrition. These *essential nutrients*, as they're called, help the body perform daily activities, do heavy physical work, and contribute to the recovery and rebuilding process after exercise. Some nutrients, known as *macronutrients*, are needed in large quantities. Other nutrients, known as *micronutrients*, are required in very small amounts but pack a big punch! In the following sections, we examine all these nutrients.

Carbohydrates: The fuel that powers movement

Carbohydrates are molecules composed of carbon, hydrogen, and oxygen. They can be simple molecules like glucose (a simple sugar) or more complex carbohydrates containing multiple linkages of sugars. In the body, carbohydrates are transported through the bloodstream in the form of glucose and stored in the muscle and liver as glycogen. One gram of glucose contains 4 kilocalories (kcals) of energy, and this energy can be created using both aerobic and anaerobic metabolism. Carbs are versatile!

REMEMBER

Fiber represents a class of carbohydrates that the body can't break down for energy because we lack the appropriate enzymes. This means that fibrous material will move through the digestive system without providing nutrient value. However, fiber still plays a role in health. It helps add bulk to fecal matter and move material through the digestive system. It can also bind to cholesterol and remove it from the body.

Glucose, glycogen, and exercise performance

The simplest form of a carbohydrate is glucose, a six-carbon molecule that can be broken down both aerobically and anaerobically to produce adenosine triphosphate (ATP), which is what our body uses for energy (see Chapter 4 for more on ATP). Glucose exists only in the blood stream, as it's being transported to the cells.

The storage form of glucose is a compact, glucose-filled molecule called *glycogen*. Glycogen is stored in both the muscle and the liver. The average person has about 2,000 kcals of glycogen stored in their body — enough to run about 15 to 20 miles (24 to 32 kilometers).

Because glucose is essential for higher-intensity exercise, carbohydrates are important for exercise and sports performance. When we exercise, muscle glycogen is used quickly, while at the same time glycogen is being broken down to glucose in the liver and dumped into the bloodstream for transport to the exercising muscle.

Glycogen depletion happens when there is a lack of muscle or liver glycogen. Without available glucose, energy production drops and the athlete fatigues. This is why *exogenous* (external) sources of glucose can mean the difference between finishing the race strong and not finishing at all (see Figure 15-1).

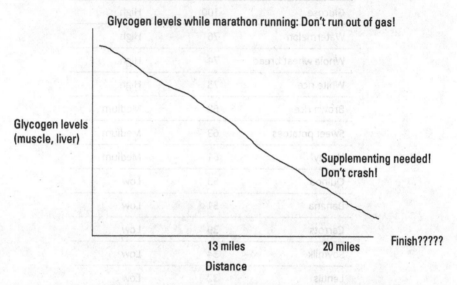

FIGURE 15-1: Glycogen use during a marathon run.

TIP The brain is a voracious consumer of carbohydrates, in the form of glucose. In fact, the brain uses about 100 to 150 grams (400 to 600 kcals) of glucose daily — something to keep in mind when you're thinking about limiting carbohydrate in your diet. The brain needs glucose.

Dosing your carbs: Glycemic index and glycemic load

If you look at carbs and glucose like a medication, you need to consider the "dosing" of the food and how fast the carbohydrate gets into the blood. Carbs that are closer to simple sugars, like glucose, are absorbed rapidly and get to the blood quickly, making blood glucose rise. More complex carbohydrates need to be broken down within the digestive system, so they take longer to make blood glucose rise. Depending on your dietary goals, you may prefer one effect or another.

To help understand how specific carbs affect blood glucose, the glycemic index (GI) was developed. The glycemic index lists foods and their associated impact on the rise of blood glucose. The simplest sugar, glucose, is used for the highest GI value of 100. All other foods fall below that level. The lower the number, the slower the rise in blood glucose. Table 15-1 shows some foods and their associated glycemic index; you can find more at https://glycemicindex.com.

TABLE 15-1 ## The Glycemic Index for Select Foods

Food	GI	Rating
Glucose	100	High
Watermelon	76	High
Whole wheat bread	74	High
White rice	73	High
Brown rice	68	Medium
Sweet potatoes	63	Medium
Honey	61	Medium
Quinoa	53	Low
Banana	51	Low
Carrots	39	Low
Soymilk	34	Low
Lentils	32	Low

You can modify the GI for a meal by intentionally combining foods. Mashed potatoes may have a high GI, but if you eat them with a vegetable and a protein-containing food, the overall GI of the meal is reduced and absorption is delayed.

Carbohydrate guidelines for performance

The acceptable nutrient range for carbohydrates is 45 percent to 65 percent of calories. So, if you're consuming 2,000 kcal per day, you should aim for 225 (2,000 × 0.45) to 325 (2,000 × 0.65) grams of carbs per day.

How much carbohydrate a person needs varies from one person to the next. If you're doing a lot of heavy-intensity work or sports, you'll need more carbs than someone who works at a desk and leads a more sedentary life.

No matter how active you are, the carbohydrates you eat should pack a punch! They should have additional nutrient value in the form of fiber, vitamins, and minerals; only a small fraction (10 percent) should come from sugars. Fruits, vegetables, and whole grains should make up most of your carbohydrate intake. This approach will ensure that you maintain muscle and liver glycogen stores while also getting the maximum in nutrient value from foods.

Getting ready for the big race: Carbohydrate loading

Because carbohydrates, in the form of stored muscle and liver glycogen, are a key fuel for high-intensity performance, the more you have stored, the longer you can maintain the work intensity. You can temporarily store more glycogen than normal, just prior to a big event. This approach is known as *carbohydrate loading* or *glycogen supercompensation*, and it's a strategy that you can use on special occasions, like before running a big race.

Follow these steps to carb load:

1. **Six days before the event, begin to taper your activity, reducing your workout volume by 40 percent to 50 percent and consume at least 50 percent of your calories from carbohydrate (at least 300 grams).**

    Continue to do this five days and four days before the event.

2. **Three days before the event, cut your activity again by 50 percent and get 70 percent of your calories from carbohydrate (at least 500 grams).**

    Continue to do this two days before the event.

    As you reduce activity, the enzymes that help make glycogen are elevated. Providing the source of carbohydrates accelerates storage of glycogen. At this point, you should feel more rested, fresh, and fast!

3. **The day before the event, rest and get 70 percent of your calories from carbohydrate.**

    The result of this six-day taper is an elevation in stored glycogen, which can remain for a few days, so make this your competition window!

Clearly, you can't do this for every event, or you'd be spending all your time tapering! So, use this approach for the most important events or activities.

THE PRE-EVENT MEAL: GETTING THE TIMING RIGHT

You may think that eating right before an event is a good idea, but think again! During exercise, your body uses stored muscle glycogen and pulls glucose from the liver by breaking down stores of liver glycogen. If you eat a meal right before an event, there is a rise in blood glucose that triggers insulin release. Insulin prevents the breakdown of liver glycogen, blocking your ability to access this important store. So, any meal needs to be consumed early enough to allow the digestive process to take place and insulin levels to come back to normal levels.

Most recommendations suggest that the pre-event meals be moderate in size and easily digestible. The meal should contain between 1 and 4 grams of carbohydrate per kilogram (or 0.45 to 1.8 grams per pound) of body weight, consumed 90 minutes to 4 hours before the event. This ensures that you'll begin the event with low insulin levels and easy access to your glycogen stores.

Remember: Elevated blood glucose causes a release of insulin. Insulin blocks the breakdown of liver glycogen! So, you don't want elevated blood glucose at the beginning of the event. Get the digestion process completed before the event begins.

Get the formula right: Carbohydrates during exercise

For activities that are moderate to high intensity and that last more than 45 minutes, muscle and liver glycogen stores are rapidly depleted. Glycogen use during heavy work can range from 60 to 90 grams per kilogram (27 to 41 grams per pound) of body weight, and by the two-hour mark may be completely gone, resulting in fatigue. You can't slow the rate of muscle glycogen loss, but you can slow down the amount of glycogen taken from the liver by providing a dietary source of glucose. This is done by digesting carbohydrates during the activity.

Sport drinks are a popular source of carbohydrates because they're formulated for the right concentration of carbohydrates and water. During exercise, the digestive system can't function as well as it does at rest, so the consumed liquids need to be mostly water, with just a pinch of carbohydrate. A solution that is 6 percent carbohydrate (60 grams per liter of fluid) works well to be absorbed quickly by the gut, while avoiding gastrointestinal (GI) distress. Because the body can use glucose at about 60 grams per hour, that would be about 1 liter of fluid per hour. You can break that down to perhaps four 250-milliliter feedings per hour.

WHAT ABOUT SPORT DRINKS AND ENERGY DRINKS?

Sport drinks are formulated to provide fuel, water, and electrolytes to the body during exercise. They are mostly water and can be absorbed easily even during exercise.

Energy drinks are not formulated to be used during exercise. Although they do contain high-glycemic sugars, they also contain caffeine and other chemicals that make the drink very thick, which makes absorption during exercise difficult and may actually draw water from the body rather than replace water!

Some people may not tolerate much fluid volume, so be prepared to change your strategy. Any drinks more than 8 percent carbohydrates are too thick and will cause GI distress.

Keep the sport drink concentration around 6 percent carbohydrate. Soda is about 11 percent and contains fructose, so that isn't a drink you want to have during the event. Keep the feedings to about 250-milliliters to prevent any stomach distress.

Carbohydrates after exercise: Recovering quickly

The body has an effective mechanism to prepare itself for replacing the stored muscle and liver glycogen. As glycogen levels drop, an enzyme called *glycogen synthase* rises. This enzyme is the key to creating glycogen — all you need is glucose along with the glycogen synthase, and you can store the glycogen. However, glycogen synthase does not stay elevated for long after exercise. So, there is a window of opportunity you have to take advantage of if you want to recover from exercise quickly and restore glycogen.

Unlike during exercise, where the sport drink needs to be very diluted, after exercise, blood flow to the gut is normal, and the drinks for recovery can contain more glucose. In fact, you want to get a hefty dose of carbohydrate soon after exercise. Within 30 minutes, 1 to 1.5 grams per kilogram (0.45 to 0.68 gram per pound) body weight of carbohydrate is recommended. So, for a 180-pound (82-kilogram) person that's between 80 and 120 grams of carbohydrate for those first 30 minutes. After that, continue the replacement every two hours out to six hours or more, depending on the extent of the exercise and depletion with a goal of more than 300 grams of carbohydrate across the 24 hours of the event. The drink should be high-glycemic sugars to accelerate the transit time into the muscle and liver to take advantage of the enzymes for making glycogen.

PROTEIN IN A RECOVERY DRINK? YES!

You may think that protein isn't needed in a recovery drink, but the body will prioritize glycogen synthesis even if you don't have any glucose! Protein taken from muscle stores can be broken down into amino acids and converted to glucose in the liver in a process known as *gluconeogenesis* (see Chapter 4). This means that repeated glycogen depletion bouts can cause muscle mass loss. One way to prevent this loss is to provide some amino acids or protein in the recovery drink. Typically, the carbohydrate-to-protein ratio should be 4:1. For example, if you're consuming 50 grams of carbohydrate in a drink, about 12 grams of protein should be in the drink as well. This will help hold off the breakdown of muscle mass by putting the ingested amino acids to work making glycogen and preserve your muscle.

TIP

CHOCOLATE MILK AS A RECOVERY DRINK?

You may have heard of chocolate milk being used as a recovery drink. How does it stack up to our recommendations? One serving of chocolate milk has 26 grams of carbohydrate and 8 grams of protein. That's a little below the 4:1 carb-to-protein ratio, but it's pretty close! Fat content varies by the type of milk (skim versus whole). The proteins in milk are complete proteins, so you'll get an array of amino acids, and the sugars in milk are quickly digested. Not too bad for a recovery drink!

WARNING

Time is important when it comes to restoring glycogen because of the dropping levels of the synthase enzyme following exercise. So, don't skip the after-event meal/drink to take a nap. Instead, prioritize eating and/or drinking something first!

Fat: Necessary in the right amounts

Fat gets a bad rap because of its link to obesity and the high number of calories in a tiny amount of high-fat food. But fat is an essential nutrient for the body, and although there may be "bad" fats, there are plenty of "good" fats that we can incorporate into the diet. In this section, we examine the different types of fats, food sources for those fats, and how they can help you during exercise. Then we offer some basic guidelines for fat intake to make a healthy diet.

CARBON, HYDROGEN, AND OXYGEN, OH MY!

TECHNICAL STUFF

Fat, or fatty acid, is a molecule composed of carbon, hydrogen, and oxygen. Fat doesn't dissolve in water, so when it's in the blood, it's bound to proteins that can carry the fat. Fat is either a solid or an oil. The most common configuration of fat is in the form of a triglyceride molecule (shown in the following figure); a triglyceride molecule is a glycerol molecule connected to three fatty acid molecules.

Triglyceride Molecule

```
    H              O
    |              ||
H — C — O ——— C —— CH2 — CH2 ----- CH2 —— CH2
    |
    H — C — O            Same as above
    |
    H — C — O            Same as above
    |
    H
```

Glycerol   Fatty acid chains (will vary in number by type)

When a fatty food is ingested, it begins to break down in the mouth. After the fat is absorbed by the body, the liver can repackage the fat to be used within the tissue. Enzymes located in different areas of the digestive system, known as *lipases*, are used to help break down fats to a point where they can be absorbed by the body.

In the mouth, *lingual lipase* begins to break down the fat while you chew. In the stomach, *gastric lipase* helps break down the fat more before it heads into the intestinal tract. In the intestines, *pancreatic lipase, bile* (a watery, salty substance that helps break fat into tiny droplets), and *intestinal lipases* break down the fat even more until you get to the smallest fat droplet known as a *chylomicron;* chylomicrons are composed mostly of triglycerides.

Because fat can't be dissolved in the plasma, the liver will wrap the triglyceride in protein. The term *lipoprotein* is used to describe this lipid-protein combination. Additional breakdown and remodeling of the lipoprotein produces a number of different particles that can move through the bloodstream:

- **Very low-density lipoproteins (VLDLs)** are mostly composed of triglycerides and cholesterol particles. They pass through the blood where cells can remove the triglycerides for energy or storage.

(continued)

(continued)

- **Low-density lipoproteins (LDLs)** contain fewer triglycerides; they contain more cholesterol and are produced in the liver. These lipoproteins can interact with arteries to both damage arterial walls and also deposit cholesterol as a plaque on the walls, which is how coronary artery disease begins. LDLs are often referred to as the "bad" cholesterol.

- **High-density lipoproteins (HDLs)** contain cholesterol and a lot of protein. HDLs can actually remove cholesterol form cell walls, so they're seen as the "good" cholesterol molecule that helps reduce your risk of heart disease.

The main types of fat

There are four main types of fats: unsaturated fat, saturated fat, cholesterol, and trans fats. We cover each of these in the following sections.

Some fats (unsaturated fats) have a positive impact on the health of the body, while others (saturated and trans fats) are linked to vascular disease.

UNSATURATED FAT

Unsaturated fats are the healthy fats found in diets that have a lot of fish and oils like olive oil and peanut oil. They help lower cholesterol and promote healthy skin and cells.

Unsaturated fats consist of carbon chains in which one or more double bonds hold the carbons together. This makes the connection weaker. For this reason, the fat is typically oil at room temperature. Monounsaturated fats have one double bond; polyunsaturated fats have two or more double bonds.

In food, unsaturated fats react with oxygen quickly, so they can break down and become rancid. Therefore, the shelf-life of these fats is not very long.

Common food sources of unsaturated fat include: avocados, dark chocolate, eggs, fatty fish (such as mackerel and salmon), nuts, olive oil, olives, and seeds.

SATURATED FAT

Saturated fats don't have the double bonds seen in unsaturated fats. Instead, they have more hydrogen-to-carbon bonds so the carbons are connected by a single bond only. Therefore, the other bonds are "saturated" with hydrogens. The term *hydrogenation* is used to denote this bonding of hydrogens to carbons. For processed foods, the advantage of hydrogenation is that it makes the foods have a long shelf life because the fat doesn't oxidize and turn rancid. This saturation also means that the fat is solid at room temperature.

WARNING

Saturated fats are linked to increased cholesterol levels and increased risk of heart disease.

Common food sources of saturated fat include: butter, coconut oil, mayonnaise, palm oil, processed meats (such as bacon, hot dogs, and sausage), red meats (such as beef, lamb, and pork), and whole-fat dairy (such as cheese, ice cream, milk, and yogurt).

CHOLESTEROL

Cholesterol is produced by the body in the liver and is essential for life. It's used to make hormones like estrogen and testosterone and helps maintain cell membranes. However, cholesterol in the form of the LDL ("bad") cholesterol increases the risk of heart disease.

TECHNICAL STUFF

Eating more cholesterol doesn't increase the risk on its own — it's the saturated and trans fats that increase the liver's production of LDL. And foods high in cholesterol often are also high in saturated fats and trans fats.

Common food sources of cholesterol include: beef, cheese, fried foods (such as fried chicken, french fries, and deep-fat fried foods), organ meats (such as heart, kidney, and liver), processed meats (such as bacon, hot dogs, and sausage), sardines, shellfish, eggs, and whole-fat dairy.

TRANS FAT

Trans fats are a form of unsaturated fat that's seen more in processed foods. The configuration of the fat is partially hydrogenated; they were initially seen as a healthy alternative to saturated fats, but data now links trans fats to heart disease. Today, trans fats are seen as one of the "bad" fats that should be limited in the diet.

Common food sources of trans fats include: biscuits, breakfast sandwiches, non-dairy creamers, fried food (such as french fries, onion rings, and deep fried chicken and seafood), doughnuts, margarine, and rolls.

The many functions of fat

Fat plays an important role in the body, and it offers numerous benefits:

>> **Energy:** Fat in the form of triglycerides provides an enormous amount of energy. One gram of fat equals 9 kilocalories (kcals) of energy, so it's a

compact source of fuel. There are more than 100,000 kcals of energy in a typical body — that'll keep you moving for a long time! Small droplets of triglycerides are stored in the muscle near the energy-producing mitochondria. Fat can only be metabolized using aerobic metabolism, so low- to moderate-intensity exercise uses a lot of fat as a primary fuel.

TECHNICAL STUFF

The metabolic process of burning fat for energy takes place in the mitochondria, and glucose is an important contributor to the steps of fat metabolism. Without glucose, acetyl coenzyme A (acetyl-CoA, a key substrate within the Krebs cycle discussed in Chapter 4) accumulates and the liver forms *ketones* (acetoacetate, an acid formed by the liver), which slows metabolic rate. Additionally, muscle begins to break down to help create glucose. So, you must have some glucose in the diet to burn fat.

>> **Nutrients:** Fatty acids such as linolenic acid (an omega-3 fatty acid) and linoleic acid (an omega-6 fatty acid) are important nutrients for skin health, vision, neurological growth, and cell growth. Fats are also important for the storage of fat-soluble vitamins (such as vitamins A, D, E, and K), as well as for obtaining these vitamins in whole foods.

>> **Insulation and padding:** Fat is stored in large components under the skin (known as *subcutaneous fat*), as well as around the internal organs (known as *visceral fat*). Subcutaneous fat serves as an insulator to keep the body warm; visceral fat can help protect the organs as a shock absorber. When fat stores are excessive, both subcutaneous fat and visceral fat increase, leading to health risks such as diabetes and heart disease.

Guidelines for fat intake

Fat is essential for both fuel for exercise and critical nutrients, the amount recommended is lower than the typical dietary intake. The current guidelines of the World Health Organization (WHO) limits fat intake to less than 30 percent of total caloric intake. Additionally, WHO recommends saturated fat intake be less than 10 percent of total caloric intake, with trans fats less than 1 percent.

Recommended diets, such as the Mediterranean diet, include fats that are high in omega-3 fatty acids and unsaturated fats and oils. These types of fats are most often associated with heart-healthy diets. A diet that includes olive oil, fresh fruits and vegetables, seafood, and nuts provides unsaturated fats, protein, and vitamins — all in low-calorie meals.

Protein: Building the body for optimal performance

Protein exists in many different forms, due to the many different combinations of the various amino acid components that make up a protein. Protein can help make muscle tissue, receptors in a cell membrane, connective tissue, or components traveling in the blood. It's vital for human existence. To understand protein, you need to understand the amino acids that help form protein.

TECHNICAL STUFF

Like fats and carbohydrates, protein is composed of carbon, hydrogen, and oxygen. However, the added ingredient for protein is nitrogen. In fact, nitrogen represents 16 percent of protein.

Amino acids: The building blocks that make protein

Amino acids are small nitrogen -containing components that are organized into specific types of proteins according to genetic instructions. Amino acids are the ingredients in the recipe for each unique protein. Genes dictate the "recipe" for a protein by indicating a specific list of amino acids that are connected to each other to form that protein. There are virtually endless combinations of amino acids, meaning there are endless types of proteins that can be made.

Because proteins are constructed with amino acids, each protein may differ in the number and types of amino acids. Some proteins have all the amino acids your body needs; others may be missing a few.

Complete proteins contain all the essential amino acids your body must obtain through the diet. These types of foods have "high-quality" protein because they give you everything you need in one food. Complete proteins come from animal foods, such as meat, fish, eggs, poultry, cheese, and milk. You have to be careful when eating complete proteins, though, because sometimes they come with other health risks, such as higher amounts of saturated fats.

Incomplete proteins don't have the full allotment of essential amino acids. But that doesn't mean they aren't good proteins. Instead, you can combine different foods and construct your own complete protein picture. Plant-based proteins are typically incomplete, but when mixing different types of plant proteins, you can get the full amino acid picture. For example, you can mix vegetables with grains, or vegetables, nuts, and seeds (like beans and peas) — and the combination would give you a complete protein meal.

The body has an ability to make some amino acids by deconstructing the amino acids you ingest, but you have to consume a minimum number of amino acids for this to occur. Amino acids are grouped into two categories:

>> **Nonessential amino acids:** These are the amino acids that the body can produce. The nonessential amino acids are: alanine, arginine, asparagine, aspartic acid, cysteine, glutamic acid, glutamine, glycine, proline, serine, and tyrosine.

NITROGEN BALANCE AND PROTEIN STATUS

There is a constant action of building up and breaking down of tissue. The nitrogen portion of protein when it's broken down can be measured in the urine, and the amount excreted can indicate whether the body is breaking down protein (*catabolism*) or building up protein (*anabolism*). The term *nitrogen balance* refers to this catabolism-anabolism relationship. When urine nitrogen levels are elevated relative to the amount of protein ingested, this indicates tissue breakdown. This situation may occur during times of heavy exercise or fasting, or when eating a very low-cab diet, because protein can be scavenged to help make glucose. Monitoring nitrogen balance during training is one way to determine if dietary protein intake is adequate to meet the needs of the exercising body. Negative nitrogen balance indicates that more dietary protein needs to be consumed to meet the demands of an exercising and recovering body.

Although nonessential amino acids can be produced by the body, that only happens if there is adequate nutrient and caloric intake. In cases of malnutrition, even nonessential amino acids become necessary in the diet because the body can't produce them.

>> **Essential amino acids:** These are the amino acids that the body can't produce; they must be obtained through the diet. The essential amino acids are: histidine, isoleucine, leucine, lysine, methionine, phenylalanine, threonine, tryptophan, and valine.

Arginine is an example of a non-essential amino acid important for the synthesis of many proteins as well as ATP production and nitric oxide. During infancy, injury, and malnutrition, the body cannot synthesize enough arginine to meet the body's needs. You may see arginine in the food supplement aisle as it may need to be taken in the diet despite the body producing it.

Knowing how much protein you need

Protein requirements vary depending on whether you're an athlete and whether you've just finished a workout. In the following sections, we explain how much protein you need.

Be sure to aim for high-quality protein, either complete proteins or combinations of proteins that ensure that you're consuming all the essential amino acids. Also, look at the protein-containing food to ensure that it isn't high in fat.

FOR HEALTH

Typically, 12 percent to 15 percent of daily dietary intake should come from protein. The recommendation is X0.36 grams per pound of body weight (0.8 grams per kilogram of body weight). For example, a 180-pound individual would need 65 grams of protein per day.

REMEMBER

These protein requirements are for healthy adults that are not subject to heavy exercise training or other activity that may require a higher protein intake. If you're training or participating in athletic activities, protein requirements are higher (see the next section). Table 15-2 identifies some sources of protein in common foods.

TABLE 15-2   ## Sources of Protein

Source	Grams of Protein
1 whole egg	6.3
½ chicken breast (3.5 ounces or 100 grams)	26.7
Cottage cheese (1 cup or 200 grams)	28
Greek yogurt (1 cup or 200 grams)	20
Lentils (½ cup or 100 grams)	9
Black beans (1 cup or 100 grams)	9
Lean beef (3 ounces or 85 grams)	25
Fish fillet (3.5 ounces or 100 grams)	30 to 40
Quinoa (1 cup or 185 grams)	8
Whey protein powder serving (1 scoop)	15 to 20

FOR ATHLETES

Both aerobic exercise and strength training have higher requirements for protein intake. Protein may be used more as a fuel during heavy exercise and is important during the recovery process after heavy exercise. Protein requirements can range from 0.5 to 0.9 grams per pound of body weight (1.2 to 2.0 grams per kilogram body weight), depending on the type, intensity, and volume of exercise. For example, a 180-pound individual would need 98 to 164 grams of protein per day.

PROTEIN POWDERS

For some people, getting enough protein through their diet may seem daunting. This is especially true if they're avoiding meat and aiming for a more plant-based diet. In this case, supplementing with protein powder may be appropriate. Protein powders may be milk-based or plant-based. Whole foods are the best source of nutrition, and protein powers don't contain all the nutrients you need. But as a supplemental source of protein, they can help you get more protein beyond what a healthy diet can provide.

Individual differences in terms of how a person responds to training can also influence protein requirements. One way of tracking too little protein intake can be to measure the urinary nitrogen (nitrogen balance). Tracking excess protein intake is more difficult. Excess amino acids are converted to glucose or fat or used as energy during exercise. Stay within the recommended intake amounts based on the level of physical activity.

AFTER EXERCISE

"Muscle is not built in the weightroom," or so the saying goes. Instead, it's built during the recovery from the muscle stress done in the gym. So, it's important to have the muscle-building materials on hand during the recovery process. This means consuming carbohydrates to fuel the building process and protein to form the protein fibers that make up the muscle.

TIP

Research has shown that the first hour after heavy exercise is a very important time for muscle protein synthesis. Whey protein seems to be absorbed the fastest during this recovery time, so it's often used in recovery protein drinks. The whey also contains the essential amino acids needed for the muscle-building process.

There are limits to how much digested amino acids can be absorbed and used for protein synthesis from a meal "dose" — around 20 to 25 grams. Keep this in mind when ingesting a meal. A very large protein meal of, say, 50 grams won't all go toward protein synthesis. Instead, perhaps as much as half the "dose" will simply be used for energy or conversion to glucose. Spreading out the meals in smaller protein doses can help maximize use for muscle building.

Water: Most of What We Are

If you looked at the fraction of water that makes up your body (60 percent to 70 percent), you may think you should be living in the ocean! The brain and heart are about 73 percent water! Muscles and kidneys are around 80 percent water.

These numbers vary by age (we dry out as we age) and even body composition (higher body fat means less water).

Water has a range of important functions that are essential to our survival:

>> It flushes the waste product from the body through the kidneys by urination.

>> It transports oxygen, carbohydrates, and fats within the bloodstream.

>> It lubricates the joints and serves as a shock absorber in the brain and tissues.

>> It maintains the metabolism of cells, keeping them growing and replicating.

>> It regulates body temperature.

>> It keeps digestion going, from ingestion to defecation.

Without water, we would quickly cease to function. Even small reductions in water can affect the body. This issue can especially be a problem for athletes during events where sweating is heavy.

A typical adult needs 11 to 15 cups (2 to 4 liters) of water every day just to survive. This amount varies by individual size, activity level, and even diet. Seventy percent of the water we consume comes from the foods we eat.

In the following sections, we explain the role of water in temperature regulation, and how to track losses in water to help inform fluid replacement during and after exercise.

Recognizing water's role in temperature regulation

During exercise, sweat loss can be as high as 13 cups (3 liters) of fluid per hour! The amount varies by body size, environment (heat and humidity), exercise intensity, and sweat gland activity. Sweat evaporation is the primary way we cool our bodies during exercise in hot environments, so sweat loss is the price we pay for maintaining normal body temperature. But replacing the water is essential for sport performance and survival.

It isn't just sweat we lose when we exercise. Body water contains the electrolytes (primarily sodium and potassium) important for nerve, muscle, and cell function. For heavy sweat loss, we must replace not only water but also electrolytes. Sport drinks are an effective solution — they contain water, glucose, and electrolytes in the proper concentration. The key is to get enough fluid during activities where you lose a lot of sweat.

You can get a head start on the sweat loss through *pre-hydration* (consuming fluids before exercise). Often people are slightly dehydrated even on regular days, so the goal of pre -hydration is to drink water/electrolyte beverages during the hours before exercise until your urine flow is a pale yellow (rather than darker yellow). The lighter the urine, the closer to full hydration.

During heavy exercise, sweat loss will be very high, and you can't replace what you've lost all at once. Often, drinking large volumes of water will cause gastrointestinal (GI) discomfort, so aim for several smaller drinks to try to keep up. Hydration during an athletic event should be about 1 cup (250 milliliters) of fluid every 15 to 20 minutes. The fluid should be cool to help transfer some heat away from the core. It should contain mostly water and about 6 percent glucose and electrolytes (sodium and potassium).

Drinking too much water is actually possible. As electrolytes are lost through sweat, if water is used as the only replacement drink, a dilution of electrolytes (especially sodium) occurs. The term *hyponatremia* refers to this low level of sodium in the blood. It leads to nausea, vomiting, and some symptoms that can be confused with heat injury. This is why it's best to replace sweat losses with a drink containing electrolytes and small amounts of glucose (like a sports drink).

After the event, you probably still won't be fully hydrated, so it's important to keep hydrating. However, after exercise, you want a higher concentration of glucose in order to quickly replace glycogen stores. So, choose the same recovery drinks mentioned for carbohydrates during recovery, with drinks that have 20 to 50 grams of carbohydrates, instead of the lighter carbohydrates drink used during exercise. These drinks will also help restore fluid balance.

AN EASY WAY TO TRACK SWEAT LOSS? BODY WEIGHT!

TIP

One way to keep an eye on fluid loss during an event is to get a pre-event nude body weight in kilograms (clothes can absorb sweat, so you don't want them involved in a pre-event/post-event weight measurement). Then repeat the measurement after exercise. Any lost weight can be assumed to be sweat loss and gives you a close approximation of the fluid you need to replace. One kilogram of weight loss is equal to 1 liter of fluid, so tracking weight loss using the metric system gives an easy computation of fluid replacement.

Micronutrients: Vitamins and Minerals

Vitamins and minerals consist of a large group of compounds and elements that serve as catalysts for many different chemical reactions in the body. They may help metabolic actions like producing energy, delivering oxygen, maintaining skin, helping with vision . . . the list is almost endless. Although micronutrients are needed in small amounts (that's why they're *micro*), these nutrients are essential for the proper functioning of the body.

Vitamins

Vitamins can be grouped into two categories: fat soluble and water soluble. The difference is the medium in which they're stored. The water-soluble vitamins are vitamin C and a number of B vitamins. Because water is constantly being filtered and removed by the kidneys, water-soluble vitamins don't last as long in the body, so you need to consume them consistently. Cooking methods that leach away the water within foods (for example, boiling) may remove some of the vitamins, so steam the food instead if you can.

Fat-soluble vitamins can be stored within fat cells, so you can get too much of them. The fat-soluble vitamins are vitamins A, D, E, and K. Table 15-3 identifies the various vitamins, their function, and some food sources.

TABLE 15-3 **Vitamins: What They Do and Where to Get Them**

Vitamin	Function	Food Sources
A	This fat-soluble vitamin is required for normal skin growth, photoceptor function in the eyes, and immune system function. It also serves as an antioxidant (which helps fight off cell damage).	Carotenoids (green leafy vegetables, apricots, carrots, sweet potatoes, squash, egg yolks, kale, spinach
B1 (thiamin)	This water-soluble vitamin can be used to prevent *beriberi* (a deficiency disease that affects the heart and nervous system). It's also important for aerobic metabolism.	Almonds, peanuts, peas, soybeans, wheat germ, whole grains
B2 (riboflavin)	This water-soluble vitamin is important in metabolism, helping to transfer hydrogens in the aerobic energy production process.	Asparagus, broccoli, chicken, dairy products, green vegetables, peanut butter, pork, sardines
B3 (niacin)	This water-soluble vitamin is important in metabolism to help transfer hydrogens in ATP production.	Almonds, chicken, enriched bread, fish, mushrooms, peanuts, pork, tuna

(continued)

TABLE 15-3 *(continued)*

Vitamin	Function	Food Sources
B5 (pantothenic acid)	This water-soluble vitamin is important in the synthesis and breakdown of fatty acids. It's also important in aerobic metabolism.	Egg yolks, peanuts, whole grain cereals and breads, chicken, fish, beef
B6 (pyridoxine)	This water-soluble vitamin is a coenzyme important in amino acid metabolism and hemoglobin formation. It also assists in converting glycogen to glucose and the synthesis of some neurotransmitters.	Banana, chicken, dried beans, egg yolks, fish, fortified cereals peanuts, spinach, tuna
B9 (folic acid)	This water-soluble vitamin is important for DNA and RNA synthesis and growth. It reduces the risk of neural tube defects for women who may become pregnant.	Banana, beets, dried beans, egg yolks, leafy green vegetables, and peas
B12 (cobalamin)	This water-soluble vitamin is essential for nucleic acid formation, DNA and RNA synthesis, and maturation of red blood cells.	Beef, dairy, egg yolks, fortified cereals, salmon, sardines, tofu, tuna
Biotin	This water-soluble vitamin is important for steps in the ATP production process of aerobic metabolism, protein breakdown, and the synthesis and breakdown of fats.	Almonds, chicken, egg yolks, peanuts, salmon, sardines, and soybeans
C	This water-soluble vitamin is an antioxidant, which helps to block damage to cells, and a treatment for *scurvy* (a deficiency disease that results in weakness, tissue damage, bleeding, and even death). It also facilitates iron absorption and helps enzymes function.	broccoli, kale, mango juice, orange juice, and tomato juice
D	This fat-soluble vitamin is important for bone health, calcium absorption, immunity, and the prevention of *rickets* (a softening or weakening of bones due to vitamin D deficiency) and *osteomalacia* (a weakening of bone due to inadequate bone mineralization). It's considered a vitamin-hormone because it is created by the body to stimulate cellular actions and has specific bone-building functions. Vitamin D can be made by the body with help from the sun. Within the skin and using ultraviolet light, a cholesterol containing precursor can be converted to vitamin D.	Egg yolks, fish, shrimp, fortified cereals, fortified milk
E	This fat-soluble vitamin serves as an antioxidant and important for immune function.	Almonds, peanuts, sunflower seeds, vegetable oils, and wheatgerm
K	This fat-soluble vitamin assists in the process of blood coagulation, as well as in protein synthesis in the bones.	Broccoli, cabbage, cauliflower, kale, spinach

In the following sections, we narrow the scope a bit on the long list of vitamins and minerals to focus on two vitamins important for the bones, blood, and energy metabolism: vitamin D and the B vitamins. Deficiencies in these vitamins often impact physical activity, so for exercise scientists, they deserve a bit more attention.

Getting enough sunlight: Vitamin D

Vitamin D is a very important vitamin for numerous functions within the body. It can function as a hormone and is essential for the maintenance and building of bone. Although you can get vitamin D in the diet, it can also be manufactured in the skin in the presence of ultraviolet (UV) radiation, or sunlight. So, going outside on a sunny day can go a long way toward supplying the vitamin D you need.

Depending on where you live, your skin may be covered up with heavy clothing for part of the year, which makes getting enough vitamin D a real problem. According to national statistics, over 40 percent of Americans have insufficient quantities of vitamin D and 22 percent have moderate deficiencies. Lack of vitamin D contributes to osteoporosis, bone fractures, diabetes, and even cardiovascular disease.

TIP

If you're not sure whether you're getting enough vitamin D, your doctor can run a simple blood test to check, and you can supplement as necessary.

Eating right to get the energy vitamins: B complex

As you can see from Table 15-3, there are a lot of B vitamins! A common theme among them: Many are important in energy metabolism and red blood cell production. For this reason, deficiencies in B vitamins can really slow you down. B vitamins are largely found in eggs, meat, dairy, and fortified whole grains. If you don't eat meat or dairy, you may be deficient in B vitamins.

Some B vitamins in particular carry added risk for anemia, as well as developmental problems. Folic acid is a key vitamin during pregnancy. When the mother's folate intake is low, the risk of neural tube defects for the baby are greatly increased. For the mother, folate deficiency anemia is possible. Fortunately, folate is found in fortified whole grains and is also available as a supplement. Vitamin B12 is another vitamin that's important for red blood cell production, and deficiencies contribute to anemia. Up to 12 percent of the U.S. population isn't getting enough vitamin B12.

Just because the B vitamins are in foods doesn't mean the body will absorb it. Alcohol can leach B vitamins from the body and reduce the body's absorption of B vitamins. Digestive disorders (such as Crohn's disease and celiac disease) and diabetes also affect B vitamin levels.

Pay attention to B vitamin availability in athletes whose diet may not be sufficient, or in people with physical conditions that get in the way of B vitamin absorption. Eating lean proteins, fruits, vegetables, and fortified grains can go a long way toward maintaining a healthy vitamin B status. A simple blood test can check your status across the different B vitamins.

Minerals

Minerals are not made by plants or animals, but instead are elements that don't contain carbon. Minerals are essential for metabolic health and normal growth. We get minerals from the foods we eat, but food quality is only as good as the soil in which it's grown, so the mineral content of food can vary even for the same food. Table 15-4 summarizes several essential minerals and their function, as well as some common food sources.

TABLE 15-4 **Minerals: What They Do and Where to Get Them**

Mineral	Function	Food Sources
Calcium	Helps with bone strength, teeth strength, and blood clotting. Also is an intracellular trigger for muscle contraction.	Dairy, fortified juices, leafy green vegetables, salmon, sardines
Copper	Helps release iron from cellular storage, transfers electrons in the aerobic energy pathway, aids in blood clotting, and serves as a scavenger of *free radicals* (molecules that damage cells).	Almonds, organ meats, peanuts, raisins, seafood, walnuts, whole-grain cereals
Iodine	Essential for the synthesis of thyroxine (a thyroid hormone). An important protein synthesis factor.	Cheese, iodized table salt, milk, yogurt
Iron	Helps with oxygen transport in the blood and muscles. Part of the liver's enzyme system for metabolizing drugs and other compounds.	Almonds, beef, broccoli, dried beans, dried peas, egg yolks, fortified cereals, spinach, tofu, walnuts
Magnesium	Is an important part of bone strength. Is an important component in 300+ enzymes and part of ATP production and metabolism.	Dairy products, leafy green vegetables, oysters, peanuts, salmon, shrimp, walnuts, whole-grain breads, whole-grain cereals
Selenium	Is a free-radical scavenger. Works with vitamin E to protect cell membranes.	Fortified cereals, lean meats, seafood, whole grains
Zinc	Is an important component in 100+ enzymes. Helps with protein synthesis and wound healing. Is part of the hormone insulin and is an immune system function factor.	Beef, chicken, dairy products, fish, oysters, peanuts, wheat germ

In the following sections, we narrow the scope a bit to cover two key minerals that the exercise scientist should know more about. Iron is a key mineral for oxygen transport and is often deficient in athletes, while calcium is essential for bone health.

Getting enough iron

Iron deficiency is the most common mineral deficiency among athletes, with rates as high as 35 percent in women and 8 percent in men. Iron is an essential mineral for the transport of oxygen in red blood cells as part of hemoglobin. It's also essential for myoglobin formation and the transport of oxygen in muscle. Finally, iron is needed in the chemical steps for the production of ATP using aerobic metabolism. Any reductions in iron can result in lowered levels of hemoglobin, myoglobin, and VO2 max (see Chapters 4 and 5).

Normal levels of hemoglobin in women are above 12 grams per deciliter (g/dl) and in men above 13 g/dl. Low iron levels contribute to *anemia,* which is a reduction in red blood cell production. Anemia lowers endurance, causes fatigue, and can also cause heart *dysrhythmias* (an abnormal heart rhythm). Anemia is seen in about 7 percent of female athletes.

Factors contributing to low iron levels include:

>> Low dietary intake

>> Blood loss in the gut

>> Menstrual cycle–related blood loss

>> Foot impact from running, damaging the red blood cells in the feet

>> Heavy training and low caloric intake

The tricky thing about iron nutritionally is that it's pretty hard for the body to absorb. In fact, only about 14 percent to 20 percent of iron is actually absorbed and made available to the body. Meat, fish, and poultry contain a peptide (known as MFP) that helps increase the absorption of iron. Plant-based iron doesn't have this peptide, so the iron has reduced rates of absorption.

How can you increase your body's iron stores? A good place to start would be to assess your current iron status. A doctor may want to use other tests along with iron status to get a clear picture of a patient's needs. An appropriate plan can then be made on a case-by-case basis. Some possible iron boosting strategies may include the following:

>> Consume iron-containing foods with fruits containing vitamin C. This combination helps increase iron absorption.

>> Add lean meats to your diet to include iron and the MFP peptide.

>> Take an iron supplement.

Athletes should track their iron status through blood measures. Iron overload is possible with excessive supplementation, so blindly supplementing is not a wise approach. Make sure the athlete has done what they can with proper assessments (by a doctor), changing their diet, and perhaps even training (reduced running on hard surfaces) to improve their iron status.

Building bone with calcium

Calcium is essential for strong bones and teeth, and it also contributes to muscle, blood vessel, and nerve function. Calcium doesn't work alone, however — nutrients such as vitamin D, phosphorous, magnesium, potassium, and protein are also very important. In addition, you need the compressive force of exercise to stimulate bone growth. But without calcium, the other nutrients just can't do the work.

Currently, 40 percent to 50 percent of the U.S. population has low calcium intake. When you add sedentary activity to the mix, you get a lot of people with weaker bones.

Calcium intake is very important during the years of peak bone growth. These are the developmental years around puberty, where the bulk of our bone mass is accumulated. Low calcium intake during these times can mean weaker bones into adulthood. Other milestone moments are during pregnancy and post-menopause, when bone growth can be greatly reduced without adequate calcium.

Calcium is best absorbed when taken in small amounts across the day. Foods that have been fortified with extra calcium work very well, because they also contain other bone-building nutrients (potassium, magnesium, and vitamin D). Calcium supplementation may be useful for those with calcium deficiency, but talk with your doctor first. Excess calcium (known as *hypercalcemia*) can lead to constipation and kidney stones. The key is eating a balanced diet that supplies all the nutrients together to maximize calcium use and bone growth. And don't forget to exercise!

5

The Part of Tens

Become familiar with the behaviors and health factors that form the foundation of physical fitness.

Uncover the link between physical activity and obesity.

Discover the many careers that a background in exercise science prepares you for.

Chapter **16**

Ten Foundations of Fitness

Sometimes, the whole idea of fitness can seem very confusing. So many plans, so many ways of exercising, so many interrelated components! However, much of fitness can be narrowed down to ten key concepts that provide you with the foundation of knowledge you need to move forward with a fitness plan. Keeping it simple helps make fitness more attainable, and this chapter is designed to help you do just that.

Training Specificity

The human body is capable of running fast, jumping high, and lifting heavy things, but it performs best when trained. Many physiologic systems of the body — from the brain and nervous system down to the chemistry of cell metabolism — are involved with any given activity. These systems adapt based on the nature of the training. So, if you're trying to achieve a specific effect (for example, running fast), you need to train specific to that activity. Sprint training won't help those aerobic muscle fibers run a marathon better; instead, it'll help them adapt to faster sprinting.

Here are some key questions to ask when it comes to training specificity:

>> Is the activity aerobic or anaerobic?

>> What is the desired velocity of the movement?

>> Are you training for speed or endurance?

>> Which energy system is the primary system used?

>> What types of muscle fibers do you hope to train?

The key is to train specific to the desired outcomes. This will drive the physiologic adaptations that match your activity.

Training Overload

No one ever got bigger muscles by lifting a pencil. The body adapts to the physical environment it's challenged with. Muscle grows when it's stressed and loaded with more work than it's used to. This is the *overload principle*, which states that a body system has to be stressed beyond its normal ability in order for it to adapt. For example:

>> When a weight lifter lifts a load that is at least 60 percent of their one-repetition maximum (1RM) to fatigue, they stress and fatigue their muscles, which adapt and grow in response.

>> When a runner adds a bit more mileage to give more stress to their cardio-vascular and muscular systems will improve their VO_2 max.

>> When a basketball player practices three-point shots, even when fatigued, they provide overload and improve their stamina during games.

REMEMBER

The process of overloading is individualized. Everyone progresses differently, and the step jumps in loading should be done with knowledge of the capability of the individual.

Reversibility: If You Don't Use It, You Lose It

The human body is a constantly changing set of systems. If you exercise and overload the body, the systems kick in to adapt and improve. But if those same systems don't get any stress or strain, they lose the positive adaptation. Being inactive doesn't just keep you in the "average" zone — your body systems will regress. For example:

>> Muscle mass is lost.

>> Bone becomes weaker.

>> The metabolic rate slows.

>> Fat mass is added.

>> Blood vessels don't grow and spread through tissue.

Astronauts going into the weightless environment of space begin losing muscle and bone mass almost immediately. Moving is a must. This is why prolonged sitting is a health risk — the systems regress and health deteriorates. This is also why any movement is a positive! You can stop the decline and change the environment to one of movement and appropriate overload.

Exercising to Build Better Bone

Strong bones are the foundation for a strong body. Although the most bone is deposited during childhood and through puberty, bone continues to be remade (broken down and built back up) through much of adulthood. Just as guitar players have callouses of thick skin on their fingertips from regularly playing guitar, you can build denser bones by regularly putting them under some stress.

REMEMBER

Bones react to compression forces by growing stronger. Gravity and weight make excellent bone builders. Each step you take places your spinal column under a compressive load, which stimulates bone growth. The reverse is also true: Lack of activity — sitting around, lying in bed, and so on — accelerates bone loss. Bone is an important part of healthy body composition (see Chapter 13).

Sticking with It: Exercise Adherence

The best laid plans don't work if you don't implement the plan. How many people set big exercise goals for the coming year, only to have it fall by the wayside within a few weeks. Sticking to an exercise program and other lifestyle changes that can lead to better health is challenging. People often know what they need to do but have trouble sticking with it.

Here are some factors that are linked with exercise adherence:

>> **The nature of the exercise program:** Is the program too difficult to sustain? Does it require the person to exercise too often?

>> **Location:** Can the person get to the location easily?

>> **Supervision:** Does the person have a trainer helping them work out? People stick with exercise programs better when someone is helping and holding them accountable.

>> **Social interaction:** Is the environment positive and supportive?

>> **Expectations:** Are the person's expectations reasonable? Have they been educated about their health and the expected rate of improvement?

>> **Feedback:** Is their progress being monitored? Are they getting feedback from a trainer? Are they using wearable technology?

As an exercise science professional, you need to know your client, understand their goals, and identify any barriers that may interfere with their ability to reach their goals. Then tailor your plan to help create a program that they enjoy and stick with.

Cross-Training to Optimize Fitness

Muscles grow and adapt when they're given tasks that cause them to create new patterns of use and adapt to tissue trauma. When you exercise the same way all the time, you're probably leaving some muscle fibers out of the action. As a result, some muscle may get strong while others stay dormant and weak, creating muscle imbalances.

For a muscle to get the full benefit of training, it needs a changing environment of stresses. Lifting weights at different speeds, varying the lifts, and engaging in training that involves a variety of activities help muscles continually adapt. New neural connections are made, more fibers are stimulated, and balance and coordination are enhanced. (Head to Chapter 11 for more information about training.)

Accepting That Fat Goes Where It Wants

As much as we humans may try, we can't control where fat gets deposited on our bodies; nor can we control where we lose fat. All we can do is control the overall amount of fat that gets deposited or lost. Here's what this information means:

>> **You mobilize and utilize fat from the stores in your body in an order determined for you.** Fat comes and goes from cells based upon gender, genetics, age, and hormones (to name just a few key factors). Men may notice that fat seems to gravitate toward the belly, whereas their legs may not have as much. Women, on the other hand, may notice that their thighs and arms seem to be happy homes for fat.

>> **You can't lose fat in a particular area of your body just by exercising that area (doing sit-ups to eliminate abdominal fat, for example).** This strategy is akin to sitting in a room next to a physics class and expecting to learn physics. Instead, you need to create a demand for fat calories to be used by engaging in activities — like walking, jogging, and swimming — that use large groups of muscles (legs, back, and hips).

Keeping Blood Sugar under Control

Chronically elevated glucose does some serious damage to blood vessels and nerves, so *glycemic control*, or keeping blood sugar in a desirable range, is wise. You can attack the issue from two directions:

>> **Slow the amount and rate at which glucose enters the blood.** Instead of eating the usual three big meals per day, eat six smaller meals. And mix the foods up (fat, protein, and carbohydrate) to slow the rate of digestion. Adding fiber to the meal helps slow the rate of glucose absorption.

>> **Take the movement of glucose out of the blood and into cells.** Normally, the hormone insulin helps move glucose out of the blood. In people with diabetes, either insulin is not produced or it doesn't do its job. The good news is that exercise can act just like insulin and move glucose into the cells (to be burned during exercise). Daily, moderate exercise both burns calories to help keep body weight down (which helps diabetes) and helps lower blood glucose. Think of exercise as the best medicine you can take for blood sugar control!

Allowing Yourself to Recover from Exercise

Improvements in fitness don't happen during the training activity. Instead, they happen during the *recovery* from the activity, when your muscles heal and grow stronger. That makes the next bout of training easier (head to Chapter 3 for details on muscle adaptations). Recovery is important both for the short term (so you can get back out there and train again) and the long term (to improve fitness).

TIP

Muscles require protein (to add structure to the muscle) and carbohydrates (to fuel the muscle-building process). Then they need time for the recovery and adaptation to take place. In addition to taking time to recover, be sure to consume adequate amounts of carbohydrates and protein within the first few hours of a heavy workout. (You can find more on sports nutrition in Chapter 15.)

Remaining Active as You Age

Some young people think that when you hit age 30, your metabolism slows down, you get fat and weak, and your life is pretty much over. As people who are well past 30, we beg to differ! If you look only at change in fitness across different age groups, you see large declines and increases in body fat. *However,* when you look at individuals who continue to exercise, these "age-related" changes seem to disappear until people start getting to ages around 60! Inactivity is not aging — get moving to stay young!

Chapter **17**

Ten Facts about Obesity and Physical Inactivity

I n 2023, one in five U.S. adults lived with obesity, and 23 states had obesity rates over 35 percent! The prevalence of obesity has grown at a staggering rate over the past 30 years, and estimates suggest that by 2050, everyone will be obese! Although that scenario is probably not going to happen (obesity rates appear to be leveling off), obesity is clearly a global epidemic.

And, boy, does it cost money! Recent estimates put the obesity bill at about $1.6 trillion annually, with obese individuals spending almost $1,800 more in annual medical costs than normal-weight individuals due to obesity-related ailments. Although physical inactivity is not the only contributor to obesity, it certainly plays a major role, as the ten points in this chapter make clear.

As One Goes Up, the Other Goes Down

Obesity is at epidemic levels in the United States and in many industrialized countries. The biggest contributors to the obesity epidemic are physical inactivity and excessive caloric intake, especially fatty and processed foods — the hallmarks of the Western diet.

As the obesity epidemic has grown, the amount of physical activity is at all-time lows. Less than half of adults and only three out of ten kids get the recommended amounts of daily activity. Physical education (PE) time in schools has been greatly reduced. Only Oregon and the District of Columbia meet the national standards for weekly PE for elementary and middle school kids. Plus, technology has helped create a climate of inactivity. Reversing this trend means flipping the equation: Increase physical activity, and bring about a drop in the obesity rate.

Just Adding Activity May Not Be Enough

Just adding some activity to an otherwise sedentary lifestyle may not be enough to ward off obesity and the problems that come with it. Some studies show that when people start an exercise program, they actually reduce their activity in other areas (like leisure time) — a scenario that's like taking two steps forward and one step back. In addition, being sedentary for long stretches of time not only adds to the obesity problem, but also negatively affects circulation, muscle mass, and blood sugar. Your body needs to feel gravity and movement throughout the day, and exercise may not be enough of a stimulus to counteract long-term sitting.

REMEMBER

No amount of activity can offset a diet that is high in excess calories. To make a substantial impact on weight loss, nutrition planning is essential. A sustainable approach to diet management is important for long-term weight loss.

Obesity and Inactivity Can Lead to Metabolic Syndrome

WARNING

As a body becomes obese, the extra fat affects a number of body systems, and the obese person ends up with a cluster of conditions: high blood pressure, higher blood sugar, a greater risk of diabetes, abnormal cholesterol levels, and so on. Obese people also are usually quite inactive, which has its own problems.

This clustering of problems due to obesity is called *metabolic syndrome*, and it's a big reason why obesity has so many healthcare costs. Medical intervention is often necessary to control blood sugar, lower blood pressure, and improve cholesterol — all of which costs money but doesn't actually do anything to help the root cause of obesity. Long term, metabolic syndrome leads to high rates of heart disease, stroke, heart failure, kidney failure, and diabetes (to name just a few issues).

Sitting Is the New Smoking

Everyone knows that smoking is bad for you. It's linked to cancer, heart disease, asthma, and a whole host of other ills. Even secondhand smoke is hard on the body. But did you know that physical inactivity puts you at just as much risk for heart disease, cancer, and a number of other ailments? In that way, physical inactivity is the new smoking.

Across the United States, the prevalence of inactivity ranges from 10 percent to 40 percent! Think of inactivity the same way you view smoking and take steps to stop it: If you have children, help them stay active and support efforts to protect (or bring back) physical education programs in schools.

Obesity Is a Tough Burden for Children

Obesity can accelerate many chronic diseases, and when kids have obesity, they start out on a difficult path. Obesity in childhood increases the chance of obesity in adulthood. About 19 percent of kids in the United States are obese, which is a significant increase over the past 30 years.

An environment with easy access to excess sugar, fast food, and large portions, coupled with a technological world of smartphones, video games, and online activities, results in reduced physical activity — the perfect storm to promote obesity.

Obesity in kids can result in low self-esteem, reduced participation in social activities, depression, bullying, and exclusion from activities. Treating obesity in kids needs to be paired with treatment for the psychosocial-related aspects of their lives.

Caloric Restriction Has Its Limits

Most dietary recommendations suggest following a caloric restriction plan for weight loss that can be maintained consistently and becomes part of your daily regimen. Nutrient-dense foods are important, especially as you seek to reduce calories. Limiting foods high in added sugars, saturated fat, and sodium are also important.

There are also dietary approaches that try to limit calories by scheduling eating differently. *Intermittent fasting* is an approach that reduces the time window for eating; it helps reduce calories and prevent the constant eating pattern that can cause excess fat deposition.

There are limits to the number calories that can be restricted. In order to obtain the necessary nutrients — and at least enough glucose to fuel the brain — 1,200 calories per day is identified as the minimum caloric intake. Can you go lower? Sure, but you risk nutrient deficiencies as well as reducing glucose availability. This leads to scavenging of protein from muscle stores to convert to glucose. Muscle mass loss and lowered metabolic rate can occur.

There Is No Secret to Losing Fat

The list of diet plans and exercise programs that are currently in the media and on the market is enormous — and confusing! Yet, if you look at all of them, you'll notice that they share a common link: limiting calories (especially calories that have no nutritional value) and increasing the burning of calories — the hallmarks of all successful diets. But you don't need a fancy diet. Here are some general guidelines you can follow to get that first pound of fat to go away:

>> **Limit your intake of calories.** Start simply by reducing portion sizes (eating on smaller plates can help). Try to eat more fiber and complex carbohydrates and drink more water; doing so helps fill you up (fat has a lot of calories without offering much tummy-filling satisfaction).

>> **Move.** Walk a mile, run a mile, walk the stairs, dance, play with the kids . . . anything! You burn calories when you move, and that movement doesn't have to wipe you out. In fact, if you want to lose weight, try to find an activity or combination of activities that keeps you moving for about an hour every day.

Fat Can Hide in Your Body

We have all pinched an inch (or more) and felt the fat that sits between our skin and the underlying muscle. But that's not the only place where fat takes hold. In fact, the fat you really need to worry about is deeper in your body. *Visceral fat* is the fat that's deep within the central part of the body (the *viscera*) and covers your organs. Here's what you need to know:

>> **High levels of visceral fat, especially stored in the upper body, are linked to higher incidences of heart disease.** Upper-body obesity (or an "apple" shape) is linked to greater risk of heart disease.

>> **Fat can migrate!** Well, sort of. The distribution of fat changes. As you age, more of your fat is stored in the visceral area — not good news. So, that same inch you pinch at age 20 is not as bad as the inch you pinch at age 50.

You Can Make a Difference in a Day

The wonderful thing about the human body is the way it adapts and responds quickly to physical activity. Despite years of inactivity, your body will respond almost immediately to strength and aerobic training. After only one bout of exercise, you'll experience these changes:

>> Your body will begin to grow larger muscles.

>> Your body will build enzymes that help use fat as a fuel.

>> You'll improve your body's ability to control blood glucose.

>> Your ability to burn fat and control your blood sugar will improve. Studies have shown that even short bursts of high-intensity activity (one to three minutes) can improve control of blood sugar.

It All Adds Up

The good news about movement and health is that the expenditure of energy is what reduces heart disease and cancer risk — not how hard you worked or how many miles you ran, but just the total amount of work.

These calories can come from any activity. Walk the dog. Take the stairs. Go dancing. Play an active video game. Any activity that gets your body moving contributes to a healthier you. So, although you may choose to work out or do some other type of structured activity, as long as you're moving, you're burning calories. So just *move!*

Chapter 18

Ten (or So) Careers for Exercise Scientists

One exciting part of exercise science is the variety of careers that relate to movement. Movement is used to train athletes, rehabilitate injury, improve quality of life, and reduce the risk of chronic disease. Your career may specialize or be flexible enough to cover a variety of fields. In this chapter, we look at some of the common careers in the exercise science field.

Cardiac Rehabilitation

Exercise is one of the best medicines available to help improve the condition of the heart and help patients regain their quality of life. As a clinical exercise physiologist working in cardiac rehabilitation, you may work with patients in the hospital immediately after a cardiac event or surgery, helping them get back on their feet and providing them with education regarding exercise, diet, and lifestyle. Following their release from the hospital, you may use exercise training and nutrition education and collaborate with their physicians to help patients regain as much heart function as possible and hopefully prevent any future event. Additional job opportunities extend in the clinical setting to pulmonary rehabilitation, cardiac catheterization labs, cancer patient exercise rehab, and bariatric care.

TIP

One organization that can connect you to this field is the American Association of Cardiovascular and Pulmonary Rehabilitation (AACVPR; www.aacvpr.org). Certifications in clinical exercise physiology are available from AACVPR and the American College of Sports Medicine (www.acsm.org).

Strength and Conditioning Specialist

Performance in athletics is greatly dependent upon proper conditioning. Conditioning involves a combination of aerobic, anaerobic, and strength exercises. For exercise scientists interested in using strength and power training to help improve performance, a job as a strength and conditioning specialist may be just right for you.

TIP

Often, these careers require a certification from the National Strength and Conditioning Association (www.nsca.com). You'll also want to have an internship or other work experience working with clients.

Wellness Specialist

Eighty percent of corporations with more than 100 employees offer some form of wellness program. Yet healthcare costs continue to spiral upward, with many of the chronic diseases (obesity, diabetes, and heart disease) leading the cost escalation. What if they had a healthier workforce? Think of the cost savings!

If you like working with people one-on-one and enjoy spending your day conducting a variety of health-related tests, providing health information, and training clients, this may be your field! Learn more by visiting the Wellness Council of America (www.welcoa.org).

Personal Trainer

Do you like working one-on-one with clients? If so, you may want to be a personal trainer. As a personal trainer, you may work at a big sports facility, onsite at a YMCA, or in a private studio. You'll have a variety of clients, coming in all shapes and sizes. Some may be in very poor shape; others may be training for a big event. You'll design aerobic and strength programs to help clients attain your goals.

TIP

Personal trainer certifications are available by exam through organizations such as the American College of Sports Medicine (ACSM) (www.acsm.org), the American Council on Exercise (www.acefitness.org), and the National Strength and Conditioning Association (www.nsca.com). ACSM also has a higher-level exercise physiologist certification, which requires a bachelor's degree in exercise science.

Sports Biomechanist

Sports biomechanists examine how athletes move and look for ways to help them improve performance. As a biomechanist, you would evaluate things like how the movement is sequenced, how much strength an athlete has, or the influence that a type of equipment may have on performance (assessing the wind resistance for a road cyclist, for example). Often, you'll use video taken during various performances and provide feedback to the athlete.

TIP

Check out more about this profession from the American Society of Biomechanics (https://asbweb.org).

Athletic Trainer

Athletic trainers are highly qualified, multiskilled healthcare professionals who work under the direction of or in collaboration with a physician. As a part of the healthcare team, services provided by athletic trainers include primary care, injury and illness prevention, wellness promotion and education, emergency care, examination and clinical diagnosis, therapeutic intervention, and rehabilitation of injuries and medical conditions.

Athletic trainers treat a range of patients and can work in a variety of settings, including the following:

>> Secondary schools, colleges, and universities

>> A physician's practice

>> Occupational health departments in commercial settings

>> Police and fire departments and academies, municipal departments, and branches of the military

>> The performing arts, including professional- and collegiate-level dance, music, and theater physical performances

Athletic training is a master's degree program, and exercise science is a perfect undergraduate program to help get you ready.

REMEMBER

Athletic trainers must be certified through the Board of Certification, and preparation for this exam requires candidates to have graduated from a Commission on Accreditation of Athletic Training Education (CAATE) accredited master's degree program.

Regardless of their practice setting, athletic trainers practice according to their education and scope of practice and state practice acts. For more information, consult the National Athletic Trainers' Association (www.nata.org).

Sport and Exercise Psychologist

Whether someone chooses to participate in some form of physical activity in the first place — and how well they perform once involved — is largely a matter of thoughts and emotions. Sport and exercise psychologists are academically trained to study two major questions:

>> How do psychological factors (like motivation, anxiety, confidence, and goal setting) impact the quality of a person's performance — or whether the person chooses to participate at all?

>> How does the quality of a person's performance — or the fact that they even participate in physical activity — affect *psychological factors* (the way that person thinks, feels, and behaves)?

TIP

To get a quick overview of what's required to be a sports and exercise psychologist, check out the web page for the Association for Applied Sport Psychology (https://appliedsportpsych.org).

Wellness Coach

All sorts of coaches exist — sport performance coaches, strength and conditioning coaches, nutritional coaches, health coaches, even mental coaches. Regardless of their individual specialties, all coaches are, in some way or another, trying to improve the lives of the people they're coaching. In general, the more that coaches know about all aspects of exercise science, the better they're able to help their clients accomplish physical activity–related goals. Wellness coaches are motivators, and they have a broad range of expertise in helping to change people's lifestyles toward long-term positive health changes.

TIP

To learn about wellness coaching, check out the National Academy of Sport Medicine (www.nasm.org/continuing-education/wellness-coach).

A BRIDGE TO GRADUATE HEALTH PROFESSIONS

The undergraduate degree in exercise science covers a wide range of fields that involve movement and/or exercise as a therapy to improve or heal the body. This makes it the perfect undergraduate degree to prepare you for graduate-degree programs and get you to the associated careers. The health profession careers include:

- Biomechanical engineer
- Epidemiologist
- Ergonomist
- Exercise physiologist (research)
- Health administrator
- Health educator
- Nurse
- Occupational therapist
- Physical therapist
- Physician assistant
- Recreational therapist
- Sport scientist

Knowledge of the body, a background in science foundation, and practical skills in human performance assessment will help lift you above the crowd of the other bachelor's-levels students trying to gain admission to these very competitive degree programs.

Graduate programs are highly selective and very competitive! You must have a high grade point average (GPA), volunteer experience, and even an internship in a related area just to compete. An added bonus would be any research opportunity you could do while an undergraduate student.

Index

C

C vitamin, 314
calcium, 316, 318
calcium carbonate, 258
calcium phosphate, 258
calories
    about, 78–79
    restricting, 329–330
    weight gain and, 278
    weight loss and, 276
cancer, exercise and, 25–26
carbaminohemoglobin, 107
carbohydrates
    about, 296
    after exercise, 301–302
    carbohydrate loading, 299–300
    during exercise, 300–301
    glucose, 296–297
    glycemic index/load, 297–298
    glycogen, 296–297
    guidelines for performance, 298–299
    heat and, 124
    muscle mass and, 78
    for weight gain, 278
carbon dioxide (CO_2), 104, 107–108, 132
carbonic acid, 107
cardiac output, 101–102, 118
cardiac rehabilitation, 333–334
cardiorespiratory system, 12
cardiovascular drift, 115
cardiovascular system
    about, 91
    blood vessels, 110–112
    delivering air to cells, 102–109
    effects of exercise on, 112–117
    heart structure, 91–93
    how the heart works, 93–102
    long-term changes to performance, 117–118
careers, 333–337
cartilage, 190–192
cartilaginous joints, 186–187
cell body, 140
cell hypoxia, 265
cells, delivering air to, 102–109
center of gravity, 178
central fatigue, 71
central nervous system (CNS), 204

cerebellum, 144
cerebral cortex, 142
chambers, heart, 92
Cheat Sheet (website), 3
chemical bonds, 64
chemistry, 8, 56
chemoreceptors, blood-flow control and, 111
chemotoxicity, 26
children, obesity in, 329
chocolate milk, 302
cholesterol, 305
chronic workload, 288
chylomicrons, 303
circulatory system, 12
circumduction, 171
closed tasks, 216
closed-feedback mechanisms, 216
closed-loop system, 145–146
closed-packed position, 193
clothing, for cold environments, 130
collagen, 206–207, 258, 260
combined loads, 181
Compendium of Physical Activities, 21
complete proteins, 307
compression, 180, 261
compressive strength, 258
concave orientation, 193
concentric contractions, 50
concussions, 183
conditioning, 254–255
conduction cooling, 123
connective tissues, 190–192, 194–195
contractile components, 206
contractile proteins, 60
contractility, 42–43
contracting the heart, 99
contractions, 34–39, 49–50
contract-relax PNF technique, 210
convection cooling, 123
convex orientation, 193
cooldown, 40, 247, 252, 255–256
cooling mechanisms, 123–124
coordinating movement, 151–156
copper, 316
core temperature, 120
core-to-shell model of heat transfer, 121
coronary artery disease, physical activity and, 26–27

G

gait, analyzing, 227–229

galvanic skin response (GSR), 284

gases, carrying in the blood, 105–108

gastric lipase, 303

general motion, 164

gliding joints, 188

Global Positioning system (GPS), 286

gluconeogenesis, 74

glucose, 13–14, 67–68, 73–74, 296–297

glucose transporter type 4 (GLUT4), 25

gluteal, 266

glycemic control, 325

glycemic index (GI), 297–298

glycogen, 61, 67, 124, 296–297

glycogen supercompensation, 299–300

glycogenolysis, 67–68

Golgi tendon organ (GTO), 48–49, 60, 146, 149–151, 204–205, 266

goniometer, 201

gradation, of muscle force, 45–47

graduate health professions, 10, 337

gyroscopes, 285

H

hamstring, 266

hardwired muscle reflexes, 47–54

headaches, as a symptom of altitude sickness, 133

health

maintaining, 254–256

protein requirements for, 309

strength training plans for, 248–249

trackers, 283

health span, exercise and, 27–29

health-enhancement aspects, of exercise, 15–16

heart

function of, 101–102

health span and, 28

how it works, 93–102

structure of, 91–93

heart disease, 26–27, 98

heart murmurs, 94

heart rate

about, 97–101

aerobic training and, 117

cold environments and, 129

heat and, 125

monitoring, 291

during steady state, 114

heart rate methods, for aerobic exercise, 242–243

heart rate reverse method, 242–243

heat, for treating injuries, 265

heat cramps, 125–126

heat exhaustion, 126–127

heat gain, mechanisms of, 121–123

heat index, 122

heat injury, 125–127

heatstroke, 127

heavy exercise, heat from, 122

hemoglobin (Hb), 105, 131

high-altitude cerebral edema, 134

high-altitude pulmonary edema, 133–134

high-density lipoproteins (HDLs), 304

hiking, for weight loss, 274

hinge joints, 188

Hippocrates, 23

hold-relax PNF technique, 209–210

hot air, 122

HRV, 289

human performance, science of, 14–15

humidity, 122

hyaline cartilage, 186, 190–191, 263

hydration, importance of, 289–290

hydrogen (H⁺) ions, 70–71, 107

hydrostatic weighing, 272–273

hypercalcemia, 318

hyperextension, 171

hypertension (high blood pressure), 27, 98

hyperthermia, 124

hypertrophy, 60, 194, 250

hypothalamus, 120, 121

hypothermia, 128–130

I

ice, for treating injuries, 265

icons, explained, 2–3

iliotibila (IT) band, 36, 266

immovable joints, 187

immune system, health span and, 29

impulse, 179

inclinometer, 201

incomplete proteins, 307

T

tasks, 215–217

Technical Stuff icon, 3

techniques, for stretching, 207–211

technology, of wearables, 283–286

temperature

  chemoreceptors and, 111

  oxygen transport and, 105

  regulating, 120–121

  role of water in regulation of, 311–312

  sensors, 147

tendonitis, 191, 260, 263

tendons, 191, 260

tensile strength, 260

tension, 47–49, 181, 197, 261

tension reflex, 48–49

terminal phase, in movement, 152

terminal stance, in walking, 228

terminal swing, in walking, 229

third-class lever, 174

three-phase model, 219–220

throwing, analyzing, 231–235

tibio-fibular joint, 187

timing

  for aerobic exercise, 240–241

  for pre-event meals, 300

Tip icon, 3

tissue stretch, 200, 203

titin, 36

torque, 179

torsion, 181, 261

touch, 146–147

training

  about, 239–240

  amount of aerobic exercise, 240

  anaerobic glycolytic system, 87–88

  ATP-phosphocreatine system, 87

  cooldown, 247

  flexibility, 251–252

  frequency of aerobic exercise, 240–241

  for improved metabolism, 85–89

  intensity of aerobic exercise, 240, 241–245

  key components of exercise sessions, 246–247

  muscles, 54–60

  oxidative (aerobic) system, 88–89

  progression, 246

  specificity of, 54–56

  strength, 247–251

  time for aerobic exercise, 240–241, 245

  tracking sleep and recovery after, 289

  type of aerobic exercise, 240–241, 245

  warmup, 246

training overload, 322

training specificity, 87, 321–322

trans fat, 305

transverse plane, 166, 171

treating injuries, 264–266

tri-axial joints, 189

tropomyosin, 36, 37

troponin, 37

trunk movement, in walking, 156

T-tubules, 35

two-joint muscles, 45

two-phase model, 220

Type 1 diabetes, 25

Type 2 diabetes, 24–25

U

unconsciousness, cold environments and, 129

underwater weighing, 272–273

uniaxial joints, 189

unipennate, 43

unsaturated fat, 304

U.S. Centers for Disease Control and Prevention (CDC), 25–26

V

valsalva maneuver, 116

valves, heart, 92

velocity, 175, 180

vena cava, 92

venous return, 94

ventilation, during steady state, 114

ventricles, 92

vertebrae, 187

vertical axis, 168

very low-density lipoproteins (VLDLs), 303

Viagra, 135

visceral fat, 268, 306, 330–331

vision, 147
vitamins, 74, 313–315
volume of oxygen (VO$_2$)
  about, 28, 79
  for aerobic exercise, 243–244
  body weight compared with, 80–81
  monitoring, 292
  during steady state, 114

W

walking
  about, 154–156
  analyzing, 227–229
  for weight loss, 274
warmup, 246, 252, 255–256
Warning icon, 3
water
  about, 310–311
  in body composition, 270
  bones and, 258
  heat and loss of, 125
  role in temperature regulation, 311–312
watts, 244
wearables
  about, 282
  reliability and validity of, 286–287
  technology of, 283–286
  types of, 282–283

weight
  about, 178–179
  for lifting, 57
  VO$_2$ compared with, 80–81
weight gain, 277–279
weight loss
  about, 274
  dietary guidelines, 275–277
  exercise guidelines, 274–275, 277
  ketogenic diet, 276–277
  resistance training and, 275
weight management, 267. See also body composition
weight mismanagement, 279
weight training, 56–59
wellness coach, 336–337
Wellness Council of America, 334
wellness specialist, 334
wicking, 124, 130
wind chill, 128–130
windlass, 228
windup, in throwing, 231–232
workload, managing, 287–288
World Health Organization (WHO), 306

Z

Z line, 36
zero degrees, 201
Zinc, 316
zone of overlap, 36

About the Authors

Steve Glass, PhD, FACSM: Steve is a full professor of exercise physiology at Grand Valley State University in Michigan, with more than 30 years' experience developing undergraduate exercise science programs and teaching courses in exercise physiology, exercise prescription, sports medicine, and cardiac rehabilitation. He has published work focusing on effort sense (rate of perceived exertion, or RPE) during activity and studying muscle activation (electromyography, or EMG) during exercise and rehabilitation, with interest in training balance and stability. He consistently links his research to student learning, and all his student collaborative research has been published in peer-reviewed journals. He has published a metabolic calculations textbook in collaboration with the American College of Sports Medicine (ACSM) and recently authored a textbook devoted to teaching cardiac rehabilitation skills (stress testing, electrocardiogram [ECG] rhythms, exercise prescription) to undergraduate students. He has been a Fellow of the American College of Sports Medicine since 1998. In his spare time, Steve is an avid exerciser and weightlifter and retired martial arts enthusiast. His current passion is ballroom, rhythm, and line dancing with his lovely wife, Julie.

Brian Hatzel, PhD, AT, ATC: Brian is a full professor in the Physical Therapy and Athletic Training Department and teaches in the Master of Athletic Training program at Grand Valley State University. He serves as the Director of Faculty Initiatives for Student Success for the university and is the founding faculty director for the Health and Wellness house (Academic Community). Brian completed his undergraduate degree at the University of Florida (exercise and sports sciences with a specialization in athletic training), his master's degree from Ball State University (exercise science–biomechanics), and his PhD from the University of Florida (athletic training/sports medicine with a minor in rehabilitation sciences). Brian has extensive experience in the clinical setting as an athletic trainer, providing care for athletes at the clinical, high school, collegiate, professional, and Olympic level. Additionally, he serves as the developer and lead consultant for a community-based throwing assessment/performance enhancement program aimed at helping athletes identify biomechanical flaws and improve performance. Brian is an active scholar in his field, and in his research, he has examined bioimpedance analysis as an injury adjunct, muscle firing characteristics of the shoulder complex, throwing athlete adaptations, glenohumeral joint arthrometry, recovery strategies from injury, and debt load implications for athletic trainers.

Rick Albrecht, PhD: Rick is a professor emeritus in the Department of Movement Science at Grand Valley State University. He holds advanced degrees in counseling psychology (MA) and in the psychosocial aspects of sport and physical activity (MA, PhD) from Michigan State University. A recipient of the Doctoral Dissertation Award presented by Division 47 of the American Psychological Association (Sport and Exercise Psychology), he was elected to member status in the American Psychological Association in 1994. Rick is a charter member of the Association of

Applied Sport Psychology and served as president of the National Council for the Accreditation of Coaching Education. He was one of five members of a team of national experts responsible for writing the second edition of the National Standards for Sport Coaches. Over the past 30 years, Rick has held a variety of faculty positions in the Department of Kinesiology and College of Human Medicine at Michigan State University and the Department of Movement Science at Grand Valley State University where he taught undergraduates majoring in pre-occupational therapy, pre-physical therapy, pre-athletic training, and physical education. His first book, *Coaching Myths: Fifteen Wrong Ideas in Youth Sports* (McFarland & Company), was the culmination of the hundreds of coaching clinics and workshops he conducted across the country.

Dedication

From Steve: This book is dedicated to my wife, Julie, for her endless encouragement and unconditional support. I hope to be as great as she thinks I am! I also dedicate this to all of the students I have taught over the past 30+ years, striving for clarity and making difficult information more easy to access. I have always enjoyed my students "aha" moments and excitement to learn.

From Brian: To my most gracious and supportive wife of 25 years, Gayle, and the most loving and amazing children ever, Alyssa, Justin, and Kayla. Thank you for supporting and encouraging me throughout my career. Even though you may not have realized it, you provided me with the focus and support I needed but often couldn't find by myself.

From Rick: To Mom and Andrea (as always).

Authors' Acknowledgments

From Steve: Thanks to Deb Feltz at Michigan State for sending the *For Dummies* folks my way. They are a team of excellent professionals who really know how to write! Thanks to Dr. Ron Knowlton, my dissertation mentor who taught me the value of words and clarity of meaning when writing. Thanks to Dr. Lenny Kaminsky and Dr. Mitch Whaley, who showed me the obligation to give back to the profession and help others gain expertise in the field. They all put up with me and guided me for many years. I will always be grateful.

From Brian: I'd like to thank my mom and dad, who taught me that nothing worthwhile is ever easy and that hard work and relationships are what define you. Thanks also to my students, who make me want to give them the best that I have to offer every day, and to the many mentors throughout my career — Kevin

Mathews, Chris Patrick, Dr. Tom Kaminski, and Jim Scott, to name just a few — who took the time to teach and had the patience to stick with me as I grew up in the field.

From Rick: I want to thank Dr. Deb Feltz, not only for getting us started on this rewarding project but because she was my graduate school advisor, dissertation director, mentor, and friend back in the early days. If it hadn't been for Deb and Dr. Vern Seefeldt, Director Emeritus of the Institute for the Study of Youth Sports, none of this would have been possible. Finally, I'd like to thank my great colleague and friend, Dr. Dana Munk at Grand Valley State University, for her continuous support and understanding as I still try to get a handle on this professor gig, even after many years of practice.

From all: We'd all like to acknowledge the support and direction we received from the folks behind the *For Dummies* series: Lindsay Berg and Shannon Kucaj, for getting us started; Elizabeth Kuball, our editor, who provided constant feedback and suggestions, kept us on track, and found the right words in the right context; our technical editor, Deborah Riebe, for her expertise; and, our illustrator, Kathryn Born, who, through expertise and patience, created images that connect the reader to the material — an outstanding achievement considering our not-so-detailed sketches!

Publisher's Acknowledgments

Managing Editor: Murari Mukundan

Executive Editor: Lindsay Berg

Editorial Assistant: Shannon Kucaj

Editor: Elizabeth Kuball

Technical Editor: Deborah Riebe, PhD, FACSM, FNAK

Production Editor: Magesh Elangovan

Illustrator: Kathryn Born

Cover Image: © kentoh/stock.adobe.com

Special Help: Carmen Krikorian, Kristie Pyles